Get **FIT** Stay **FIT**

Get **FIT**
Stay **FIT**

WILLIAM E. PRENTICE, PH.D., P.T., A.T.,C.

Professor, Coordinator of the Sports Medicine Specialization,
Department of Exercise, and Sports Science
The University of North Carolina
Chapel Hill, North Carolina

Sixth Edition

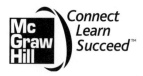

Mc Graw Hill

Connect
Learn
Succeed™

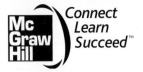

The McGraw·Hill Companies

Connect
Learn
Succeed™

GET FIT, STAY FIT, SIXTH EDITION

Published by McGraw-Hill, a business unit of The McGraw-Hill Companies, Inc., 1221 Avenue of the Americas, New York, NY 10020. Copyright © 2012 by The McGraw-Hill Companies, Inc. All rights reserved. Previous editions © 2009, 2007, and 2004. Printed in the United States of America. No part of this publication may be reproduced or distributed in any form or by any means, or stored in a database or retrieval system, without the prior written consent of The McGraw-Hill Companies, Inc., including, but not limited to, in any network or other electronic storage or transmission, or broadcast for distance learning.

Some ancillaries, including electronic and print components, may not be available to customers outside the United States.

This book is printed on acid-free paper.

2 3 4 5 6 7 8 9 0 DOC/DOC 1 0 9 8 7 6 5 4 3

ISBN 978-0-07-352385-9
MHID 0-07-352385-2

Vice President & Editor-in-Chief: *Michael Ryan*
Vice President & Director of Specialized Publishing: *Janice M. Roerig-Blong*
Publisher: *David Patterson*
Senior Sponsoring Editor: *Debra B. Hash*
Marketing Manager: *Caroline McGillen*
Project Manager: *Erin Melloy*
Design Coordinator: *Brenda A. Rolwes*
Cover Designer: *Studio Montage, St. Louis, Missouri*
Cover Image: *© Ultimate Group, LLC/ Alamy*
Buyer: *Sherry L. Kane*
Media Project Manager: *Sridevi Palani*
Compositor: *Aptara®, Inc.*
Typeface: *10/12 Palatino*
Printer: *R. R. Donnelley, Crawfordsville*

All credits appearing on page or at the end of the book are considered to be an extension of the copyright page.

Library of Congress Cataloging-in-Publication Data

Prentice, William E.
    Get fit, stay fit / William E. Prentice. — 6th ed.
        p. cm.
    Includes bibliographical references and index.
    ISBN-978-0-07-352385-9
        1. Physical fitness. 2. Exercise. 3. Health. I. Title.
    RA781.P67 2011
    613.7—dc23   2011018755

www.mhhe.com

CONTENTS

PREFACE

If you believe what you hear, see, and read in the media, you would think that every person in America has become a "fitness junkie." It is true that millions of people exercise in some way, shape, or form on a somewhat consistent basis. But the fact is that for the vast majority of Americans the thought of going out and "exercising" never even crosses their minds. Through TV and DVDs, on the Internet, in magazines or newspapers, our society is constantly bombarded by images that suggest the importance of being physically fit and healthy. It seems that people in your generation, in contrast to all the previous ones, are finally starting to realize that there really is a reason for living a healthy lifestyle and for incorporating regular exercise into that lifestyle.

Get Fit, Stay Fit is a text designed to tell you not only how you can go about getting yourself fit, but also why it is to your advantage to make fitness and exercise a regular part of your lifestyle. It begins by discussing the basic principles of fitness that apply to any type of exercise program, and then explains how being fit relates to a healthy lifestyle. Specific techniques and guidelines for developing cardiorespiratory endurance, for improving muscular strength and endurance, for increasing flexibility, and for maintaining appropriate body weight and composition are described in detail so that you can put together a personalized fitness program based on your individual needs. This book also provides recommendations and suggestions on selecting and using the exercise equipment available to help you get fit, as well as tips for making your exercise program as safe and free of injury as possible.

FEATURES

- *Practical application chapters are dedicated to starting your own fitness program (3), practicing safe fitness (9), and becoming a wise consumer (10). These chapters cut through the confusion and provide essential information on how to start up, equip yourself, and safely execute an individual fitness program.*
- *Special boxes—Fit Lists, Health Links, and Safe Tips—highlight, summarize, and provide quick reference to important information.*
- *Lab Activities assist in evaluating a number of personal measures of fitness as well as providing guidelines for increased health.*
- *Key terms are in color and are defined in boxes to help build a working vocabulary of concepts, terms, and principles necessary for understanding, beginning, and maintaining any fitness program.*
- *Chapter pedagogy also includes chapter objectives, key terms, definition boxes, bulleted summaries, and suggested readings to enhance the learning process.*
- *All exercise safety information and illustrations have been updated to provide proper fitness techniques for a safe and effective fitness program.*

- *Each chapter contains an expanded list of reviewed Web sites relevant to the chapter topic. Using the power of the World Wide Web as a resource, students will be able to obtain further information to take their studies beyond the classroom.*
- *An updated and expanded list of references provides a significant resource for students as well as instructors for further study of key issues and topics.*

NEW TO THIS EDITION

Throughout the text in this sixth edition, multiple photos have been added to emphasize specific points in the text.

Highlights of the changes in each chapter are as follows:

CHAPTER 1

- *Changed the approach to the wellness continuum to better reflect the philosophy that fitness is only one aspect of that continuum*
- *Updated information on Healthy People 2020*
- *Changed skill-related components to performance-related components*
- *Better emphasis on the target audience which is the average, non-athlete college student*
- *Updated the photos to reflect ordinary individual doing more normal activities*

CHAPTER 2

- *Added financial wellness to our list of wellness components*
- *Added more emphasis on spiritual wellness*
- *Added new information on the effects on cortisol on the stress response*
- *Added new information on a Type C personality*
- *Updated recommendations on levels of cholesterol*
- *Added information on the benefits of exercise as a cancer treatment*
- *Changed "Recreational Drugs" section to "Abused Illegal Drugs"*

- *Added new information on abused prescription drugs*
- *Added new information on OxyContin*
- *Added a new chart estimating the number of alcoholic drinks that will cause a specific level of impairment*

CHAPTER 3

- *Updated information on the warm-up*
- *Added new information on a dynamic warm-up*
- *Updated information on recommendation for how you should exercise*
- *Added new Fit List on the 2008 Physical Activity Guideline for Americans from the Centers for Disease Control*

CHAPTER 4

- *Updated the discussion of the FIT Principle*
- *Provided updated recommendations for the intensity of activity*
- *Provided updated recommendations for the frequency of activity*
- *Updated the method of calculating lower and upper limits of target heart rate range*
- *Updated ACSM recommendations for high, moderate, and low intensity exercise*
- *Added new expanded table on guidelines for continuous training*
- *Updated photos that show various training techniques for improving cardiorespiratory endurance*

CHAPTER 5

- *Emphasized that in females strength gains occur primarily as a result of increased neuromuscular efficiency rather than increases in the size of a muscle.*
- *Added many new and additional photos on different strength training techniques*
- *Added a new HealthLink on progressive resistance exercise*

CHAPTER 6

- *Reorganized the discussion of the various stretching techniques to differentiate ballistic stretching versus dynamic stretching*
- *Emphasized the emergence of dynamic stretching as a widely used technique*
- *Added many new and additional photos on different stretching techniques*

CHAPTER 7

- *Added new 2010 Dietary Guidelines for Americans*
- *Replaced MyPyramid with the new MyPlate program*
- *Clarified the discussion of LDL versus HDL cholesterol*
- *Added new information on vegetarian diets*
- *Clarified information on potassium in the diet and lost in sweat*
- *Added a new table comparing the amount of calories, carbohydrates, sodium, and potassium in a variety of fluid replacement drinks.*
- *Identified additional specific food sources for the various types of nutrients*
- *Clarified and added new information regarding interpreting food labels*

CHAPTER 8

- *Added new information on caloric expenditure following exercise in the recovery period*
- *Emphasized getting help and treatment for eating disorders*

CHAPTER 9

- *Addressed misconception that a large percentage of heat is dissipated from the head*
- *Added new recommendations for wearing lightweight microfiber garments that allow for better evaporation of sweat*

CHAPTER 10

- *Added new information on using an incline treadmill*
- *Emphasized the importance of choosing good Web sites when seeking information on fitness*

ANCILLARY

TEST BANK

The Test Bank for *Get Fit, Stay Fit* contains more than 300 multiple choice, true-false, fill-in, and short essay test questions for convenience in preparing examinations. The Test Bank can be found on the Instructors Resource website: www.mhhe.com/getfit6e.

ACKNOWLEDGMENTS

In revising *Get Fit, Stay Fit,* my developmental editor Gary O'Brien and my project manager Jill Eccher have been instrumental in the development of the sixth edition, and have provided a great deal of help and support. The reviewers provided many constructive recommendations about content and organization. Their input and suggestions have been greatly appreciated and are reflected throughout the text. They include the following:

Joseph Cole
Trevecca Nazarene University

Joseph Coti
Southwestern Michigan College

Megan Franks
Lone Star College-North Harris

Paula Polittle
Concordia University

And finally, as always, this is for my wife Tena and our boys, Brian and Zach, who each day make my life more worthwhile.

By writing this book, I have tried to provide you with all the details you need to know about getting yourself fit and to stress the importance of developing a healthy lifestyle. But the bottom line is that to get fit, you need to stop reading about it and start doing it. There is no better time than now!

William E. Prentice

Getting Fit Why Should You Care?

Objectives

After completing this chapter, you should be able to do the following:

- Explain why fitness is an important aspect of a healthy lifestyle.
- Give several reasons why being fit should be important to you.
- Discuss the physical, social, and psychological benefits of being fit.
- List the component parts of physical fitness.
- Determine your reasons for wanting to become physically fit.

So, you've finally decided it's time to get fit. Why is that? People have many different reasons and motivations for beginning a physical activity program. Have you decided that it's time to improve your overall health and well-being? Are you concerned about the way you look to your friends? Are you tired of being a couch potato? Are you interested in fitness primarily because you are required to take this fitness class? Whatever your motivation happens to be, consistently engaging in physical activity can not only make you physically fit but also can have many positive benefits on your style of living.

WHY SHOULD YOU CARE ABOUT BEING PHYSICALLY ACTIVE?

Have you noticed that it is virtually impossible to go through a day without being exposed to something involving some aspect of wellness or fitness? We eat, sleep, go to class, and some of us even try to include some form of physical activity in our busy schedules. Fitness information comes from many sources. "Experts" give advice on television or radio and in magazines, books, and newspapers. Even our friends and classmates are willing to give opinions on the

KEY TERMS

physical fitness	*caloric expenditure*
wellness	*performance-related*
health-related	*components*
components	*speed*
cardiorespiratory	*power*
endurance	*neuromuscular*
muscular strength	*coordination*
muscular endurance	*balance*
flexibility	*agility*
body composition	*reaction time*
caloric intake	

best ways to work out or on how to lose weight. Furthermore, the image of the attractive, healthy, physically active person is used to market everything—clothing, food, cosmetics, health care products, sports equipment, weight loss programs—the list goes on.

Our society is characterized by a fast-paced lifestyle, with obligations and stresses that affect our physical and emotional well-being. A common misconception is that daily living activities incorporate enough physical activity to maintain overall health. Surveys indicate that virtually all adults believe that physical activity is a critical aspect of health and wellness and that regular physical activity is essential for themselves and for their children. Still, despite this increased interest in fitness and wellness, the U.S. Department of Health and Human Services reports that only 24 percent of adults participate in a minimum of 30 minutes of light-to-moderate physical activity at least five times per week and only 12 percent are active seven times per week. Approximately 60 percent of the population is somewhat active but fails to achieve exercise intensity levels necessary for improving cardiorespiratory endurance.

Unfortunately, approximately 25 percent of American adults are essentially sedentary and do not engage in any type of leisure-time physical activity. Technological advances, such as the automobile, television, elevators, escalators, and moving sidewalks, eliminate the need for physical exertion and contribute to a sedentary lifestyle. The 1996 *Surgeon General's Report of Physical Activity and Health* reviewed mounting evidence that relates physical

activity to reduced risks of a variety of health problems. According to the Center for Disease Control (CDC) regular physical activity substantially reduces the risk of dying of coronary heart disease and decreases the risk for stroke, colon cancer, diabetes, and high blood pressure. It also helps to control weight; contributes to healthy bones, muscles, and joints; helps to relieve the pain of arthritis; reduces symptoms of anxiety and depression; and is associated with fewer hospitalizations, physician visits, and medications. Being fit means that the various systems of your body are healthy and function efficiently to enable you to engage in work, in activities of daily living, and in recreational pursuits and leisure activities; also to be healthy, to resist hypokinetic diseases, and to meet emergency situations (Figure 1-1).

Fitness is not entirely dependent on physical activity. It is an important aspect of choosing to live a healthy lifestyle. Fitness affects the total person, including intellect, emotional stability, physical conditioning, and stress levels. In addition to fitness, the journey toward

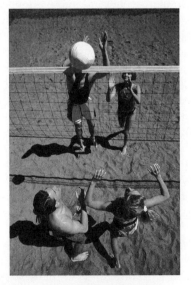

FIGURE 1-1. PHYSICAL FITNESS.
Being fit allows you to engage in both activities of daily living and recreational pursuits and leisure activities.

physical fitness: Being physically fit means that the various systems of your body are healthy and function efficiently to enable you to engage in work, in activities of daily living, and in recreational pursuits and leisure activities; also to be healthy, to resist hypokinetic diseases, and to meet emergency situations.

achieving a healthy lifestyle includes proper medical care, eating the right foods in the right amounts, appropriate physical activity that is adapted to individual needs and physical limitations, satisfying work, healthy play and recreation, and proper amounts of rest and relaxation. Engaging in physical activity to get yourself fit allows you to satisfy your needs regarding mental and emotional stability, social consciousness and adaptability, spirituality and morality, and physical health consistent with your heredity. This is the definition of the term **wellness,** which will be discussed in chapter 3.

EXERCISE AND PHYSICAL ACTIVITY

Are exercise and physical activity the same? The answer is, not necessarily. Clearly there exists a continuum, with a sedentary lifestyle at one end and aggressive fitness programs at the other end. So what exactly constitutes exercise? If an activity is harder (more intense) than what an individual normally does on a daily basis, this would be considered exercise. For example if you usually go for a walk each morning always at the same pace and for the same amount of time, then your morning walks would be considered physical activity, not exercise. Exercise must challenge the body's physiological systems, forcing them to work harder than they are accustomed to working. Over time, exercise will cause these physiological systems to improve and function more efficiently and thus they will adapt to the imposed demands. What may be considered exercise for one person may not be for another.

> **wellness:** Satisfying your needs regarding mental and emotional stability, social consciousness and adaptability, spiritual and moral fiber, and physical health consistent with your heredity

Perhaps the distinction between the two is specific to an individual's current fitness status and lifestyle.

HEALTHY PEOPLE 2020 OBJECTIVES

Every 10 years, the U.S. Department of Health and Human Services (HHS) re-evaluates major risks to health and wellness, changing public health priorities, and emerging trends and innovations related to our nation's health preparedness and prevention over the past decade. Healthy People 2020 takes into consideration scientific insights and new knowledge of current data. Healthy People 2020 is a set of health objectives for the nation to achieve over the next decade. It can be used by many different people, states, communities, professional organizations, and others to help them develop programs to improve health. Healthy People 2020 builds on initiatives pursued over the past 3 decades. The 1979 surgeon general's report, *Healthy People,* and *Healthy People 2000: National Health Promotion and Disease Prevention Objectives* both established national health objectives and served as the basis for the development of state and community plans. Like its predecessors, Healthy People 2020 was developed through a broad consultation process, built on the best scientific knowledge and designed to measure programs over time. The 28 focus areas of Healthy People 2020 were developed by leading federal agencies with the most relevant scientific expertise. Additionally, comments on the draft objectives were received through a series of regional and national meetings and on an interactive Web site. The Secretary's Council on National Health Promotion and Disease Prevention Objectives for 2020 also provided leadership and advice in the development of national health objectives.

As in Healthy People 2010, the leading health indicators will be used to measure the health of the nation over the next 10 years. Each of the 10 leading health indicators has one or more objectives from Healthy People 2020 associated with it. As a group, the leading health indicators reflect the major health concerns in the United States during the early 21st century. The leading health indicators were selected on the basis of their ability to motivate action, the availability of data to measure progress, and their importance as public health issues. The leading health indicators are:

- Physical activity
- Overweight and obesity
- Tobacco use
- Substance abuse
- Responsible sexual behavior
- Mental health
- Injury and violence
- Environmental quality
- Immunization
- Access to health care

Healthy People 2020 offers a simple but powerful idea: Provide health objectives in a format that enables diverse groups to combine their efforts and work as a team. It is a road map to better health for all. The initiative has partners from all sectors. Health Link Box 1-1 lists the Healthy People 2020 objectives for improving health, fitness, and quality of life through physical activity.

THE PHYSICAL BENEFITS OF BEING PHYSICALLY ACTIVE

Human beings are designed to be active creatures. Although changes in civilization have resulted in a decrease in the amount of activity needed to accomplish the basic tasks associated with living, the human body has not changed. Therefore, it is important to be aware of the requirements for good health and recognize the importance of vigorous physical activity in your life (Figure 1-2). If you do not, your health, productivity, and effectiveness are likely to suffer. Health Link Box 1-2 summarizes 10 physical benefits associated with physical activity.

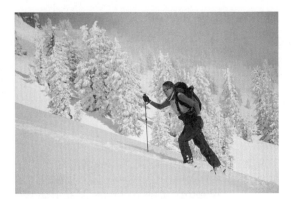

FIGURE 1-2. PHYSICAL BENEFITS.
Physical activity is important in achieving good health.

THE SOCIAL REWARDS OF BEING PHYSICALLY ACTIVE

If you are willing to participate in physical activities that help keep you fit, you benefit from the outlets, companionship, and feelings of belonging inherent in such activities. Physical activity can provide a great mechanism for exploring strategies to resolve conflicts, act fairly, comply with rules and fair play, and generally develop a moral and ethical code of behavior. Participation in physical activity provides an opportunity for socializing (Figure 1-3). Physical fitness affects

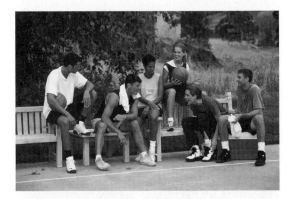

FIGURE 1-3. SOCIAL REWARDS.
Participating in physical activity provides an opportunity for socializing.

HEALTH LINK 1-1

Healthy People 2020 Objectives to Improve Health, Fitness, and Quality of Life Through Daily Physical Activity

- Reduce the proportion of adults who engage in no leisure-time physical activity.
- Increase the proportion of adults that meet current Federal physical activity guidelines for aerobic physical activity and for muscle strength training.
- Increase the proportion of employed adults who have access to and participate in employer-based exercise facilities and exercise programs.
- Increase the proportion of physician office visits for chronic health diseases or conditions that include counseling or education related to exercise.
- Increase the proportion of adults who perform physical activities that enhance or maintain flexibility.
- Increase the proportion of adolescents that meet current physical activity guidelines for aerobic physical activity and for muscle-strengthening activity.
- Increase the proportion of children and adolescents that meet guidelines for television viewing and computer use.
- Increase the proportion of the Nation's public and private schools that require

- daily physical education for all students.
- Increase the proportion of adolescents who participate in daily school physical education.
- Increase the proportion of adolescents who spend at least 50 percent of school physical education class time being physically active.
- Increase the proportion of the Nation's public and private schools that provide access to their physical activity spaces and facilities for all persons outside of normal school hours (that is, before and after the school day, on weekends, and during summer and other vacations).
- Increase the proportion of States and school districts that require regularly scheduled elementary school recess.
- Increase the proportion of school districts that require or recommend elementary school recess for an appropriate period of time.
- Increase the proportion of trips made by walking.
- Increase the proportion of trips made by bicycling.

the entire person, and rich dividends come to the person who concentrates on the development of the body as well as the mind.

THE PSYCHOLOGICAL BENEFITS OF BEING PHYSICALLY ACTIVE

Physical activity generally has a positive influence on a person's psychological health throughout a lifetime cycle by improving health and enhancing function and quality of life. Some of the psychological benefits include enhanced motivation, increased self-perception and esteem, improved mood states, emotional well-being, reduction of stress and anxiety, and creation of a realistic body image. Physical activity has a positive impact on mental health and appears to alleviate the symptoms of depression, anxiety, and, to a lesser extent, panic disorder.

HEALTH LINK 1-2

Physical Benefits of Being Physically Active

1. Regular, vigorous activity increases muscle size, strength, and power and develops endurance for sustaining work and resisting fatigue.
2. Exercise strengthens the heart muscle and improves the efficiency of the vascular system in delivering oxygenated blood to the working tissues and in using it, thereby improving cardiorespiratory endurance.
3. Exercise improves the functioning of the lungs by deepening the respiration process.
4. Exercise helps to keep the digestive and excretory organs in good condition.
5. Muscular exercise enhances nerve–muscle coordination.
6. Exercise helps a person to maintain a healthy body weight by reducing the percentage of total body weight that is made up of fat tissue.
7. Exercise contributes to improved posture and appearance through the development of proper muscle tone, greater joint flexibility, and a feeling of well-being.
8. Physical activity generates more energy and thus contributes to greater individual productivity for both physical and mental tasks.
9. The person who is fit has more strength, energy, and stamina; an improved sense of well-being; better protection from injury (because strong, well-developed muscles safeguard bones, internal organs, and joints and keep moving parts limber); and improved cardiorespiratory function.
10. It is often the case that people who become physically active will pay more attention to such things as proper nutrition, rest, and relaxation and may also drink less alcohol and stop smoking because they do not want to undo the benefits gained through physical activity. They are likely to be committed to engaging in health-promoting, rather than health-harming, behavior.

www.health.gov/healthypeople/

Many people use regular exercise, especially of a recreational nature, as a means of mental relaxation. Exercise can play a significant role in reducing stress. It diverts attention from stress-producing thoughts to a more relaxing and positive focus. Exercise may also help us to feel better about ourselves and to feel that we are more capable of handling potential stress-producing situations. Exercise controls the release of a hormone called cortisol in response to stress. Prolonged cortisol release due to chronic stress can result in significant negative physiological changes. Some people say that engaging in physical activity gives them an "exercise high." It is true that exercise causes the release of chemicals called endorphins in the brain that can positively affect your attitude and outlook.

It has also been shown that regular physical activity and increased physical fitness increase *serotonin* levels in the brain, which lead to improved mood and feelings of well-being. Serotonin is an important neurotransmitter (brain chemical) that contributes to a range of functions, including sleep and wake cycles, libido, appetite, and mood. Lack of serotonin has also been linked to depression.

THE BENEFITS OF EXERCISE IN THE AGING PROCESS

For the traditional student, at this point in your life it is likely that your physical health is, for the most part, fine. However, a fact that we wish we could change, but unfortunately cannot, is that aging begins immediately at birth and involves a lifelong series of changes in physiological and performance capabilities. These capabilities increase as a function of the growth process throughout adolescence, peak sometime between the ages of 18 and 30 years, then steadily decline with increasing age. Interestingly, this decline may be caused by the sociological constraints of aging as much as by biological effects. It is possible to maintain a relatively high level of physical function if you maintain an active lifestyle (Figure 1-4).

In most cases, after age 30, qualities such as muscular endurance, coordination, and strength begin to decrease. Furthermore, as we age, recovery from vigorous exercise requires a longer amount of time. Regular physical activity, however, tends to delay and in some cases prevent the appearance of certain degenerative processes. If you were active as a child, became fit as a teenager, and continue to stay fit throughout your life, it is very likely that you will have greater strength, flexibility, and cardiorespiratory health and a lower percentage of body fat than if you chose a more sedentary lifestyle. The good news is that it is NEVER too late to make a positive change in your style of living.

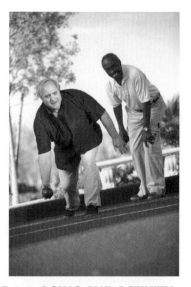

FIGURE 1-4. AGING AND ACTIVITY.
Maintaining an active lifestyle as you age can help to maintain a relatively high level of physical function.

WHAT COMPONENTS OF FITNESS ARE IMPORTANT TO YOU?

Engaging in physical activities can have a positive effect on many different physical attributes. For the vast majority of people in our society, regardless of age, the focus should be on those components of fitness that are concerned with the development of qualities necessary to maintain a healthy lifestyle and to function efficiently physically. Those fitness components include cardiorespiratory endurance, muscular strength, muscular endurance, flexibility, and body composition. Collectively, they are referred to as **health-related components.** Fit List Box 1-1 summarizes the fitness components.

Cardiorespiratory endurance is the ability to persist in a physical activity requiring oxygen for physical exertion without experiencing undue fatigue (Figure 1-5). If you go out

> **health-related components:** components of a healthy lifestyle, including muscular strength, muscular endurance, cardiorespiratory endurance, flexibility, and body composition
>
> **cardiorespiratory endurance:** the ability to persist in a physical activity requiring oxygen for physical exertion without experiencing undue fatigue

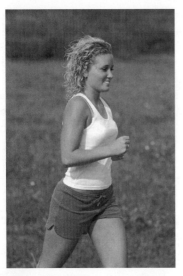

FIGURE 1-5. CARDIORESPIRATORY ENDURANCE.
Perhaps the most essential fitness component for both good health and skill-related performance.

and run 2 miles or swim 2,000 yards, you are displaying cardiorespiratory endurance. The functioning of the heart, lungs, and blood vessels is essential for distribution of oxygen

FIT LIST 1-1

Fitness Components
Health-related fitness components
• Cardiorespiratory endurance
• Flexibility
• Muscular strength
• Muscular endurance
• Body composition
Performance-related fitness components
• Speed
• Power
• Agility
• Neuromuscular coordination
• Balance
• Reaction time

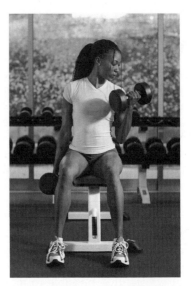

FIGURE 1-6. MUSCULAR STRENGTH.
The ability to generate force against resistance.

and nutrients and removal of wastes from the body. For performance of vigorous activities, efficient functioning of the heart and lungs is necessary. The more efficiently they function, the easier it is to walk, run, work, and concentrate for longer periods. Exercise of this nature involves the heart, the vessels supplying blood to all parts of the body, and the oxygen-carrying capacity of the blood.

Muscular strength is the ability or capacity of a muscle or muscle group to exert force against resistance (Figure 1-6). It refers to a muscle's ability to exert maximal force in a single effort. Strength is needed in all kinds of work and in physical activity, and strong muscles provide better protection of body joints, resulting in fewer sprains, strains, and muscular difficulties. Furthermore, muscle strength helps in maintaining proper posture and provides greater endurance, power, and resistance to fatigue.

muscular strength: the ability or capacity of a muscle or muscle group to exert force against resistance

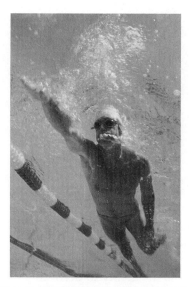

FIGURE 1-7. MUSCULAR ENDURANCE.
The ability to perform muscular contractions repeatedly over a period of time.

Muscular endurance is the ability of muscles to perform or sustain a muscle contraction repeatedly over a period of time (Figure 1-7). Muscular endurance is closely related to muscular strength. If you are strong, you will be more resistant to fatigue because relatively less effort will be required to produce repeated muscular contraction.

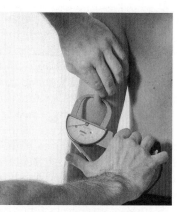

FIGURE 1-9. MEASURING BODY COMPOSITION.
Exercise can reduce the percentage of total body weight that is fat tissue.

Flexibility is the ability to move the joints in your arms, legs, and trunk freely throughout a full, nonrestricted, pain-free range of motion (Figure 1-8). It may be improved by engaging regularly in stretching. Flexibility is essential in carrying on many daily activities and can help to prevent muscle strain and muscular problems such as backaches. It is important for maintaining good posture. It is also important for performance in most active sports.

Body composition refers to the different types of tissues that make up your body. These primarily include bones, muscles, tendons, ligaments, skin, and fat (Figure 1-9).

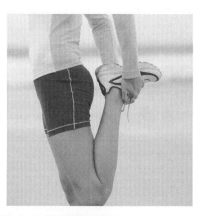

FIGURE 1-8. FLEXIBILITY.
The ability to move freely through a full range of motion.

muscular endurance: the ability of muscles to perform or sustain a muscle contraction repeatedly over a period of time

flexibility: the ability to move the joints in your arms, legs, and trunk freely throughout a full, nonrestricted, pain-free range of motion

body composition: the percentage of fat in the body relative to the percentage of all the other tissues

Body composition particularly refers to the percentage of fat in the body relative to the percentage of all the other tissues. An excess of fat in the body is unhealthy because it causes the body to expend more energy for movement, and it may reflect a diet in which an individual is consuming more calories than he or she needs. The demand on the cardiorespiratory system is greater when the percent of body fat is high. Furthermore, it is believed that obesity contributes to degenerative diseases such as high blood pressure and **atherosclerosis.** It has also been linked to diabetes and certain cancers. Obesity can also result in psychological maladjustments and may shorten life. A balance between caloric intake and caloric expenditure is necessary to maintain proper body fat content. Adequate exercise, therefore, is effective in controlling body fat. **Caloric intake** is the total number of calories consumed in a 24-hour period regardless of the type of foods ingested. **Caloric expenditure** is the number of calories burned off in a 24-hour period from basal metabolism and exercise.

Performance-related fitness components are also important for any physically active individual. These components deal more with performance in physical activities than with basic health and include speed, power, neuromuscular coordination, balance, agility, and reaction time.

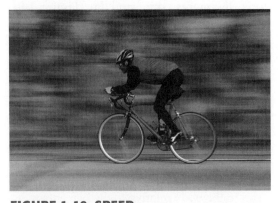

FIGURE 1-10. SPEED.
Speed is an important component in many competitive athletic situations.

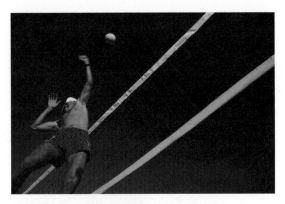

FIGURE 1-11. POWER.
Spiking a volleyball requires the ability to generate large amounts of force very quickly.

Speed is the ability to perform a particular movement very rapidly. It is a function of distance and time (Figure 1-10). Speed is an important component for successful performance in many competitive athletic situations.

Power is the ability to generate great amounts of force against a certain resistance in a short period (Figure 1-11). Power is a function of both strength and speed. The

atherosclerosis: a process by which fatty plaques are deposited along arterial walls

caloric intake: the number of calories consumed in the diet

caloric expenditure: the number of calories expended through basal metabolism and exercise

performance-related fitness components: Relate more to performance than basic health

speed: the ability to perform a particular movement very rapidly; it is a function of distance and time

power: the ability to generate great amounts of force against a certain resistance in a short period of time

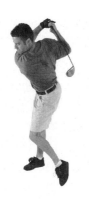

FIGURE 1-12. NEUROMUSCULAR COORDINATION.
The ability to integrate the senses with motor function to produce coordinated movement.

ability to drive a golf ball, hit a softball, or kick a ball a long distance requires some element of power.

Neuromuscular coordination is the ability to integrate the senses—visual, auditory, and proprioceptive (knowing the position of your body in space)—with muscle function to

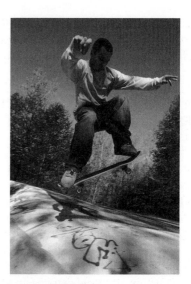

FIGURE 1-14. AGILITY.
The ability to change direction of movement quickly and accurately.

produce smooth, accurate, and skilled movement (Figure 1-12).

Balance is the ability to maintain some degree of equilibrium while moving or standing still (Figure 1-13).

Agility is the ability to change or alter—quickly and accurately—the direction of body movement during activity. Agility to a large extent depends on coordination. Agility may be improved with increased flexibility and muscular strength (Figure 1-14).

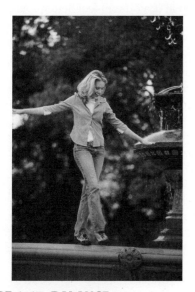

FIGURE 1-13. BALANCE.
The ability to maintain equilibrium when moving or stationary.

> **neuromuscular coordination:** the ability to integrate the senses with muscle function to produce smooth, accurate, and skilled movement
>
> **balance:** the ability to maintain some degree of equilibrium while moving or standing still
>
> **agility:** the ability to change or alter—quickly and accurately—the direction of body movement during activity

Reaction time is the time required to produce an appropriate and accurate physiological or mechanical response to some external stimulus.

DETERMINING YOUR REASONS FOR WANTING TO BE FIT

Perhaps the most important thing that you have learned by this point in your life is that people are different. These differences are evident in all aspects of our being. Certainly, each person has his or her individual reasons for choosing to live a healthy lifestyle and to engage in regular exercise as part of that lifestyle. Before you begin your personal fitness program, it may be helpful to determine your personal reasons for wanting to get fit and your present level of activity.

Regardless of whether you are just starting an individualized fitness program or if you are already exercising, you should first consider exactly what it is that you are trying to accomplish. The exercise program you choose should be one that results in the development of the desired fitness component(s). This means that activities selected should be specific to goals. For example, if your goal is increasing stamina or endurance, this may be achieved effectively by engaging in activities such as running, swimming, skating, or cycling—all activities that maximize the use of the circulatory system. Lab Activity 1-1 will help you to determine your individual reasons for wanting to become physically fit.

DETERMINING HOW FREQUENTLY YOU ENGAGE IN PHYSICAL ACTIVITY

Before you begin any type of fitness program, it is essential to establish some baseline information about your existing exercise habits. It is important to appraise your daily schedule regularly to determine if you are devoting the proper amount of time to keeping yourself fit.

Lab Activity 1-2 will help you determine your current levels of physical activity. There is little question that incorporating consistent, regularly scheduled exercise into your lifestyle may be difficult, especially in light of existing demands on your time.

HOW LONG WILL IT TAKE YOU TO GET FIT?

There is no shortcut to fitness; it takes time. You should not expect results in a matter of hours or even days. After a month of appropriate activity on a regular basis, some improvement should be noted, depending on what your physical condition was when you started. After an extended period of gradual improvement, you may reach a plateau at which you experience no improvement but instead seem to stay at the same level of fitness. This is a natural phenomenon. In time, with regular workouts, improvement will occur; after several months, the desired results will be attained. Make a commitment to your fitness program and keep at it; you will feel better, and this will in turn motivate you to continue. It may be helpful to keep a journal that will document what physical activities you do each day. What were you hoping to accomplish during this exercise session? Did you enjoy that activity? How did you progress relative to the previous session? Once you have attained a desirable physical fitness level, you will be strongly motivated to maintain this level through regular workouts.

Any fitness program requires effort to produce results. Too often, people look for the easy way to achieve their goals. Steam baths, sauna baths, fitness machines, massages, and gimmicks such as body wraps or fad diets may

reaction time: the length of time required to react to a stimulus

be relaxing or produce short-term effects, but it is necessary to exert effort to achieve the lasting benefits of physical fitness. The body must do the work. You can't sit and be fit!

The purpose of the chapters that follow is to provide you with knowledge about and understanding of the various aspects of fitness. They are designed to show the importance of its essential ingredients. They will explain how you can assess, develop, and maintain your fitness. Finally, they will show you how to plan, develop, and implement a personalized physical activity program based on your individual interests.

Summary

- Being fit means that the various systems of your body are healthy and function efficiently to enable you to engage in work, in activities of daily living, and in recreational pursuits and leisure activities; also to be healthy, to resist hypokinetic disease, and to meet emergency situations.
- Being physically active produces various physiological, social, and psychological benefits.
- Engaging in regular exercise throughout your lifetime can delay many of the degenerative processes associated with aging.
- Most people should focus on those components of fitness that are concerned with maintaining a healthy lifestyle, including cardiorespiratory endurance, muscular strength, muscular endurance, flexibility, and body composition.
- Other components of fitness are more closely related to performance in physical activities than to good health and include speed, power, neuromuscular coordination, balance, agility, and reaction time.
- Before starting a fitness program, it is helpful to examine your attitude toward

physical fitness, your reasons for wanting to be physically fit, and your present level of activity.
- There is no short-cut to becoming physically fit. It requires time, hard work, and determination.

Suggested Readings

American College of Sports Medicine. 2003. *Fitness book.* Champaign, IL: Human Kinetics.

Baumann, A. E. 2004. Updating the evidence that physical activity is good for health: An epidemiological review 2000–2003. *Journal of Science and Medicine in Sport* 7(1 Supplement): 6–19.

Blair, S. N., Y. Cheng, and S. Holder. 2001. Is physical activity or physical fitness more important in defining health benefits? *Medicine and Science in Sports and Exercise* 33(6 Suppl.): S379–99.

Bouchard, C. 2010. *Physical activity and obesity.* Champaign, IL: Human Kinetics.

Brown, D. W., D. R. Brown, and G. W. Heath. 2004. Associations between physical activity dose and health-related quality of life. *Medicine and Science in Sports and Exercise* 36(5):890–96.

Buckworth, J., and R. K. Dishman. 2002. Interventions to change physical activity behavior. In *Exercise psychology,* edited by J. Buckworth. Champaign, IL: Human Kinetics.

Centers for Disease Control and Prevention. 1977. Guidelines for school and community programs: Promoting lifelong physical activity. *CAHPERD Journal/Times* 60(2):7–12.

Corbin, C. B. 2002. Physical activity for everyone: What every physical educator should know about promoting lifelong physical activity. *Journal of Teaching in Physical Education* 21(2): 128–44.

Corbin, C. B., R. P. Pangrazi, and G. C. Le Masurier. 2004. Physical activity for children: current patterns and guidelines. *President's Council on Physical Fitness and Sports Research Digest* 5(2):1–8.

Dwyer, G., and S. Davis. 2009. *ACSM's health-related fitness assessment manual.* Baltimore: Lippincott, Williams and Wilkins.

Epstein, L. H., and J. N. Roemmich. 2001. Reducing sedentary behavior: Role in modifying physical activity. *Exercise and Sport Sciences Reviews* 29(3):103.

Erikssen, G. 2001. Physical fitness and changes in mortality: The survival of the fittest. *Sports Medicine* 31(8):571–76.

Fleck, S. J. and W. J. Kraemer. 2004. Integrating other fitness components. In Fleck, S. J. (ed.), *Designing Resistance Training Programs* edited by S. J. Fleck. 3rd ed. Champaign, IL: Human Kinetics.

Halvorson, R., Sonnemaker, B. 2010. Fun, fast and furious: Three trends shaping today's fitness landscape *IDEA Fitness Journal* 7(5):36.

Haskell, W., I. Lee, and R. Pate. 2007. Physical activity and public health: Updated recommendation for adults from the American College of Sports Medicine and the American Heart Association. *Medicine and Science in Sports and Exercise.* 39(8):1423–34.

Hawkins, S. A., M. G. Cockburn, A. S. Hamilton, and T. M. Mack. 2004. An estimate of physical activity prevalence in a large population-based cohort. *Medicine and Science in Sports and Exercise* 36(2):253–60.

Heyward, V. H., ed. 2010. *Advanced fitness assessment and exercise prescription.* 6th ed. Champaign, IL: Human Kinetics.

Introduction to health-related fitness concepts. 2005. In *National Association for Sport and Physical Education, physical best activity guide.* 2nd ed, Champaign, IL: Human Kinetics.

Jackson, A. W. 2004. *Physical activity for health and fitness.* Champaign, IL: Human Kinetics.

Jonas, S. 2010. What are health and wellness?, *AMAA Journal* 23(1):10.

Kilpatrick, M., E. Hebert and J. Bartholomew. 2005. College students' motivation for physical activity: Differentiating men's and women's motives for sport participation and exercise. *Journal of American College Health* 54(2):87.

Krems, C., P. M. Luehrmann, and M. Neuhaeuser. 2004. Physical activity in young and elderly subjects. *Journal of Sports Medicine and Physical Fitness* 44(1):71–76.

Mack, D., P. Wilson, and K. Gunnell. 2007. Healthy Campus 2010: Progress toward the reduction of gender disparities in physical activity objectives. *Journal of Sport and Exercise Psychology* 29 (Supplement):S184.

McKormack-Brown, K., D. Thomas, and J. Kotecki. 2005. *Physical activity and health: An interactive approach.* Boston: Jones & Bartlett.

Melville, D. S., and B. J. Cardinal. 2002. Physical activity and fitness recommendations for physical activity professionals: Highlights of a position statement. *Strategies* 15(5):19.

Nelson, T., S. Gortmaker, and S. Subramanian. 2007. Vigorous physical activity among college students in the United States. *Journal of Physical Activity and Health* 4(4):495.

Seefeldt, V., R. M. Malina, and M. A. Clark. 2002. Factors affecting levels of physical activity in adults. *Sports Medicine* 32(3):143–68.

Sharkey, B. J., ed. *Fitness and health.* 6th ed. Champaign, IL: Human Kinetics. 2006.

Short, F. 2005. Health-related physical fitness and physical activity. In J. Winnick. *Adapted physical education and sport.* 4th ed. Champaign, IL: Human Kinetics.

Sparling, P. B., and T. K. Snow. 2002. Physical activity patterns in recent college alumni. *Research Quarterly for Exercise and Sport* 73(2):200–205.

Stone, W. J. and D. A. Klein. 2004. Long-term exercisers: What can we learn from them? *ACSM's Health & Fitness Journal* 8(2):11–14.

Strand, B., Egeberg, J., Mozumdar, A. 2010. The prevalence and characteristics of wellness programs and centers at two-year and four-year colleges and universities. *Recreational Sports Journal* 34(1):45.

Trudeau, F., Laurencelle, L., Shephard, R. 2009. Is fitness level in childhood associated with physical activity level as an adult? *Pediatric Exercise Science* 21(3):329.

U.S. Department of Health and Human Services, Office of Disease Prevention and Health Promotion. 2010. *Healthy People 2020,* Washington, DC: U.S. Government Printing Office.

Walkuski, J., and C. Masterson. 2005. Developing health-related fitness: it takes more than a week! FITNESSGRAM: part 2. Strategies 18(3):35–38.

Williams, A. The wellness culture: Self-responsibility at last., *IDEA Fitness Journal* 6(9):28.

Zick, C., K. Smith, and B. Brown. 2007. Physical activity during the transition from adolescence to adulthood. *Journal of Physical Activity and Health* 4(2):125.

SUGGESTED WEB SITES

American College of Sports Medicine

ACSM promotes and integrates scientific research, education, and practical applications of sports medicine and exercise science to maintain and enhance physical performance, fitness, health, and quality of life. **www.acsm.org**

American Council on Exercise

The American Council on Exercise (ACE) is committed to promoting active, healthy lifestyles and their positive effects on the mind, body, and spirit. **www.acefitness.org**

Canada's Physical Activity Guide Web site

Physical Activity Guide for older adults. **www.phac-aspc.gc.ca/pau-uap/paguide/**

CDC's Nutrition and Physical Activity Program

This site provides science-based activities for children and adults that address the role of nutrition and physical activity in health promotion and the prevention and control of chronic diseases. **www.cdc.gov/nccdphp/dnpa**

Guide to Physical Activity

This guide advocates an increase in physical activity as an important part of a weight management program. **www.nhlbi.nih.gov/health**

Healthy People 2020

Healthy People 2020 challenges individuals, communities, and professionals to take specific steps to ensure that everyone can enjoy good health, as well as long life. **www.healthypeople.gov/**

International Society for Aging and Physical Activity

The ISAPA is an international not-for-profit society promoting research, clinical practice, and public policy initiatives in the area of aging and physical activity.
www.isapa.org

National Center on Physical Activity and Disability

This site provides references for articles, books, videos, Web sites, vendors for specialized products and services, recreational programs, and other information available on physical activity and disability.
www.ncpad.org

National Institute for Fitness and Sport

NIFS is a nonprofit organization committed to enhancing human health, physical fitness, and athletic performance through research, education, and service.
www.nifs.org

Name _____   Section _____   Date _____

PURPOSE   To determine how important it is for you to engage in a physical fitness activity.

PROCEDURE   Determine how important each of the following is to you. Check the appropriate box for each item. Then total your checked responses, multiply by the appropriate weighted factor (1–5), and add together.

	Rating				
Factor	Extremely Important 5	Very Important 4	Important 3	Not So Important 2	Of Little Concern 1
Lose weight	☐	☐	☐	☐	☐
Feel better	☐	☐	☐	☐	☐
Lessen the risk of heart attack	☐	☐	☐	☐	☐
Have a better self-image	☐	☐	☐	☐	☐
Be more successful in sports	☐	☐	☐	☐	☐
Have more strength	☐	☐	☐	☐	☐
Relieve stress	☐	☐	☐	☐	☐
Increase efficiency for study, work, and other responsibilities	☐	☐	☐	☐	☐
Help my sleep pattern	☐	☐	☐	☐	☐
Reduce tension	☐	☐	☐	☐	☐
Increase energy	☐	☐	☐	☐	☐
Have a better looking figure	☐	☐	☐	☐	☐
Contribute to my health	☐	☐	☐	☐	☐
Have a greater resistance to illness and disease	☐	☐	☐	☐	☐
Improve cardiorespiratory function	☐	☐	☐	☐	☐
Increase flexibility	☐	☐	☐	☐	☐
Improve my posture and appearance	☐	☐	☐	☐	☐
Improve my outlook on life	☐	☐	☐	☐	☐
Increase my social outlets	☐	☐	☐	☐	☐
Outlet for frustration/anger	☐	☐	☐	☐	☐
Total	—	—	—	—	—

After considering each item, analyze your basic motivation for becoming involved in some fitness activity.

"Extremely important" $\dfrac{}{\text{Total}} \times \dfrac{5}{\text{factor}} = \underline{}$

"Very important" $\dfrac{}{\text{Total}} \times \dfrac{4}{\text{factor}} = \underline{}$

"Important" $\dfrac{}{\text{Total}} \times \dfrac{3}{\text{factor}} = \underline{}$

"Not so important" $\dfrac{}{\text{Total}} \times \dfrac{2}{\text{factor}} = \underline{}$

"Of little concern" $\dfrac{}{\text{Total}} \times \dfrac{1}{\text{factor}} = \underline{}$

Sum Total _____

INTERPRETATION

Total Score

85–100	Physical fitness has extreme importance to you.
70–84	You believe being physically fit is very important.
50–69	Physical fitness is important but not a very high priority.
35–49	You do not believe physical fitness has as much importance in your life as it does for others.
20–34	You are not concerned about being physically fit.

Based on this assessment, to what extent do you believe physical fitness is important?

Name _____   Section _____   Date _____

PURPOSE It is important to regularly appraise your daily schedule to determine if you are devoting the proper amount of time to keeping fit.

PROCEDURE For this activity, keep a daily record for one week using the form that follows.

	Mon.	Tues.	Wed.	Thurs.	Fri.	Sat.	Sun.
Physical Activity Type of activity							
Duration (min)							
Intensity 3 = High 2 = Moderate 1 = Mild							
Time of Day							
Recreational Activity Type of Activity							
Duration (min)							
Health Requirements (i.e., sleeping, eating) Type of Activity							
Duration (hrs)							

What was the total number of hours that you engaged in physical activity during the week?
_____
_____

Did you choose to engage in the same type of physical activity each day? _____

What was the average length of time that you participated in a physical activity during each session? _____
_____

19

Daily Fitness Schedule

What was your best estimate of the average intensity of the physical activity during each session?

_____

_____

What was the best time of day for you to engage in physical activity? _____

Was it at the same time every day? _____

The American College of Sports Medicine recommends that you engage in physical activity at least 3 times per week at a moderate intensity level for a minimum of 20 minutes per session. Are you meeting these minimal recommendations? _____

If not, how can you change your lifestyle to make time to meet these recommendations?

_____

_____

_____

CHAPTER 2

Creating a **Healthy** Lifestyle

Objectives

After completing this chapter, you should be able to do the following:

- Discuss the importance of creating a healthy style of living and how fitness fits into this lifestyle.
- Recognize the impact of stress on the healthy lifestyle and identify stress management techniques.
- Identify risk factors present in your lifestyle that may predispose you to coronary artery disease.
- Explain how unhealthy lifestyle practices may contribute to the development of cancer.
- Explain why alcohol, drugs, and tobacco are considered deterrents to fitness.

WHY SHOULD YOU BE CONCERNED ABOUT YOUR LIFESTYLE?

Being physically active is critical to a healthful style of living but is perhaps no more important for total well-being than is your social, emotional, mental, or spiritual stability. Fitness can affect each of these components in either a positive or a negative manner.

Choosing a healthy lifestyle encourages you to prevent illness by improving your positive well-being in various ways, including (1) developing yourself physically, (2) expressing your emotions effectively, (3) having good relations with those persons around you, (4) being concerned about your decision-making abilities (5) having a healthy sense of drive to succeed in your career, (6) having an interest in a variety of problems in the environment in which we live, (7) paying attention to ethics, values, and spirituality and, (8) being comfortable with your financial situation. These are the eight elements or domains of wellness (Fit List 2-1). All of these

KEY TERMS

stress management	*lipoproteins*
coronary artery	*hyperlipidemia*
disease	*stress*
cancer	*tobacco use*
coping	*drug abuse*
relaxation techniques	*alcoholism*

FIT LIST 2-1

The Elements or Domains of Wellness

Social Wellness Refers to your level of social interaction and how it pertains to your health. Some of the most powerful predictors of long-term physical and psychological well-being surround friendship. This area of wellness focuses on caring about others, the value of close friendships, group associations, and our willingness to seek out others during stressful times. In general, people who are closely connected with others enjoy better long-term physical and psychological health.

Physical Wellness Promotes physical fitness and long-term bodily health. In addition to exercise, this component promotes good eating habits and seeks the avoidance of other risky daily behaviors such as drug and alcohol abuse, or unsafe sex. In general, people who are committed to fitness, good eating, and respect for one's body usually have better long-term physical and psychological health.

Emotional Wellness Refers to the psychological and emotional outlook that people hold concerning their lives. High levels of emotional wellness are associated with an optimism and enthusiasm about life, as well as an ability to acknowledge the stress sometimes felt, and a willingness to talk with others about it. In general, having these qualities is associated with better long-term physical and psychological health.

Career Wellness Includes planning strategies and the nourishment of attitudes that are most often associated with success in college, a career, parenting, and other dimensions of life. Our general sense of motivation, dedication, honesty, and responsibility will impact our attitude and commitment to whatever tasks we undertake, and, in turn, directly impact our degree of happiness and self-satisfaction. Having a healthy sense of drive to succeed, determination to see a project through to its end, and an adherence to responsible and ethical standards is associated with better long-term physical and psychological health.

Intellectual Wellness Is a state of mind, a way of approaching the world of ideas unrelated to I.Q. or college board scores. The more that people are intellectually excited by what they are doing, the healthier they are. This component of wellness considers such things as our enjoyment of exploring new ideas, generating creative solutions to problems, playing with new sights and sounds, and approaching novel situations with an open mind.

Environmental Wellness Encompasses the ways we think and act in preserving our living planet. Behaviors and attitudes that promote environmental wellness may or may not affect your health directly. Nevertheless, it is certain that having an interest in a variety of problems in our society and in the world in general will directly affect the quality of life for all of us.

Spiritual Wellness Is not concerned with just the nature of your religious beliefs or specific religious practices. Rather, it deals with broad spiritual experiences that most of us have had that may or may not be related to religion. Having a sense of interconnected respect for all life forms or becoming lost in meditation, poetry, music, or prayer can have profound positive physical and psychological consequences.

Financial wellness Is having a balance of the physical, mental, and spiritual aspects in our dealings with money. Maintaining that balance consists of being comfortable with where your money comes from and being realistic about how it is being spent. Financial wellness is knowing your financial situation and dealing with it in such a way that you are prepared for unexpected financial challenges.

http://www.smu.edu/education/wellness/Choices1Resources.asp

elements of self are interwoven into the fabric of your being. One element affects the others, and you are only as strong as your weakest link. The bottom line in your effort to create a healthy style of living is to achieve a balance between all of the elements, with no more emphasis on any single element than on the others.

A key component of wellness is knowing how to plan to be well. Steps include assessment of your lifestyle, setting goals, planning your program, implementing the program, rewarding yourself for achieving goals and reassessing your goals and plan.

Those who adhere to this approach believe it is the responsibility of the individual to work toward achieving a healthy lifestyle and thus realize an optimal sense of well-being. A healthy lifestyle should reflect the integration of such components as regular and appropriate physical activity, **stress management,** and elimination of controllable risk factors such as alcohol, smoking, and drug abuse. Many diseases, such as **coronary artery disease** or **cancer,** may ultimately be the result of an unhealthy lifestyle.

This chapter focuses on various lifestyle choices or practices that potentially interfere with or are deterrents to wellness, achieving a healthy lifestyle and, in particular, physical fitness.

WHAT IS THE EFFECT OF STRESS ON A HEALTHY LIFESTYLE?

It is important for the health-conscious, physically active individual to understand the potential effect of stress on the body. Stress has been linked to many diseases. It may also interfere with performance of daily tasks or the attainment of one's goals (Figure 2-1). Most importantly, poorly managed stress greatly reduces the quality of one's life.

The term *stress* comes from the Latin word *stringere*, meaning "to draw tight." The term refers to the responses that occur in the body as a result of what is called a stressor, or stimulus. Stress occurs when the internal balance or equilibrium of the body systems is disrupted.

Everyone experiences stress, and some stress is needed to perform the daily tasks of life and, more importantly, to stimulate growth and development. Stress can be beneficial. However, too much stress, especially when it exists for a prolonged period and is unrelieved, can result in physical and mental illness. Stress is caused or triggered by stressors that may be physical, social, or psychological and negative or positive

stress management: involves techniques that attempt to reduce both the quantity and the quality of stress in your life

coronary artery disease: disease that results from the accumulation of fatty deposits (atherosclerotic plaque) within the coronary arteries

cancer: a collection of abnormal cells that tends to invade and ultimately take over normal tissue

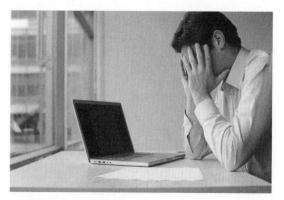

FIGURE 2-1. STRESS.
Stress can interfere with social, emotional, spiritual, and intellectual aspects of your life and prevent you from attaining your goals.

in nature. Human reactions to positive stressors are called *eustress*; that is, stress that is beneficial. The term *distress* denotes detrimental responses or negative stressors. Often, only a fine line distinguishes whether a situation or action causes eustress or distress. For example, moderate physical training is a stressor that can make you stronger and more fit. However, if you do too much too soon, it can produce distress in the form of soreness or injury.

Sometimes the difference between eustress and distress is only a matter of interpretation; do you interpret the stressor as a threat or a challenge? Although we may habitually respond in ways that seem automatic and beyond our control, we can choose to examine the way we think and then work on changing counterproductive thinking or beliefs. In many instances, the way we react to stressful situations is learned from our parents.

Stress should not, however, be considered solely a physiological phenomenon. Stress has also been viewed from a psychological or cognitive perspective. Current research suggests that the stress response is not a simple biological response. It is an interrelated process that includes the presence of a stressor, the circumstances in which the stressor occurs, the interpretation of the situation by the person, that person's typical reaction, and the resources the person has available to deal with the stressor.

For example, some people may find downhill skiing fun and exciting. They look forward to taking winter vacations to ski the slopes. Other people may have tried to ski, but their dislike of cold weather and fear of injury make skiing a distressing activity. Therefore the stress response in a given situation depends on the individual's perceptions. Individuals under stress usually exhibit certain warning signs and symptoms that may vary from person to person. Health Link 2-1 lists the potential signs of stress.

HEALTH LINK 2-1

Signs of Stress

Irritability and depression
Heart palpitations
Dryness of throat and mouth
Impulsive behavior
Inability to concentrate
Feelings of weakness or dizziness
Crying
Anxiety
Emotional tension
Nervous tics
Vomiting
Easily startled by small sounds
Nervous laughter
Trembling hands
Stuttering or other speech problems
Insomnia

Breathlessness
Sweating
Frequent urination
Diarrhea and indigestion
Migraine headaches
Premenstrual tension or missed
　　menstrual cycles
Pain in back
Increased smoking
Loss of appetite
Nightmares
Fatigue

www.futurehealth.org/stresscn.htm
www.cdc.gov/nasd/docs

THE PSYCHOLOGICAL OR COGNITIVE RESPONSE TO STRESS

Once the stress process is initiated by the presence of a stressor, psychological or thought processes that determine how the stressor is perceived take over. An individual's perceptions of a particular situation can cause a response that may vary from arousal to anxiety. The degree to which a particular situation elicits an emotional response depends greatly on how the individual views the situation and how well prepared he or she feels to handle the situation.

THE PHYSIOLOGICAL RESPONSE TO STRESS

Every organ system in the body is affected by the stress response (Figure 2-2). The physiological response to stress follows a three-stage pattern of alarm, resistance, and exhaustion.

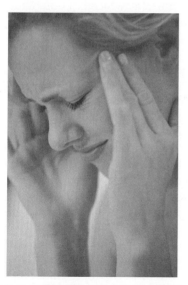

FIGURE 2-2. PHYSIOLOGICAL STRESS RESPONSE.
Stress can have a significant impact on every organ system and thus will alter normal physiological body functions.

There are two regulatory systems in the body that govern the stress response: the nervous system and the endocrine system. Differences between the nervous and endocrine systems are found in terms of how quickly they respond to a stressor and how long their responses are sustained. The endocrine system secretes hormones that prepare the body to deal with a stressful situation. These hormones may remain in the bloodstream for several weeks. The endocrine system's response to stress endures, whereas the nervous system's response is short-lived. This suggests that the endocrine system is more important to investigate for any connection between stress and disease.

During the alarm stage, the body undergoes physiological changes that are collectively referred to as the fight-or-flight syndrome (e.g., increased heart rate, blood pressure, respiratory rate). These physiological changes are primarily a nervous system response to prepare the body for vigorous muscular action. In the resistance stage, the body adjusts to stress and appears to return to its normal state of internal balance. If stress persists for a long time, exhaustion sets in. The person becomes less able to resist stress. Sustained stress can affect various body systems so that illness and even death may result. Health Link 2-2 summarizes specific physical disorders associated with stress.

▶ Exercise and Stress Reduction

In Chapter 1, many positive reasons for engaging in exercise were discussed. The physical, psychological, and social benefits that exercise provides can all have a positive effect on minimizing stress. In fact, engaging in physical activity is widely used as a means for reducing or alleviating stress. It is well known that exercise can decrease stress hormones like cortisol. Many people who exercise report the feeling of a "high" both during and immediately following exercise. This euphoric feeling may be

HEALTH LINK 2-2

Stress and Specific Physical Disorders

Heart Disease Personality	Having the characteristics of a Type A personality is a risk factor for coronary artery disease.
High Blood Pressure	Individuals who are under stress are more likely to have high blood pressure. This may have some relationship to personality type.
Immune System	Chemicals released during the stress response suppress the immune system, which involves a network of organs, tissues, and white blood cells that fight disease.
Digestive System	Stress can cause heartburn, diarrhea, gastritis, and gas. Stress will not cause an ulcer but can make an ulcer feel worse.
Headaches	Tension headaches and migraine headaches are both more likely to occur with increased stress.
Skin Problems	Certain skin conditions such as acne, herpes simplex, psoriasis, hives, and eczema are likely to appear or worsen with increased stress.
Muscles	Stress causes increased tension, particularly in the muscles of the neck and upper back, that can lead to the development of painful trigger points.
Respiratory Problems	Stress can worsen asthma, especially the type of asthma that is exercise induced.
Diabetes	Stress can affect blood sugar levels, which is a potentially dangerous problem for a diabetic.

attributed to the release of opiate-like chemicals called endorphins in the brain. Moderate or vigorous exercise will cause your brain to release endorphins while "burning off" cortisol. Consistent exercise also lowers both resting blood pressure and cholesterol, both of which can help to minimize the insidious damage caused by stress.

PERSONALITY AND STRESS

In identifying people who are at risk for developing cardiovascular disease, researchers believed that there was a connection between behavior pattern and risk of heart disease. People were classified as being either "type A" or "type B" personalities. The type A person is always "on the go," never satisfied with his or her level of achievement, appears tense, suffers from a sense of time urgency, and is competitive and impatient. In contrast, the type B person is more easy-going and relaxed, more patient, and satisfied with his or her level of achievement. The type A person was believed to have a higher risk of developing cardiovascular disease. However, recent research suggests that only those individuals who have hostile or angry behavior patterns are at risk. Therefore, identifying the sources of anger and hostility in these people and helping them with behavior modification may allow them to cope more effectively with stress. Recently, a "type C" personality has been identified. This individual may be characterized as someone who responds to stress with depression and a sense of hopelessness. Type C personalities have a tendency to be eager to please, introverted, conforming and compliant. There is some evidence that suggests type C personalities are more prone to developing cancer.

COPING WITH STRESS AND STRESS MANAGEMENT

Life is filled with many challenges, some of which represent potential obstacles in the path of your career and life goals. **Coping** is an attempt to effectively manage or control stress so that it does not dominate your life. By coping with stress, you use techniques that alter the physiological and psychological consequences of stress (Figure 2-3). Some of these methods show short-term usefulness but are ultimately harmful because the source of the stress has not been properly handled. Examples of negative or harmful ways of coping with stressful situations include overeating or starvation or increasing consumption of alcohol, tobacco, or caffeine.

Other people cope by employing various defense mechanisms, which serve to protect the ego. These mechanisms preserve harmony within a person and provide some sense of adequacy. For example, a commonly used defense mechanism is projecting blame for failure on someone or something else. Defense mechanisms are not necessarily the most effective way to deal with stress. They may bolster the ego, but they can also circumvent managing real problems.

Various methods of coping are beneficial because they allow people to achieve self-fulfillment. People learn to manage conflicts, sources of pressure, and frustration without experiencing harm to their bodies.

It is important to develop and incorporate into your lifestyle any techniques that will help you effectively reduce stress. Fit List 2-2 identifies some general guidelines for reducing stress. Lab Activity 2-1 will help you become more aware of your response to stress and how you cope with stress.

Stress management involves more than simply reducing the total quantity of stress in your life; it also means being able to change the quality of stress in your life. Uncontrolled stress can result in physical and psychological disorders that pose a real threat to well-being. To manage stress effectively you must realize that you are responsible for your own emotional and physical well-being. Your perception of events (but not the events themselves) is under your control. You do not need to allow other people's behavior to affect your ability to maintain a relatively stable emotional and physical condition. Besides using physical activity, learning to control thought processes can be an effective method of managing stress. Collectively referred to as relaxation techniques, these methods have been demonstrated to be helpful.

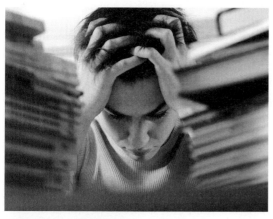

FIGURE 2-3. COPING.
Coping with stress means incorporating a variety of relaxation and coping strategies that over time will alter the physical and psychological consequences of stress.

coping: an attempt to effectively manage or control stress by using techniques that alter the physiological and psychological consequences of stress

FIT LIST 2-2

Suggestions for Managing and Coping with Stress

1. First try to be honest with yourself about all the things that are going on in your life, and then share your worries with someone you love, trust, or respect.

2. When you are feeling hassled and little things upset you that shouldn't, take a deep breath, count to 10, and then put everything in perspective. Ask yourself, "Is this the worst thing that is ever going to happen to me? Has anyone I love been hurt or affected? Will this still make me mad tomorrow?"

3. Become a better time manager. Keep a prioritized list of things to be done each day. Break down large, time-consuming projects into small chunks and reward yourself when you complete each part. Accept the fact that there is only so much time each day and that as long as you're working consistently, what you don't get done today you can finish tomorrow.

4. Work on developing healthy lifestyle habits that will enhance your resistance to stress (e.g., exercise), and avoid negative addictions such as smoking and drinking.

5. Keep a diary of things that seem to cause you stress so that over a period of time you can identify patterns or situations that cause problems. Then figure out how you can eliminate these stress-inducing situations.

6. Try to be positive and optimistic. If you constantly look for what's wrong with you or others around you, you will always find something, which often makes you feel even worse. Instead, focus on the positive aspects of all situations and try to find a little something that is good about each situation.

7. Laugh at yourself and try to maintain a sense of humor no matter what the situation.

8. Accept the fact that you can't control everything in your life and realize that your way is not always going to be the best way. Try to relax and accept other ways of doing things.

9. Develop a network of people—both family and friends—whom you love and trust, and put a degree of faith in their support when things get tough. Live your life for the good times that you share with these people, but make sure they will be there for your when things aren't so good.

10. Try to constantly focus on the pleasant aspects of your life and on the things that you can do to improve your situation.

11. Don't procrastinate. If you constantly put off things that you don't want to deal with or that are unpleasant, and you know that sooner or later you are going to have to address them, your level of frustration escalates, and you feel more stressed. Deal with every situation as soon as you can.

12. Learn how to improve your focus, relax, and reduce your stress through meditation, prayer, affirmations, or specific spiritual practices that support your connection to a higher power or belief in your own meaning or purpose.

►Relaxation Techniques

Relaxation is essentially a mental phenomenon concerned with the reduction of tensions that could originate from muscular activity but are more likely to result from psychological responses to our hectic lifestyles. **Relaxation techniques** may be broadly classified as either muscle-to-mind techniques, which

relaxation techniques: techniques for reducing tensions that could originate from muscular activity but are more likely to result from psychological responses to hectic lifestyles

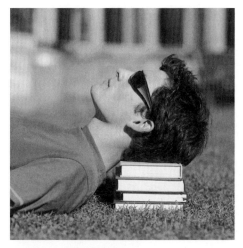

FIGURE 2-4. RELAXATION.
Relaxation techniques can be used to reduce tension associated with stress.

FIT LIST 2-3

Relaxation Techniques

Muscle-to-mind techniques

- Progressive relaxation
- Massage
- Biofeedback

Mind-to-muscle techniques

- Yoga
- Meditation
- Imagery
- Autogenic training

control the level of stimulation going to the brain from the muscles (progressive relaxation, massage, and biofeedback), or mind-to-muscle techniques, which control the level of stimulation along the nerve pathways coming from the brain to the muscles (yoga, meditation, imagery, and autogenic training) (Figure 2-4). Fit List 2-3 summarizes these relaxation techniques.

Progressive Relaxation. Progressive relaxation involves alternately tensing (5 to 10 seconds) and relaxing (45 seconds) the muscles, moving through the body in a systematic fashion to tense and relax all major muscle groups. Concentrate first on the large muscle groups in the arms, legs, trunk, and neck. Then ease tension in the forehead, eyes, face, and even the throat through a program of progressive relaxation. The program teaches the person to relax his or her whole body to the point of negative exertion. The result is a release of tension, which is an antidote to fatigue; the result is also an inducement to sleep.

Massage. Massage can be useful as a stress-reducing technique, as it induces relaxation. You can massage your neck, face, head, and shoulders, or massage can be done by another person (Figure 2-5). To many, touch is a useful form of nonverbal communication and can be reassuring.

Biofeedback. Biofeedback is a common form of stress management and relaxation therapy. Its main goals are to teach concentration, relaxation, awareness, and self-control. A machine monitors various body functions and relays the information to the subject in the form of either sounds or lights. Biofeedback helps people become aware of tensions they had not previously perceived and learn to reduce them, eventually without relying on the monitoring machines.

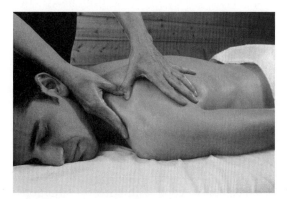

FIGURE 2-5. MASSAGE.
Massage is a good stress-reducing technique.

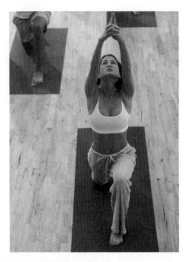

FIGURE 2-6 YOGA.
Yoga is an effective technique for calming the body psychologically and reducing stress.

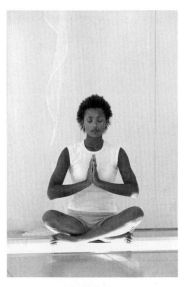

FIGURE 2-7 MEDITATION.
Meditation involves sitting quietly and mentally focusing on a word or object to reduce stress.

Yoga. Yoga uses several positions for the body through which the practitioner may progress, beginning with the simplest and moving to the more complex (Figure 2-6). The purpose of the various positions is to increase mobility and flexibility of the body. Slow, deep, diaphragmatic breathing can help alleviate stress and lower blood pressure and heart rate. Deep breathing has a calming effect on the body. It also increases production of endorphins, the body's own natural, morphine-like painkilling substances.

Meditation. Meditation uses mind-focusing exercises to control or concentrate one's attention. In most forms, meditation involves sitting quietly for a certain period, usually 15 to 20 minutes, and concentrating on a single word or image while breathing slowly and rhythmically to produce decreases in respiratory rate, heart rate, blood pressure, and muscle tension (Figure 2-7).

Imagery. Imagery can be used as a means of relaxation to cope with stressful situations. Images are pictures formed within the mind. The procedure is to sit relaxed, close your eyes, and concentrate on a particular image. With practice, you can learn to project your own body image into this picture and ultimately to perform various tasks within the mind, learning to cope with all possible variations of a situation that may be stress-producing before confronting the situation in real life.

Autogenic Training (Hypnosis). Autogenic training involves a series of specific exercises and autohypnosis that are designed to achieve a deep mental and physical state of relaxation.

HOW CAN YOU PREVENT CORONARY ARTERY DISEASE?

Cardiovascular disease ranks as the number one killer of men and women worldwide, including in the United States. It is responsible for 40 percent of all the deaths in the United States, more than all forms of cancer combined. The term *cardiovascular disease* encompasses a broad range of diseases that affect the heart and the flow of blood, the most

FIT LIST 2-4

Cardiovascular Diseases

- Coronary artery disease
- Heart attack
- Heart failure
- High blood pressure (hypertension)
- Stroke
- Arrhythmias
- Peripheral arterial disease (PAD)
- Pericarditis
- Congenital heart disease
- Cardiomyopathy

common of which are coronary artery disease, heart attack, heart failure, high blood pressure, and stroke. Other less common forms of cardiovascular disease include congenital heart disease, arrythmias, peripheral artery disease, pericarditis, and cardiomyopathy (see Fit List 2-4).

Coronary artery disease (CAD) by itself ranks as the second leading cause of death in the United States behind cancer. The lifestyle you choose plays a major role in determining whether you develop CAD. Coronary artery disease results from the accumulation of fatty deposits (atherosclerotic plaque) within the coronary arteries (Figure 2-8). The coronary arteries supply blood to the heart muscle, which functions properly only when provided with a steady blood supply. The deposition of fatty plaque often begins early in life, and the continued, gradual deposition of plaque can lead to a significant narrowing of the coronary arteries, or *atherosclerosis.* The partial or complete blockage of one or more of the major

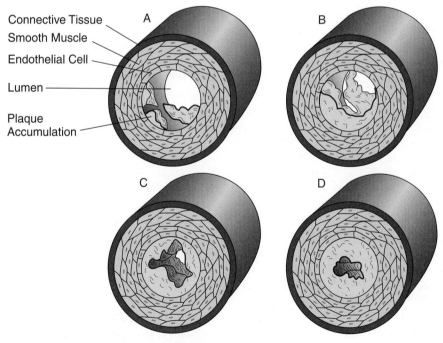

FIGURE 2-8. THE DEVELOPMENT OF ATHEROSCLEROSIS.
(A) Normal coronary artery. (B) Beginning stages of atherosclerosis; fatty plaque is deposited in vessel walls. (C) Advanced stage of atherosclerosis. (D) Completely blocked coronary artery.
Modified from Hahn, D. and W. Payne. 1991. Focus on health, *St Louis: Mosby.*

coronary arteries can lead to a condition called *myocardial ischemia,* in which the heart muscle fails to receive an adequate supply of oxygen. This can produce symptoms such as chest pain (angina pectoris) and, if severe, can precipitate a heart attack. A heart attack can occur suddenly and without warning. The factors that ultimately lead to a cardiac arrest are present early in life but mostly go undetected until they manifest as a potentially life-threatening heart attack.

RISK FACTORS

Coronary artery disease is related to personal lifestyle health habits known as *risk factors.* These risk factors cannot be labeled as causes but are instead characteristics that increase the probability of one's having CAD. The risk factors are summarized in Health Link 2-3.

Risk factors may be divided into those risk factors *that cannot be changed,* risk factors *that can be changed,* and *contributing risk factors* whose significance and prevalence have yet to be precisely determined. Some of them can be changed, treated, or modified, and some cannot. Each of these risk factors is related to CAD in an additive fashion; the greater the number of risk factors present, the greater the likelihood of developing CAD. Also, each of these factors is, at least in part, a function of individual lifestyles and behavior patterns. This observation holds out hope that it may be possible to prevent premature CAD through modification of the risk factors. With the exception of age, gender, race, and heredity, each of the other risk factors can be altered through lifestyle modification.

▶ Risk Factors That Cannot be Changed

Family History. A history of CAD in the family is considered a predisposing risk factor when parents or siblings experienced evidence of the atherosclerotic disease process before the age of 55 to 60 years.

Age. As age increases, so do the chances of a person's having some type of CAD.

Gender. More females than males die from CAD each year, although males tend to develop CAD at a younger age.

Race. African Americans have a higher incidence of hypertension than caucasians.

▶ Risk Factors That Can be Changed

Cigarette Smoking. Of all the risk factors listed, perhaps none is as great a risk factor as

HEALTH LINK 2-3

Risk Factors for Coronary Artery Disease

Risk Factors That Cannot be Changed
Family History
Age
Gender
Race

Risk Factors That Can be Changed
Cigarette smoking
Hypertension

High blood-cholesterol level
Physical inactivity

Contributing Risk Factors
Obesity
Diabetes
Stressful living

American Heart Association, www.americanheart.org

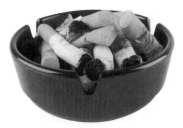

FIGURE 2-9. SMOKING.
Of all the risk factors, cigarette smoking perhaps is the greatest.

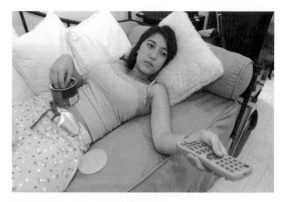

FIGURE 2-10. INACTIVITY.
Physical inactivity increases the chances of developing coronary artery disease.

cigarette smoking (Figure 2-9). It should be noted that all cigarette smokers have a much higher risk than nonsmokers. Recently it has also been shown that individuals exposed to secondhand smoke (the smoke from a cigarette that enters the environment) are also at higher risk for coronary artery disease and lung cancer.

Hypertension. Blood pressure is the pressure that the blood exerts against the inner wall of the arteries. Individuals with chronic high blood pressure are three to four times more likely to develop CAD and seven times more likely to develop a stroke than those with normal blood pressure.

Men and women who have a systolic blood pressure between 120 to 139 mmHg *or* a diastolic blood pressure of 80 to 89 mmHg are now considered "prehypertensive"—a category that includes about 45 million Americans. Blood pressure levels above 140/90 mmHg are considered high, and those over 160/100 are severely high.

High Blood-Cholesterol Level. Cholesterol is a fatty substance transported in the bloodstream, and if present in excessive amounts, it adheres to the walls of the arteries. This contributes to the deposition of atherosclerotic plaque. Thus cholesterol levels are directly related to the incidence of CAD. The higher the cholesterol level, the greater the risk of CAD. **Lipoproteins** are carriers of cholesterol. Low-density lipoprotein (LDL) deposits cholesterol into the arterial wall, whereas high-density lipoprotein (HDL) seems to be able to remove the cholesterol deposited by LDL from the arterial walls. Thus the more HDL present, the better off you are, because it appears to be an antirisk factor.

Recommended cholesterol levels are as follows:

- Total >200mg/dl (milligrams per deciliter)
- LDL >100 mg/dl
- HDL< 60 mg/dl

Research has shown that individuals who engage in regular physical activity can increase HDL levels.

Physical Inactivity. Those individuals who lead a relatively sedentary style of living are more likely to suffer from CAD and are less likely to survive a heart attack than are those who maintain an active lifestyle (Figure 2-10). Recent evidence indicates that individuals who expend a minimum of 2,000 calories of energy a week in physical activity, significantly reduce death rates from heart disease when compared with those who do not exercise.

It goes without saying that each of these four risk factors can be reversed by making

lipoproteins: a compound of fat and protein that carries cholesterol

changes in your lifestyle that include quitting smoking, altering diet, reducing stress, and exercising more to lower blood pressure and reduce cholesterol.

▶ Contributing Risk Factors

Obesity. Obesity is related to CAD only in that people who are obese tend to have higher blood pressures as well as **hyperlipidemia.** Also, obese individuals are more likely to develop a form of diabetes. Obesity reduces the ability to engage in exercise, thus impacting on another risk factor—physical inactivity. All of these are risk factors for CAD.

Diabetes. Diabetes mellitus is defined as a condition in which blood sugar levels are not properly controlled by the hormone insulin. In type I diabetes, which usually occurs in young people, the pancreas produces little or no insulin. In type II diabetes, which has an onset in adulthood, the pancreas produces insulin, but the body is unable to use it. Adult-onset diabetes produces abnormalities in lipoproteins, which seems to accelerate atherosclerosis. Increased blood sugar may also, over time, damage some of the blood vessels not only in the heart but also in the brain, thus potentially predisposing an individual to have a stroke. Other potentially detrimental effects of poorly controlled diabetes include insulin shock and diabetic coma. Many older, overweight individuals develop adult-onset diabetes. With weight loss, blood sugar levels often return to normal.

Stressful Living. **Stress** increases blood pressure, thus forcing the heart to work harder.

> **hyperlipidemia:** an excessively high level of fat in the blood
>
> **stress:** the responses that occur in the body when the internal balance or equilibrium of the body systems is disrupted

EFFECTS OF EXERCISE AND DIET ON RISK FACTORS

As physical activity levels increase, the number of deaths attributed to CAD decrease. These findings are consistent for both men and women. Even moderate levels of physical fitness that are attainable by most adults appear to provide some protection against early death.

Like exercise, diet can affect many of the risk factors identified. There is little doubt that adopting a healthful style of living, which incorporates good exercise and dietary habits, has the greatest influence in reducing the incidence of CAD. In fact, several research studies have demonstrated that diets low in fat and cholesterol in combination with comprehensive lifestyle changes including moderate aerobic exercise, stress reduction techniques, peer support, smoking cessation, and nutritional supplementation can collectively cause significant overall regression of coronary atherosclerosis, and a decrease in both blood cholesterol and blood pressure.

WHAT IS CANCER?

Cancer is the second leading cause of death in adults, falling behind cardiovascular disease. Cancer is a condition in which cellular behavior becomes abnormal. The cells no longer perform their normal functions. In general, cancer cells do not multiply at an increased rate. Instead, whatever causes the cancer alters the cell's genetic makeup and changes the way the cell functions. This abnormal cell then divides, forming additional cancer cells, and over a period of time this tumor, or collection of abnormal cells, tends to invade and ultimately take over normal tissue.

Tumors are either benign or malignant. Benign tumors typically pose only a small threat

HEALTH LINK 2-4

American Cancer Society's Cancer Warning Signals

Change in bowel or bladder habits
A sore that does not heal
Unusual bleeding or discharge
Thickening or lump in breast or elsewhere
Indigestion or difficulty in swallowing

Obvious change in wart or mole
Nagging cough or hoarseness

Modified from the American Cancer Society, *Cancer facts and figures*, New York, 2002, The Society. www.cancer.org

to tissue and tend to remain confined in a limited space. Malignant tumors, however, are cancerous, grow out of control, and spread within a specific tissue. Unfortunately, malignancies can invade surrounding tissues and spread via the blood and lymphatic systems (metastasize) throughout the entire body, thus making it difficult to control the cancer.

Malignancies are classified according to the types of tissues in which they occur as well as according to the rate at which they affect the tissue. Although different types of cancer cells share similar characteristics, each is separate and distinct. Some types are relatively easy to cure, whereas others are difficult to cure and even life threatening. Outdoor exposure to sun without sunscreen protection can lead to skin cancer, which is the most common type of cancer; fortunately, it is one of the easiest to detect and cure.

Males and females have different incidences of other types of cancers. In the male, the highest incidence of cancer is in the prostate, followed closely by lung, colon/rectal, and urinary tract cancers and leukemias/lymphomas. In the female the highest incidence is found in the breast, followed by colon/rectal, lung, and uterine cancers and leukemias/lymphomas.

The precise causes of cancer are not easily identified. Researchers have identified more than 100 types of cancer with genetic origins. Certain cancers appear to occur along family lines. The onset of most cancer has also been attributed to certain environmental factors, including viruses, exposure to ultraviolet light, radiation, alcohol use, and certain chemicals, including tobacco. A fatty diet has also been linked to cancer. Probably a combination of heredity and environmental factors is responsible for the development of cancer.

The American Cancer Society has identified warning signs of cancer, which are listed in Health Link 2-4. Unquestionably, early detection and treatment of cancer markedly improve the patient's chances of beating the disease.

EFFECTS OF EXERCISE AND DIET ON CANCER

Physical activity has been associated with a reduced risk of certain types of cancer. Moderate exercise has been shown to produce certain enzymes that reduce the formation of free radicals formed with incomplete oxidation of nutrients. These free radicals enhance the risk of chronic illnesses including cancer. There appears to be overwhelming research-based evidence that supports the benefits of exercise as a possible treatment for cancer. Several studies have examined the relationship between exercise, rehabilitation, and quality of life in cancer patients. These studies have found that overall, exercise has a positive effect on physical and psychological functioning of cancer patients while undergoing treatment.

Eating a healthy diet also has the potential to reduce the risk of cancer. The American

Cancer Society recommends the following dietary precautions:

- Reduce total fat intake
- Eat more high-fiber foods
- Eat foods rich in Vitamins A and C
- Include vegetables in your diet (broccoli, brussels sprouts)
- Avoid smoked, salt-cured, and charred foods
- Limit alcohol consumption
- Avoid obesity

WHAT LIFESTYLE HABITS ARE DETERRENTS TO FITNESS?

Physical fitness involves more than exercise. To be physically fit means that a person must develop lifestyle habits that exclude negative practices such as smoking, abusing drugs, and drinking excessive amounts of alcohol.

TOBACCO USE

▶Facts:

- Smoking cigarettes has been labeled "the single most preventable cause of disease and death in the United States" by the Surgeon General.
- Coronary heart disease (CHD) and stroke caused by smoking are the first and third leading causes of death in the United States.
- A smokers' risk of developing CHD is two to four times greater than that of non-smokers.
- Smoking-related heart disease results in more deaths per year than smoking-related lung cancer
- Lung cancer, attributed to smoking, is the leading cause of cancer death among both men and women in the United States.
- Smoking also increases the risk of many other types of cancer, including cancers of the throat, mouth, pancreas, kidney, bladder, and cervix.

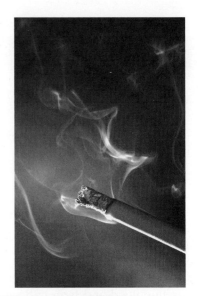

FIGURE 2-11. CIGARETTES.
Cigarettes along with smoke are not only addicting but also pose a major threat to health and well-being.

The United States government is currently waging an all-out war against tobacco. Over the years many steps have been taken to educate the nation's 60 million smokers about the dangers of tobacco. Yet millions of Americans continue to smoke (Figure 2-11).

▶Why Do People Smoke?

The pleasure derived from smoking may be due as much to the social ritual that is associated with it as to the physiologic effects. Certainly, many young people who begin to smoke do so because they regard it as symbolic of adulthood. Some use smoking as a form of rebellion. Still others use smoking as a form of weight control. It has been suggested that the habit-forming nature of tobacco is to a large extent psychologically and socially determined. As millions of smokers know, smoking is a

tobacco use: the use of cigarettes, cigars, pipes, or smokeless tobacco

habit that becomes more difficult to break the more and the longer one smokes. Nicotine is physically addictive. Although a smoker does not suffer the harsh withdrawal symptoms typical of certain addictive drugs, nervousness and irritability are commonly experienced when smoking is stopped.

▶ What Is In Tobacco Smoke?

A single cigarette contains approximately 4,000 chemicals. The major components of tobacco smoke are carbon monoxide, nicotine, and tars, all of which have harmful effects on the body. The more deeply the smoker inhales and the shorter the length to which the cigarette is smoked, the more nicotine is absorbed.

Nicotine. Nicotine, a colorless, oily compound, is extremely poisonous in concentrated form. Nicotine affects the body in a variety of ways. Small doses have a stimulating effect upon various brain centers. It constricts the blood vessels of the skin, resulting in a clammy, pallid appearance and a reduction of skin temperature. Nicotine also increases the blood pressure and the heart rate. It has a numbing effect on the taste receptors of the tongue, hence the loss of interest in food by many heavy smokers. Beginning smokers may experience some slight toxic effects such as nausea and vomiting, but, as the smoker builds up a tolerance, these generally disappear.

Carbon Monoxide. Approximately 1 percent of cigarette smoke is composed of carbon monoxide. A highly poisonous gas, carbon monoxide is also a component of automobile exhaust. Many individuals are killed each year by the inhalation of this gas in closed areas such as garages. The carbon monoxide in cigarette smoke reduces the oxygen carrying capacity of the red blood cells and therefore causes a reduction of oxygen in the body. This is one of the reasons why smokers complain of "shortness of breath" after mild exercise.

Tar. Tobacco tar is a dark, sticky substance that can be condensed from cigarette smoke. It is the substance discussed in advertisements

concerning "low tar and nicotine." Certainly "low tar" is not better than "no tar." Tar is extremely toxic and is carcinogenic (causing cancerous lesions) on test animals. The chemicals in cigarette tar are believed to contribute to the development of lung cancer.

▶ Passive Smoke

Passive inhalation of smoke ("secondhand") by nonsmokers also has dangers. Both smokers and nonsmokers are exposed to smoke containing carbon monoxide, nicotine, ammonia, and cyanide. Obviously smokers inhale the greater quantity of contaminated air. However, it has been estimated that for each pack of cigarettes smoked, the nonsmoker sharing a common air supply will inhale the equivalent of three to five cigarettes. According to a review of passive smoking research, passive smoking may be responsible for as many as 15,000 premature deaths among exposed nonsmokers. It is also true that significant numbers of individuals exposed to passive smoke develop nasal symptoms, eye irritation, headaches, cough, and in some cases allergies to smoke. For these reasons and others, many state, local, and private sector policies have been established that restrict or ban smoking in public areas. There is little doubt that passive smoking poses a significant health threat to the nonsmoker.

▶ Smokeless Tobacco

Unfortunately, the use of smokeless chewing tobacco has seen a tremendous increase in recent years. Once a pinch or pouch of chewing tobacco is placed "between the cheek and gum," nicotine is absorbed through the mucous membranes, and within a short period of time the level of nicotine in the blood is equivalent to that of a cigarette smoker. The user of chewing tobacco experiences the nicotine effects without exposure to the tar and carbon monoxide associated with a burning cigarette. Certainly the use of smokeless tobacco has eliminated many of the risks associated with cigarette smoking. However, inadvertently swallowed saliva contains carcinogens that must be eliminated through the digestive and urinary systems, thus predisposing the user to the risks of cancer. Additionally, the use of chewing tobacco increases the risk of periodontal disease in the gums, destroys the enamel on teeth, and causes the development of white blotches on the mucous membranes of the mouth, which are thought to be associated with development of cancer in the mouth.

▶ Curbing the Use of Tobacco

Many steps have been taken to caution the nation's 60 million smokers about the dangers of tobacco. A warning from the U.S. surgeon general is printed on each package of cigarettes. Television commercials for cigarettes have been banned. Group therapy sessions have been organized to help people stop smoking. Patches that deliver nicotine through the skin are often prescribed along with group sessions to help smokers "kick the habit." Special cigarette holders and filter tips have been devised to cut down on tar and nicotine. Some states have outlawed smoking in all public buildings. Municipalities are acting to ban smoking altogether in public places. In many states it is illegal to sell tobacco products to individuals under 18 years of age. Yet millions of Americans, including many college students, continue to smoke. Many adults belong to the hard core group of smokers who will never quit the habit. However, a major focus is on educational efforts to prevent young people from choosing to begin to smoke.

DRUG USE AND ABUSE

Drug abuse differs from drug use and drug misuse. Drug use refers to the taking of any drug for medical purposes. Drug misuse refers to the irresponsibility that many individuals show in the use of drugs. People who ignore medical advice about proper use of a prescribed drug or lend prescriptions to others are displaying a misuse of drugs. Drug abuse may be defined as the use of drugs for nonmedical reasons; that is, with the intent of getting "high"—altering mood or behavior.

After time, the body builds a tolerance to the usual level of certain drugs. Therefore, after abusing one of these drugs for a certain period, a person no longer gets the same "high" unless the dosage is increased. This is one reason that chronic drug abusers continually need to increase their number of "fixes" or doses of a drug.

Habituation is defined as psychological dependence as a result of continued use. People can be habituated to the use of alcohol, cigarettes, or drugs. They can become habituated to almost anything if they feel that it is helping them. In other words, drug abuse can become a habit if the individual feels psychologically that it is helping him or her in some way.

The term *addiction* means physical dependence. An addicted individual's body (1) needs a drug to function, (2) builds a tolerance to that drug, and (3) in most cases suffers from withdrawal symptoms. Withdrawal symptoms are the unpleasant physical problems that occur when the drug is taken away.

Drugs are most commonly abused because of their effects on mood and behavior. For example, a drug may produce a feeling of euphoria, often called a "high." These drugs are often referred to as psychoactive or psychotropic drugs. However, certain drugs, when abused, can distort the personality to such a degree that the individual may become dangerous to self or society. Research has indicated that most individuals who abuse psychoactive drugs have the type of personality that is often impressionable, escapist, or

> **drug abuse:** the use of drugs for nonmedical reasons; that is, with the intent of getting "high"—altering mood or behavior

fragile. Persons with stronger personalities may experiment with drugs but are less likely to become dependent on them because the drugs do not satisfy their needs.

Drug abuse can cause both personal and family problems such as domestic violence, crime, and relationship difficulties.

▶ Abused Illegal Drugs

Obviously, many drugs are abused in our society. Often referred to as "recreational drugs" these are not only a deterrent to a healthy lifestyle, but their use or possession is also illegal. Among the more common illegal drugs are marijuana, cocaine, crystal methamphetamine, and ecstasy.

Marijuana. When used in small doses, marijuana produces a "high" feeling and sense of relaxation lasting for several hours after use. The immediate effects of use are relaxation and feelings of heightened awareness of visual, auditory, and tactile sensations. It also results in changes in perception, mood, consciousness, cognition, and behavior. Problems associated with long-term use include the development of anxiety, psychosis, depression, restlessness, irritability, loss of motivation, sleep disturbances, and possible damage to the lungs (Figure 2-12).

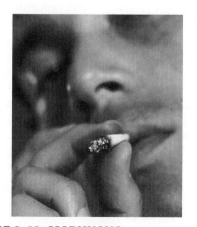

FIGURE 2-12. MARIJUANA.
Marijuana use can cause a variety of physical and social problems.

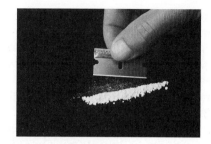

FIGURE 2-13. COCAINE.
Cocaine is one of the most widely used recreational drugs.

Cocaine. Cocaine has become one of the most popular drugs of abuse during recent years (Figure 2-13). Cocaine is a stimulant with effects of short duration. Cocaine use produces immediate feelings of euphoria, excitement, decreased sense of fatigue, and heightened sexual drive. Cocaine may be snorted, taken intravenously, or smoked ("free-based"). Crack is a rocklike crystalline form of cocaine that is heated in a small pipe and then inhaled, producing an immediate rush. The initial effects are extremely intense, and because they are pleasurable, users rapidly develop strong psychological dependence, regardless of whether they can afford this expensive habit.

Long-term effects include nasal congestion and damage to the membranes and cartilage of the nose if snorted, bronchitis, loss of appetite leading to nutritional deficiencies, convulsions, impotence, and cocaine psychosis with paranoia, depression, hallucinations, and disorganized mental function. An overdose can cause abnormal heart rhythms, which can result in death.

Crystal Methamphetamine. This drug is used by individuals of all ages and is increasingly gaining in popularity as a club drug. It is a colorless, odorless, and highly addictive synthetic stimulant. Crystal methamphetamine resembles small fragments of glass or shiny blue-white "rocks" of various sizes. Like powdered methamphetamine it is abused because of the long-lasting euphoric effects it produces. But it has a higher purity level and may produce even longer-lasting and more intense physiological effects than the powdered form of the drug. It may either be smoked using glass pipes similar to pipes used to smoke crack cocaine or it may be injected. A user who smokes or injects the drug immediately experiences an intense sensation followed by a high that may last 12 hours or more.

Crystal methamphetamine use is associated with numerous serious physical problems, which may include rapid heart rate, increased blood pressure, and damage to the small blood vessels in the brain that can lead to stroke. Overdoses can cause increased temperature, convulsions, and death. People who use crystal methamphetamine may have episodes of paranoia, anxiety, violent behavior, confusion, and insomnia. The drug can produce psychotic symptoms that persist for months or years after an individual has stopped using the drug.

Ecstasy. Considered the most commonly used designer drug, Ecstasy is a close derivative of methamphetamine and can be described as a hallucinogenic stimulant. Designer drugs are illicit variations of other drugs. Ecstasy is most often found in tablet, capsule, or powder form and is usually consumed orally, although it can also be injected. Ecstasy can cause euphoria and feelings of well-being, enhanced mental or emotional clarity, anxiety, and paranoia. Heavier doses can cause hallucinations, sensations of lightness and floating, depression, paranoid thinking, and violent, irrational behavior. Physical reactions can include loss of appetite, nausea, vomiting, blurred vision, increased heart rate and blood pressure, muscle tension, faintness, chills, sweating, tremors, insomnia, convulsions, and loss of control over voluntary body movements. Some reactions have been reported to persist up to 14 days after taking Ecstasy.

▶ Abused Perscription Drugs

Certainly the abuse of illegal drugs is a major concern. However, several government agencies have indicated that more people are abusing prescription drugs than the typical illegal drugs discussed previously. It has been estimated that one out of five teens have abused prescription drugs. A majority of abused prescription drugs are obtained from family and friends, most coming from the home medicine cabinet. But prescription drugs are also sometimes sold on the street like other illegal drugs. Some people think that prescription drugs are safer and less addictive than street drugs. But prescription drugs are only safe for the individuals who actually have prescriptions for them. The prescription drugs that are commonly abused in the United States fall into several broad categories including pain relievers, depressants, and stimulants.

ADHD Medications. The abuse of medications commonly used for treating attention deficit and hyperactivity disorder (ADHD) is a relatively new phenomenon, but one that has become a major cause for concern, especially in the college population. These medications usually are amphetamines such as Ritalin, Adderall, and Dexedrine. They are stimulants but they also decrease an individual's distractibility and facilitate concentration and focus. Reasons for abusing or misusing stimulant medication include improving attention, partying, reducing hyperactivity, and improving grades. Some individuals are illegally or illicitly obtaining the medications for their own use or for sale. Common signs and symptoms include shakiness, rapid speech or movements, difficulty sitting still, difficulty concentrating, lack of appetite, sleep disturbance, and irritability.

OxyContin (Oxycodone) OxyContin is a perscription drug used to treat moderate to severe pain. Oxycodone is in a class of medications called opiate (narcotic) analgesics. It works by altering the way the brain and nervous system respond to pain.

While this is an extremely effective medication it has become perhaps the most widely abused prescription drug. The drug is relatively inexpensive but may be sold on the street at 20 times the value. Tablets may be crushed, then snorted, chewed, or injected to obtain a heroin-like high. It is rare to become addicted to OxyContin when the drug is used as recommended. However, due to pharmacy break-ins, growing levels of illegal use, and increased media reports of OxyContin abuse, prescriptions are heavily regulated.

ALCOHOL ABUSE

The consumption of alcohol in American society is commonplace (Figure 2-14). The reasons some people abstain and some drink moderately, while others imbibe heavily, have never been completely explained. Studies seem to indicate that alcohol meets individual need patterns. It is felt that situations and environmental conditions that produce tension and insecurity may cause some to resort to drinking.

People who are uncomfortable and lack poise at social gatherings use drinking as a social lubricant. Alcohol gives them courage and helps them feel at ease. Unfortunately, some people have failed to develop wholesome interpersonal relationships. Alcohol provides a temporary means of escape from those experiences that frustrate and worry them. Drinking does not solve the problem but instead offers a temporary means of escape from reality. Although there are some conflicting views as to its cause, there appears to be agreement that some of the causes are psychological. Some psychologists believe that individuals who are emotionally disturbed, have compulsive personalities, or exhibit obsessive-compulsive behavior are more prone to alcoholism.

▶ What Is Alcoholism?

Alcoholism is called a disease because an alcoholic is sick, totally dependent on the substance and the abuse of it. The National Council on Alcoholism defines an alcoholic as "a person who is powerless to stop drinking, and whose drinking seriously alters his (or her) normal living pattern." Many persons may ask, "Why do some people become alcoholics while others in the same situation or environment do not?" Why is it that only 10 to 15 percent of the more than 100 million drinkers become alcoholics? These are valid questions for which there are no absolute answers. Many potential alcoholics do not become alcoholics. Unfortunately, alcoholism is a chronic condition that does not go away. It is progressive and incurable as long as the alcoholic keeps on drinking. If he or she stops drinking, the disease can be arrested. But most experts believe that the alcoholic must not drink again. Otherwise that person will be right back where he or she was when the decision was made to stop drinking. Alcoholics are sensitive to alcohol and all other sedatives. The brain of an alcoholic produces a substance called THIQ, which is extremely addicting. Years of abstinence will not eliminate the ability to produce THIQ. It is always present and renders the alcoholic powerless to quit once she or he begins drinking.

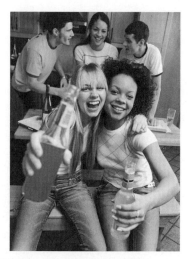

FIGURE 2-14. ALCOHOL ABUSE.
Alcohol is widely used and abused by both college and high school students.

alcoholism: a disease in which a person is powerless to stop drinking and drinking seriously alters his or her normal living pattern

HEALTH LINK 2-5

Fact: Alcohol Use Even in Low Levels Can Cause Impairment.

Use this simple chart to estimate your Blood Alcohol Concentration (BAC)

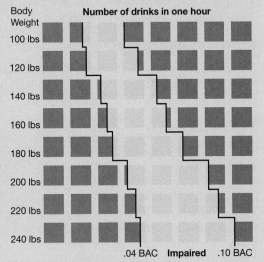

Body Weight — Number of drinks in one hour

100 lbs
120 lbs
140 lbs
160 lbs
180 lbs
200 lbs
220 lbs
240 lbs

.04 BAC   Impaired   .10 BAC

Procedure: This chart represents the number of drinks it would take to bring your blood alcohol concentration to a particular level in one hour.

1. Locate the line that corresponds to your body weight.

2. From left to right, each square represents one drink.
3. The first dark line to the right indicates an alcohol concentration of .04 (indicating impairment).
4. The second dark line to the right indicates an alcohol concentration of .10 (legal intoxication in most states).

To calculate concentration during a longer period of time:

1. Add the total amount of drinks consumed.
2. From that total, subtract 1 drink for each hour of drinking. In other words, your body will burn off 1 drink per hour.

Guide Each of the following drinks contain the same amount of alcohol:

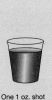
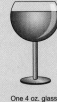
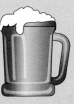

One 1 oz. shot of whiskey   One 4 oz. glass of wine   One 12 oz. mug of beer

▶ What Are the Effects of Alcohol?

Alcohol is classified as a drug that depresses the central nervous system. Alcohol is absorbed from the digestive system into the bloodstream very rapidly. Factors that affect how rapidly absorption takes place include the number of drinks consumed, the rate of consumption, the alcohol concentration of the beverage, and the amount of food in the stomach. Some alcohol is absorbed into the blood through the stomach, but the greater part is absorbed through the small intestine. Alcohol is transported through the blood to the liver, where it can be metabolized at a rate of 2/3

ounce per hour. An excess causes an increase in the level of alcohol circulating in the blood. As blood alcohol content (BAC) levels continue to increase, predictable signs of intoxication appear. At 0.1 percent the person loses motor coordination, and from 0.2 to 0.5 percent the symptoms become progressively more profound and perhaps even life threatening. Women tend to absorb more alcohol and at a faster rate than do men of the same body weight. Intoxication persists until the remainder of the alcohol can be metabolized by the liver. There is no way to accelerate the liver's metabolism of alcohol ("sober up"); it just takes time. Health Link 2-5 gives you an

HEALTH LINK 2-6

Warning Signs for Excessive Alcohol Use

Do you:

- Drink more frequently than you did a year ago?
- Drink more heavily than you did a year ago?
- Plan to drink, sometimes days in advance?
- Gulp or "chug" your drinks, perhaps in a contest?
- Set personal limits on the amount you plan to drink but then consistently disregard these limits?
- Drink at a rate greater than two drinks per hour?
- Encourage or even pressure others to drink with you?
- Frequently want a nonalcoholic beverage but then end up drinking an alcoholic drink?
- Drive your car while under the influence of alcohol or ride with another person who has been drinking?
- Use alcoholic beverages while taking prescription or over-the-counter medications?
- Forget what happened while you were drinking?
- Have a tendency to disregard information about the effects of drinking?
- Find your reputation fading because of alcohol use?

National Institute on Alcohol Abuse and Alcoholism, www.niaaa.nih.gov

estimation of the number of drinks that will cause a specific level of impairment.

▶Alcohol-Related Diseases

Alcohol consumption can directly or indirectly cause numerous physical problems. Gastritis, an inflammation of the stomach, can result from excessive alcohol consumption. Alcoholics suffer from malnutrition because they lose interest in food and are unable to purchase proper foods. Also, alcohol provides considerable calories but lacks important nutrients.

Alcohol is poisonous to cells. The most common cause of liver disorders, cirrhosis (a scarring and hardening of liver tissue), is a result of chronic alcoholism. Over the years alcohol has been linked to cancer, especially cancer of the liver, larynx, esophagus, and tongue. These represent only a few of the diseases caused when excessive amounts of alcohol are consumed for extended periods of time.

How can you tell whether you currently have or are developing a drinking problem? You must identify the warning signs that let you know that the potential for such a problem exists. Health Link 2-6 will give you some idea of the warning signs.

CREATING A HEALTHY LIFESTYLE: YOUR PERSONAL RESPONSIBILITY

Some people today think of health as the responsibility of doctors, hospitals, clinics, insurance companies, and the government. It is important to realize, however, that health cannot be purchased or the responsibility relegated to some other person or agency. Health is an obligation on the part of each individual, and it is erroneous to equate more health services with better health. Instead, individuals must take responsibility for their own health.

The decisions that people make relative to their lifestyle have an effect on their health. They are the ones who decide what to eat and when and whether to exercise, drink, engage in drug abuse, smoke, or see a doctor. Thus the decisions they make leave an imprint on their health and well-being. In many cases people who become sick have only themselves to blame.

The call to attain the optimal level of health for ourselves and our loved ones is a lifetime challenge. No one can do the job for us, nor should they. This is a responsibility each person should assume to the extent he or she is able, with pride and conviction. Lab Activity 2–2 will help you determine whether you are living a healthy lifestyle.

SUMMARY

- Creating a healthy lifestyle incorporates aspects of intellectual, physical, social, emotional, and spiritual health in a manner that allows you to enjoy the highest level of health and well-being possible.
- Everyone experiences stress, and some stress is needed to perform the daily tasks of life and for growth and development. Stress involves physiological and psychological responses.
- Coping skills to ward off stress are those procedures that allow a person to deal with reality in a positive way. Several relaxation techniques for coping with stress exist, including the progressive relaxation technique, biofeedback, yoga, breathing exercises, meditation, imagery, massage, and autogenic training.
- Coronary artery disease (CAD) results from atherosclerosis. The major risk factors that predispose a person to CAD, which cannot be changed, are family history, age, gender and race. Risk factors that can be changed include cigarette

smoking, hypertension, lack of physical activity, and high blood-cholesterol levels. Obesity, diabetes, and stressful living would be considered contributing risk factors.

- Cancer is the second leading cause of death in adult Americans. Early detection and treatment are critical for reducing the likelihood of death.
- It is important to recognize that using alcohol, tobacco, or other drugs is a deterrent to health and wellness.
- Creating a healthy style of living is a personal responsibility.

SUGGESTED READINGS

American Cancer Society. 2010. *2009 cancer facts and figures.* Atlanta: American Cancer Society.

American Heart Association. 1998. *Primary prevention of coronary heart disease: Guidance from Framingham.* Dallas: American Heart Association.

Bassuk, S. S., and J. E. Manson. 2004. Preventing cardiovascular disease in women: How much physical activity is "good enough"? *President's Council on Physical Fitness and Sports research digest* 4(5):1–7, 9.

Baylen, C., and H. Rosenberg. 2006. A review of the acute subjective effects of MDMA/ecstasy. *Addiction* 101(7):933.

Begg, C. B. 2001. The search for cancer risk factors: When can we stop looking? *American Journal of Public Health* 91(3):360–64.

Bellenir, K. 2004. *Smoking concerns sourcebook: Basic consumer health information about nicotine addiction and smoking cessation, featuring facts about the health effects of tobacco use.* Detroit: Omnigraphics, Inc.

Brehm, B. A. 2002. Heart disease: Lifestyle is key to prevention. *Fitness Management* 18(5):30.

Brubaker, P., L. A. Kaminsky, and M. H. Whaley. 2002. *Coronary artery disease: Essentials of prevention and rehabilitation programs.* Champaign, IL: Human Kinetics.

Burak, L. J. 2001. Smokeless tobacco education for college athletes. *Journal of Physical Education, Recreation and Dance* 72(1):37–38, 53.

Carr, A. 2010. *The easy way to stop smoking : Join the millions who have become non-smokers using Allen Carr's easy way method,* New York, Sterling Publishers

Chen, D., and A. Park. 2007: Components of mental resilience: Effects of comprehensive stress management and prevention. *Journal of Sport and Exercise Psychology* 29:S17.

Cooper, C. B. 2001. Smoking and exercise. *ACSM's Health and Fitness Journal* 5(2):27, 31.

Courneya, K. S., and J. R. Mackey. 2001. Exercise during and after cancer treatment: Benefits, guidelines, and precautions. *International Sports Medicine Journal* 1(5):206–10.

Davis, M., McKay, M., Eshelman, E. 2008. *Relaxation & stress reduction workbook,* Oakland, CA, New Harbinger Publications, Inc.

Dickey, R. A., and J. J. Janick. 2001. Lifestyle modifications in the prevention and treatment of hypertension. *Endocrine Practice* 7(5):392–99.

Do Lee, C., and S. N. Blair. 2002. Cardiorespiratory fitness and smoking-related and total cancer mortality in men. *Medicine and Science in Sports and Exercise* 34(5):735–39.

Esselstyn, C. 2008. *Prevent and reverse heart disease : The revolutionary, scientifically proven, nutrition-based cure,* New York, Penguin Group.

Exercise and acute cardiovascular events: Placing the risks into perspective. 2007. *Medicine and Science in Sports and Exercise* 39(5):886–97.

Gill, J. 2004. *Personalized stress management: A manual for everyday life and work.* Otsego, Michigan: Pagefree Publishing Inc.

Green, G. A., F. D. Uryasz, T. A. Petr, and C. D. Bray. 2001. NCAA study of substance use and abuse habits of college student-athletes. *Clinical Journal of Sport Medicine* 11(1):51–56.

Greene, R. 2002. *Get with the program!: Getting real about your weight, health, and emotional well-being.* New York: Simon and Schuster Adult Publishing.

Hajek, P., Taylor, T., McRobbie, H. 2010. The effect of stopping smoking on perceived stress levels. *Addiction* 105(8):1466.

Heart disease risk high, knowledge low. 2004. *IDEA Personal Trainer* 15(2):10.

Heyward, V. H. 2010. Assessing and managing stress. In *Advanced fitness assessment and exercise prescription,* 5th ed., edited by V. H. Heyward, pp. 251–58, 347–48. Champaign, IL: Human Kinetics.

High-intensity exercise best to reduce stress. 2004. *Fitness Business Canada* 5(4):46–47.

Hildebrand, K. M., D. J. Johnson, and K. Bogle. 2001. Comparison of patterns of alcohol use between high school and college athletes and non-athletes. *College Student Journal* 35(3):358–65.

Howard-Pitney, B., and M. A. Winkleby. 2002. Chewing tobacco: Who uses and who quits? Findings from NHANES III, 1988–1994. *American Journal of Public Health* 92(2):250–56.

Iritani, B., D. Hallfors, and D. Bauer. 2007. Crystal methamphetamine use among young adults in the USA. *Addiction* 102(7):1102.

Kavanagh, T. 2001. Exercise in the primary prevention of coronary artery disease. *Canadian Journal of Cardiology* 17(2):155–61.

Keller, J. 2004. Nine risk factors to blame for 90% of heart attacks. *IDEA Fitness Journal* 1(5):13.

Kinney, J. 2008. *Loosening the grip: A handbook of alcohol information.* New York: McGraw-Hill.

Koehler, G. 2001. Stress management: Exercises for teachers and students. *Strategies* 15(2):7–10.

Ksir, C., Hart, C., Oakley, R. *Drugs, society, and human behavior,* New York, McGraw-Hill.

LaFountaine, J., M. Neisen, and R. Parsons. 2006. Wellness factors in first year college students., *American Journal of Health Studies* 21(3/4):214.

Lee, I. 2010. Physical activity and cardiac protection. *Current Sports Medicine Reports* 9(4):214.

Lee, I. M., and R. S. Paffenbarger, Jr. 2001. Preventing coronary heart disease: The role of physical activity. *Physician and Sports Medicine* 29(2):37–40, 43–46, 49, 52.

Luskin, F., and K. Pelletier. 2005. *Stress free for good: 10 scientifically proven life skills for health and happiness.* New York: Harper Collins Publishers.

Meade, T. W. 2001. Cardiovascular disease: Linking pathology and epidemiology. *International Journal of Epidemiology* 30(5):1179–83.

Meyer, H. E., A. J. Sogaard, A. Tverdal, and R. M. Selmer. 2002. Body mass index and mortality: The influence of physical activity and smoking. *Medicine and Science in Sports and Exercise* 34(7):1065–70.

Monroe, M. 2006. What is wellness? *IDEA Fitness Journal* 3(8):103–6.

Nieman, D. C. 1998. *The exercise-health connection.* Champaign, IL: Human Kinetics.

Perkinson, R. 2003. *The alcohol and drug abuse patient workbook.* Thousand Oaks, CA. Sage Publications.

Pescatello, L. S., B. A. Franklin, and R. Fagard. 2004. American College of Sports Medicine position stand: Exercise and hypertension. *Medicine and Science in Sports and Exercise* 36(3):533–53.

Prentiss, C. 2005. *Alcoholism and addiction cure : A holistic approach to total recovery,* Malibu, CA, Power Press.

Prudhomme, B., and K. Becker-Blease. 2006. Stimulant medication use, misuse, and abuse in an undergraduate and graduate student sample. *Journal of American College Health* 54(5):261.

Robbins , G., Powers , D., Burgess , S. 2010. *Wellness way of life,* New York, McGraw-Hill.

Slattery, M. L., and J. D. Potter. 2002. Physical activity and colon cancer: Confounding or interaction? *Medicine and Science in Sports and Exercise* 34(6):913–19.

Smoking cessation in young adults. 2007. *American Journal of Public Health* 97(8):1354.

Stork, T. 2010. *The doctor is in: A 7-step prescription for optimal wellness,* New York, Simon and Schuster Adult Publishing.

The war on cancer: Are we winning or losing? 2004. *Tufts University Health & Nutrition Letter* 22(2):8.

Thune, I., and A. S. Furberg. 2001. Physical activity and cancer risk: Dose-response and cancer, all sites and site-specific. *Medicine and Science in Sports and Exercise* 33(6 Suppl):S530–50.

Wannamethee, S. G., and A. G. Shaper. 2001. Physical activity in the prevention of cardiovascular disease: An epidemiological perspective. *Sports Medicine* 31(2):101–14.

Williams, A. 2009. The wellness culture: Self-responsibility at last., *IDEA Fitness Journal* 6(9):28.

Woolf, S., and S. Maisto. 2007. Rethinking substance abuse: What the science shows, and what we should do about it. *Addiction* 102(11):1841.

Your Personal Stress Inventory

Response	Never	Rarely	Some-times	Often	Very Often
Behavioral Responses to Stress					
1. I eat compulsively or too fast.	N	R	S	O	A
2. I light up a cigarette.	N	R	S	O	A
3. I drink alcohol or use mood-altering drugs.	N	R	S	O	A
4. I grind my teeth.	N	R	S	O	A
5. I clench my fists.	N	R	S	O	A
6. I pace, walk rapidly, or rush.	N	R	S	O	A
7. I tap my feet.	N	R	S	O	A
8. I sleep a lot or have trouble falling asleep.	N	R	S	O	A
9. I sulk and don't talk to people.	N	R	S	O	A
10. I snap back or get angry with others.	N	R	S	O	A
Total Number O's and A's Circled:				_____	_____
Cognitive (Thinking) Responses to Stress					
1. I can't concentrate on what I'm doing.	N	R	S	O	A
2. I forget things or I get confused.	N	R	S	O	A
3. My thoughts seem to race.	N	R	S	O	A
4. This isn't where I want to be in my life.	N	R	S	O	A
5. I worry a lot.	N	R	S	O	A
6. I have recurring, troublesome thoughts.	N	R	S	O	A
7. I can't turn off my thoughts at night and relax.	N	R	S	O	A
8. I have trouble sleeping because of things on my mind.	N	R	S	O	A
9. Things must be perfect.	N	R	S	O	A
10. I must do it myself.	N	R	S	O	A
Total Number O's and A's Circled:				_____	_____

Continued

Your Personal Stress Inventory

Response	Never	Rarely	Some-times	Often	Very Often
Emotional (Feelings) Responses to Stress					
1. I feel depressed, sad, and unhappy.	N	R	S	O	A
2. I can't say no without feeling guilty.	N	R	S	O	A
3. I feel worthless, disappointed in myself and life.	N	R	S	O	A
4. I don't get a sense of accomplishment most days.	N	R	S	O	A
5. I feel trapped.	N	R	S	O	A
6. I can't seem to share my feelings with my family/friends.	N	R	S	O	A
7. I feel exploited, used by others.	N	R	S	O	A
8. I'm afraid of things that didn't used to bother me.	N	R	S	O	A
9. I feel cynical and disenchanted.	N	R	S	O	A
10. I feel agitated, irritated, short-tempered, impatient.	N	R	S	O	A
Total Number O's and A's Circled:				_____	_____

Scoring Interpretation

Total the number of circled responses in the columns indicating frequent reactions to stress (O: Often and A: Always). Those reactions will most likely be the first to alert you that you are experiencing excessive stress.

Notice which category (physical, behavioral, cognitive, or emotional) has the most O's and A's. For example, if you have more frequent reactions in the physical category, you may want to become aware of those tension spots and learn about relaxation or biofeedback techniques to reduce stress.

By simply becoming aware of your signs of stress, you'll be taking a major step toward better managing your stress level.

Name   Section   Date

PURPOSE   All of us want good health. But many of us do not know how to be as healthy as possible. Health experts now describe lifestyle as one of the most important factors affecting health. In fact, it is estimated that as many as seven of the ten leading causes of death could be reduced through common-sense changes in lifestyle. That's what this brief test, developed by the Public Health Service, is all about. Its purpose is simply to tell you how well you are doing to stay healthy. The behaviors covered in the test are recommended for most Americans. Some of them may not apply to persons with certain chronic diseases or handicaps or to pregnant women. Such persons may require special instructions from their physicians.

PROCEDURE   1. Circle the appropriate response for each question.
2. Add the total number of points for each section.

Behavior	Almost Always	Sometimes	Almost Never
Tobacco Use If you *never smoke* or use tobacco products, enter a score of 10 for this section and go to the next section on Alcohol and Drugs.	10	0	0
1. I avoid smoking cigarettes and chewing tobacco.	2	1	0
2. I smoke only low tar and nicotine cigarettes or I smoke a pipe or cigars.	2	1	0
Smoking Score: _____			
Alcohol and Drugs			
1. I avoid drinking alcoholic beverages *or* I drink no more than 1 or 2 drinks a day.	4	1	0
2. I avoid using alcohol or other drugs (especially illegal drugs) as a way of handling stressful situations or the problems in my life.	2	1	0

Continued

51

Behavior	Almost Always	Sometimes	Almost Never
3. I am careful not to drink alcohol when taking certain medicines (for example, medicine for sleeping, pain, colds and allergies) or when pregnant.	2	1	0
4. I read and follow the label directions when using prescribed and over-the-counter drugs.	2	1	0
Alcohol and Drugs Score:_____			
Eating Habits			
1. I eat a variety of foods each day, such as fruits and vegetables, whole grain breads and cereals, lean meats, dairy products, dry peas and beans, and nuts and seeds.	4	1	0
2. I limit the amount of fat, saturated fat, and cholesterol I eat (including fat in meats, eggs, butter, and other dairy products, shortenings, and organ meats such as liver).	2	1	0
3. I limit the amount of salt I eat by cooking with only small amounts, not adding salt at the table, and avoiding salty snacks.	2	1	0
4. I avoid eating too much sugar (especially frequent snacks of stick candy or soft drinks).	2	1	0
Eating Habits Score: _____			
Exercise Habits			
1. I maintain a desired weight, avoiding overweight and underweight.	3	1	0
2. I do vigorous exercises for 15–30 minutes at least 3 times a week (examples include running, swimming, brisk walking).	3	1	0

Health Style: A Self-Test

Behavior	Almost Always	Sometimes	Almost Never
3. I do exercises that enhance my muscle tone for 15–30 minutes at least 3 times a week (examples include yoga and calisthenics).	2	1	0
4. I use part of my leisure time participating in individual, family, or team activities that increase my level of fitness (such as gardening, bowling, golf, and baseball).	2	1	0
Exercise/Fitness Score: _____			
Stress Control			
1. I have a job or do other work that I enjoy.	2	1	0
2. I find it easy to relax and express my feelings freely.	2	1	0
3. I recognize early and prepare for events or situations likely to be stressful for me.	2	1	0
4. I have close friends, relatives, or others whom I can talk to about personal matters and call on for help when needed.	2	1	0
5. I participate in group activities (such as church and community organizations) or hobbies that I enjoy.	2	1	0
Stress Control Score: _____			
Safety			
1. I wear a seat belt while riding in a car.	2	1	0
2. I avoid driving while under the influence of alcohol and other drugs.	2	1	0
3. I obey traffic rules and the speed limit when driving.	2	1	0
4. I am careful when using potentially harmful products or substances (such as household cleaners, poisons, and electrical devices).	2	1	0
5. I avoid smoking in bed.	2	1	0
Safety Score: _____			

Health Style: A Self-Test

What Your Scores Mean to YOU

Scores of 9 and 10: Excellent! Your answers show that you are aware of the importance of this area to your health. More importantly, you are putting your knowledge to work for you by practicing good health habits. As long as you continue to do so, this area should not pose a serious health risk. It's likely that you are setting an example for your family and friends to follow. Because you scored very high on this part of the test, you may want to consider other areas where your scores indicate room for improvement.

Scores of 6 to 8: Good. Your health practices in this area are good, but there is room for improvement. Look again at the items you answered with a "Sometimes" or "Almost Never." What changes can you make to improve your score? Even a small change can often help you achieve better health.

Scores of 3 to 5: Fair. Your health risks are showing! Would you like more information about the risks you are facing and about why it is important for you to change these behaviors? Perhaps you need help in deciding how to successfully make the changes you desire. In either case, help is available.

Scores of 0 to 2: Poor. Obviously, you were concerned enough about your health to take the test, but your answers show that you may be taking serious and unnecessary risks with your health. Perhaps you are not aware of the risks and what to do about them. You can easily get the information and help you need to improve, if you wish. The next step is up to you.

What am I doing to become as healthy as possible? _____

_____

What steps can I take to feel better? _____

_____

What changes do I need to make in my lifestyle? _____

_____

YOU Can Start Right Now!

The test you just completed offers numerous suggestions to help you reduce your risk of disease and premature death. Here are some of the most significant.

Avoid Cigarettes and Other Tobacco Products   Cigarette smoking is the single most important preventable cause of illness and early death. It is especially risky for pregnant women and their unborn babies. Persons who stop smoking reduce their risk of getting heart disease and cancer. So if you're a cigarette smoker, think twice about lighting that next cigarette. If you choose to continue smoking, try decreasing the number of cigarettes you smoke and switching to a low tar and nicotine brand. If you chew, stop the habit.

Follow Sensible Drinking Habits   Alcohol produces changes in mood and behavior. Many people who drink are able to control their intake of alcohol and to avoid undesired, and often harmful, effects. Heavy, regular use of alcohol can lead to cirrhosis of the liver, a leading cause of death. Also, statistics clearly show that mixing drinking and driving is often the cause of fatal or crippling accidents. So if you drink, do it wisely and in moderation. **Use care in taking drugs.** Today's greater use of drugs—both legal and illegal—is one of our most serious health risks. Even some drugs prescribed by your doctor can be dangerous if taken when drinking alcohol or before driving. Excessive or continued use of tranquilizers (or "pep pills") can cause physical and mental problems. Using or experimenting with illicit drugs such as marijuana, LSD, heroin, cocaine, and PCP may lead to a number of damaging effects or even death.

Eat Sensibly Overweight individuals are at greater risk for diabetes, gallbladder disease, and high blood pressure. So it makes good sense to maintain proper weight. But good eating habits also mean holding down the amount of fat (especially saturated fat), cholesterol, sugar, and salt in your diet. If you must snack, try nibbling on fresh fruits and vegetables. You'll feel better—and look better, too.

Exercise Regularly Almost everyone can benefit from exercise—and there's some form of exercise almost everyone can do. (If you have any doubt, check first with your doctor.) Usually, as little as 15–30 minutes of vigorous exercise three times a week will help you have a healthier heart, eliminate excess weight, tone up sagging muscles, and sleep better. Think how much difference all these improvements could make in the way you feel!

Learn to Handle Stress Stress is a normal part of living: Everyone faces it to some degree. The causes of stress can be good or bad, desirable or undesirable (such as a promotion on the job or the loss of a spouse). Properly handled, stress need not be a problem. But unhealthy responses to stress—such as driving too fast or erratically, drinking too much, or prolonged anger or grief—can cause physical and mental problems. Even on a very busy day, find a few minutes to slow down and relax. Talking over a problem with someone you trust can often help you find a satisfactory solution. Learn to distinguish between things that are "worth fighting about" and things that are less important.

Be Safety Conscious Think "safety first" at home, at work, at school, at play, and on the highway. Buckle seat belts, and obey traffic rules. Keep poisons and weapons out of the reach of children, and keep emergency numbers by your telephone. When the unexpected happens, be prepared.

Where Do You Go From Here?

Start by asking yourself a few frank questions: Am I really doing all I can to be as healthy as possible? What steps can I take to feel better? Am I willing to begin now? If you scored low in one or more sections of the test, decide what changes you want to make for improvement. You might pick that aspect of your lifestyle where you feel you have the best chance for success and tackle that one first. Once you have improved your score there, go on to other areas.

If you already have tried to change your health habits (to stop smoking or exercise regularly, for example), don't be discouraged if you haven't yet succeeded. The difficulty you have encountered may be due to influences you've never really thought about—such as advertising—or to a lack of support and encouragement. Understanding these influences is an important step toward changing the way they affect you.

There's Help Available In addition to personal actions you can take on your own, there are community programs and groups (such as the YMCA/YWCA or the local chapter of the American

Heart Association) that can assist you and your family to make the changes you want to make. If you want to know more about these groups or about health risks, contact your local health department or the address below. There's a lot you can do to stay healthy or to improve your health—and there are organizations that can help you. Start a new HEALTHSTYLE today!

National Health Information Clearinghouse
PO Box 1133
Washington, DC 20013-1133
1-800-336-4797

Starting Your Own **Fitness** Program

Objectives

After completing this chapter, you should be able to do the following:

- Identify the basic principles of a fitness program.
- Discuss the importance of the warm-up and cool-down periods.
- Determine your individual goals for your fitness program.
- Identify precautions for beginning a fitness program.

A t this point, you should have some idea about why you need to get fit. Your individual reasons and motivations have been identified in Chapter 1. Beginning a fitness program is simple. In addition, you can do several things to ensure that your program is successful and yet fun and enjoyable.

THE PROGRAM SHOULD BE FUN AND ENJOYABLE

Enjoying yourself may be one of the most critical factors for a successful fitness program over the long run. The activity you select must be one that you enjoy and that provides motivation to continue for a lifetime (Figure 3-1). For example, a quick look at the streets on a sunny day will show that running is a popular form of physical activity. There is no question that a running program eventually will result in significant improvement in cardiorespiratory endurance. Personally, I hate to run and would prefer to do any other activity.

If I were to select running as my fitness activity because it is "in" and not because I enjoy doing it, then chances are that I would not stick with it for long. This is not to say that there is not some potential value in doing some things you don't enjoy with the understanding that "enjoyment" will come later. For example, while golfing can be extremely frustrating initially, with practice, it can become a rewarding and enjoyable activity as you improve. You should enjoy getting into good physical condition, and a successful fitness program will be considered fun rather than work.

KEY TERMS

overload   *specificity*

SAID principle   *warm-up*

progression   *cool-down*

consistency

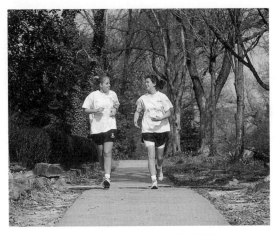

FIGURE 3-1. EXERCISE PROGRAMS.
An exercise program should be fun and enjoyable.

ADHERING TO AN EXERCISE PROGRAM

Motivation plays an important role in your ability to stick with an exercise program. You should select the type of activity that will allow

FIT LIST 3-1

Suggestions for Making Physical Activity Fun

Some students find physical activity dull. Here are some ways to make it more inviting.

- Exercise to music.
- Exercise with classmates.
- Keep your program simple.
- Instill variety into activity: for example, dancing, hiking, tennis, and swimming.
- Reward yourself when fitness goals are met.
- Don't become upset when goals are not met and benefits are not immediate.
- Keep a record of things such as your weight and the distance you jog.
- Take a break whenever you wish.
- Plan the program to fit into your daily life.

you to do two things: (1) achieve the ultimate goals of physical fitness improvement that you have established for yourself, and (2) maintain your interest and motivation for a long time (weeks, months, even years). The physical benefits of engaging in regular physical activity listed in Health Link 1-2 on page 6 in Chapter 1 should provide sufficient motivation for anyone to engage in a physical activity program. Fit List 3-1 provides some suggestions that can make your program fun and enjoyable.

WHAT ARE THE BASIC PRINCIPLES OF A FITNESS PROGRAM?

Regardless of the type of physical activity in which you choose to participate, certain principles should be incorporated into every program. These principles and guidelines apply to anyone who is physically active. Paying attention to these basic principles will help to create an effective yet safe environment for physical activities. Fit List 3-2 summarizes these principles.

OVERLOAD

To achieve the greatest benefits from an exercise program, you should recognize the principle of **overload** (Figure 3-2). For a physical

FIT LIST 3-2

The Basic Principles of a Fitness Program

- Overload
- Progression
- Consistency
- Specificity
- Diminishing Returns
- Reversibility
- Individuality
- Safety

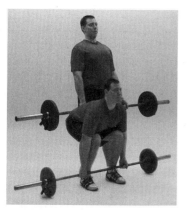

FIGURE 3-2. OVERLOAD.
To see improvement in any physiologic system you must use the principle of overload.

component of fitness to improve, the system must work harder than it is used to working. The system must experience stress so that over a period of time it will improve to the point where it can easily accommodate additional stress. The **SAID principle** (an acronym for *specific adaptation to imposed demands*) states that when the body is subjected to stresses and overloads of varying intensities, it will gradually adapt, over time, to overcome whatever demands are placed on it. Even though overload is a critical factor for getting fit, the stress must not be great enough to produce damage or injury. The body needs to have a chance to adjust to the imposed demands. Therefore overload is a gradual increase in the frequency, intensity, and time or duration (FIT) of the

> **overload:** exercising at a higher level than normal
>
> **SAID principle:** when the body is subjected to stresses and overloads of varying intensities, it will gradually adapt, over time, to overcome whatever demands are placed on it

physical activity that is a part of the fitness program. (The FIT formula will be discussed in detail in Chapter 4.) This is one of the most critical factors in any activities program. For example, if you are on a running program to improve cardiorespiratory endurance and you go out and run 1 mile in 15 minutes, the cardiorespiratory system will be able to accommodate this distance and intensity very easily. However, if the long-range goal of your fitness program is to run the New York Marathon, it is foolish to believe that you could finish a race of this distance and intensity by running only one 15-minute mile a day. If you gradually overload the system by running farther at a faster pace, you will force the cardiorespiratory system to work more efficiently to keep up with increased physical demands. In weight training, adding more weight and decreasing the number of sets and repetitions will help in developing muscular strength. Therefore, by overloading the system over a long period, one should expect to produce significant improvement in that system's ability to handle a stressful exercise session.

Certainly, some individuals take the principle of overload to an extreme and do too much physical activity. They become obsessed with working out and either exercise too often, at too high an intensity, or for too long without proper rest. These individuals are likely to develop overuse type musculoskeletal injuries. Overtraining may also lead to staleness or burnout, which may be characterized by chronic physical and emotional exhaustion, weight loss, and inability to sleep or rest properly.

PROGRESSION

A little today and a little more tomorrow is a good principle to follow in any fitness program. You should start gradually and add a little each day. The rate of **progression** should be within your capabilities to adapt physically. In other words, the workout should gradually become a little longer or more intense until you reach the desired level of physical fitness. If you try to progress too rapidly, it is likely that you may develop some type of injury (see Chapter 9). There comes a time in many fitness programs when *improving* fitness levels becomes less important than *maintaining* fitness levels. Progression is closely related to overload. Without overloading the system, progression does not occur. Progression is also important for motivation. Interest level in an activity remains high as long as you continue to see improvement in your physical ability. Even though weight increases may be minimal in strength training, a progression of even 1 pound is often enough to maintain interest and motivation.

CONSISTENCY

One of the biggest problems with beginning a fitness program is finding time during the day to fit in an hour or so of activity. This is particularly true for students who have many demands on their time. Nevertheless, it is important to select a specific period for exercising each day and stick to it.

The best time of day for you to exercise is whenever you have the time and are motivated to do so. The important point is to set aside some time for a fitness program and make it part of your daily routine for **consistency.** The least desirable times are probably after a meal, when activity may make you uncomfortable, and just before bedtime, when the activity is so invigorating that it is difficult to fall asleep. The number of days per week you are involved with a specific activity will vary depending on several personal factors. However, it is recommended that you try to work out at least 3 days per week to see minimal improvement.

SPECIFICITY

The type of physical changes that occur is directly related to the type of training undertaken. To realize the maximum gains desired, activities and programs should be selected and designed with **specificity** to achieve this aim. Once again, according to the SAID principle, a particular physical system will respond and adapt over time to whatever specific demands are placed on it. For example, to develop flexibility in a specific joint, stretching exercises must be incorporated that progressively lengthen the muscles and tendons that surround that joint.

The training must be specific not only to the activity, but also to individual abilities (tolerance to training stress, recoverability, and the like). Training loads must be increased over time, allowing some workouts to be less intense than others, and an individual must train often enough not only to keep a detraining effect from happening, but also to force an adaptation.

DIMINISHING RETURNS

The greatest gains in fitness will be seen early on in an exercise program. After the initial increase, gains will continue, but at a slower pace. The fitness benefits that an individual acquires from exercising are only sustained if he or she maintains the exercise program. Therefore people should continue to exercise throughout their lifetime to prevent these gains from being lost.

progression: gradually increasing the level and intensity of exercise

consistency: engaging in fitness activities on a frequent and regular basis

specificity: the type of physical changes that occur are directly related to the type of training used

REVERSIBILITY

In adults, it is likely that some or all of the gains made in strength, flexibility, cardiorespiratory endurance, and the like during an exercise program will be lost if the program is stopped. However, in children and teenagers who are still growing, it is possible that some of the gains achieved from increased loading during an exercise program may be retained after the exercise program is discontinued.

INDIVIDUALITY

When you become involved in a fitness program, it is important to remember that no two persons are exactly the same. People have different ideas about their goals for a fitness program, motivation, and state of physical fitness (Figure 3-3). A fitness program for one person will not necessarily satisfy the needs of another person. Furthermore, not all people involved in similar activities will progress at the same rate, nor will they be able to overload their systems to the same degree. Exercise is good, but it must be adapted to individual needs and abilities. Just as a medical prescription must be related to a person's health needs, so should a physical fitness prescription. A person's exercise prescription needs to be based on his or her objectives, needs, functional capacity, and interests.

SAFETY

Another factor to consider when planning a fitness program is safety. The purpose of your fitness program should be to improve selected components of fitness through physical exercise. Unfortunately, injuries often occur as the result of poorly planned activity programs. The rule of thumb to follow is to start out slowly and progress according to your own capabilities. Adhering to the rule "train—don't strain" can certainly reduce the likelihood of injury. If you are unsure of how to get started or perhaps of how quickly to progress in a personal fitness program, seek professional advice from persons with some expertise in fitness.

SHOULD YOU DO A WARM-UP ROUTINE BEFORE YOU EXERCISE?

Absolutely! It is important to **warm up** before you begin any type of workout for several reasons. It has been suggested that a warm-up routine increases body core temperature,

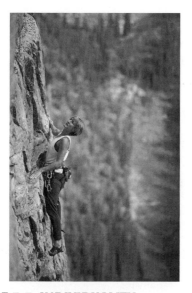

FIGURE 3-3. INDIVIDUALITY.
When it comes to fitness, people have different ideas about their goals and the types of activities they choose to engage in.

warm-up: designed to increase body temperature, stretch ligaments and muscles, and increase flexibility

stretches ligaments and muscles, and increases flexibility. A good, short warm-up routine can also be an effective motivator. If you get satisfaction from warming up, you probably will have a stronger desire to participate in an activity. By contrast, a poor warm-up routine can lead to fatigue and boredom, limiting your attention and ultimately resulting in a poor program. Also, there is some evidence that a good warm-up routine may improve certain aspects of performance.

The function of the warm-up routine is to prepare your body physically for a workout. The purpose is to gradually stimulate the cardiorespiratory system to a moderate degree. This produces an increased blood flow to exercising muscles and results in an increase in muscle temperature.

Moderate activity speeds up your metabolism, producing an increase in your body temperature. Furthermore, an increase in the temperature of muscle allows the muscle to stretch to a greater degree thus reducing the chance of injury.

A good warm-up routine should begin with 2 or 3 minutes of slow walking, light jogging, or cycling to increase your metabolism and warm up the muscles. Breaking into a light sweat is a good indication that the muscle temperature has increased (Figure 3-4). The latest approach to the warm-up is to use an active or "dynamic" warm-up to prepare for physical activity. A dynamic warm-up involves continuous movement using hopping, skipping, and bounding activities with several different footwork drills and patterns. It enhances coordination and motor ability as it revs up the nervous system. It prepares the muscles and joints in a more activity-specific manner than static stretching. The dynamic warm-up forces individuals to focus and concentrate. It should include exercises that address all the major muscle groups. The entire dynamic warm-up can be done in as little as five minutes or as

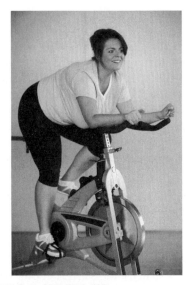

FIGURE 3-4. WARM-UP.
A warm-up routine should include an activity to increase body core temperature.

long as 20 minutes, depending on the goals, age, and fitness level of the group. You should begin your activity immediately following the warm-up routine. Fit List 3-3 summarizes the components of a dynamic warm-up.

FIT LIST 3-3

Components of a Dynamic Warm-Up

- Continuous movement—hopping, skipping, bounding, jogging
- Different footwork drills and movements
- Revs up nervous system
- Enhances coordination and agility
- Warms up the muscles and increases metabolism
- Prepares muscles and joints in a more activity orientated fashion

WORKOUT

The type and length of workout in which you choose to engage are determined by your reasons for engaging in a fitness program and by the goals you have established for yourself. Thus the workout will differ significantly between individuals. Recommendations for workouts to accomplish specific fitness goals are presented throughout the text.

COOL-DOWN

After a vigorous workout, a **cool-down** period is essential. The cool-down period prevents pooling of blood in the arms and legs, thus maintaining blood pressure and enabling the body to cool and return to a resting state. The cool-down period should last about 5 to 10 minutes. During the cool-down period, you may engage in stretching activities. Static stretching has been recommended during the cool–down period for helping improve range of motion. Although the value of warm-up routine and workout periods is well accepted, the importance of a cool-down period is often ignored. Again, experience and observation indicate that people who stretch during the cool-down period tend to have fewer problems with muscle soreness after strenuous activity.

WHAT ARE THE GOALS OF YOUR FITNESS PROGRAM?

When designing an individualized physical fitness program, you must first decide what it is you are trying to accomplish and then

> **cool-down:** prevents pooling of blood and enables the body to cool and return to a resting state

select those specific components of fitness that ultimately help you to reach your goal. For example, the goals of fitness improvement for a person who plays Frisbee occasionally on weekends will differ considerably from those of a person preparing to compete in varsity soccer. Goals are different for an individual who engages in one hour of walking versus three hours of hiking versus two days of backpacking. Riding your bicycle to the store is significantly different than riding your bicycle in an event like Ride to the Beach for Cancer. The majority of people who are not athletes should be more concerned with fitness components related to good health such as cardiorespiratory endurance, flexibility, muscular strength, muscular endurance, and body composition. Improvement in these five specific areas enhance a person's ability to perform daily tasks without undue fatigue, as stated in our definition of physical fitness.

On the other hand, the soccer player must be concerned not only with the components that have been mentioned above but also with components such as strength, speed, power, balance, and agility. The soccer player who does not include activities in the training regimen that specifically address these various performance-related fitness components likely will be unsuccessful in a competitive situation.

HOW SHOULD YOU EXERCISE?

It has been well documented that engaging in regular, moderate-intensity physical activity will result in substantial health benefits. Recommendations from various organizations as to exactly how people should exercise seem to be constantly evolving. For years, an exercise period of 30 to 60 minutes' duration at an intensity of 60 to 90 percent of maximum heart rate performed three or more times per week was the recommended standard for promoting

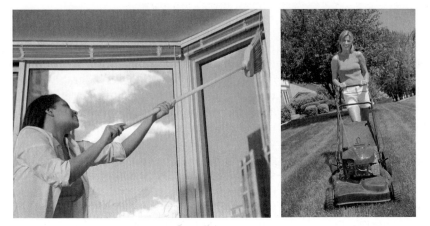

FIGURE 3-5. HOUSEWORK AND YARDWORK.
Moderate or intermittent exercise may include activities such as doing housework or moving the lawn.

to improving health than the specific type of activity performed.

The total amount of activity could be measured either in minutes of physical activity performed or in the number of calories expended. Moderate-intensity activity expends about 150 calories over a total of 30 minutes of exercise (which can be performed periodically over the course of a day). The intensity of the activities should correspond to walking "briskly" at a pace of 3 to 4 miles per hour. Engaging in this amount of activity can decrease the risk of coronary artery disease by 50 percent and the risk of colon cancer, diabetes, and hypertension by 30 percent.

In 2002, the National Academies of Science Institute of Medicine recommended that to maintain cardiovascular health at a maximal level, regardless of weight, adults and children should spend a total of at least 1 hour each day in moderately intense physical activity, which was double the daily minimum goal set by the 1996 Surgeon General's Report. The goal of 1 hour per day of total activity stems from studies of how much energy is expended on average each day by individuals who maintain a healthy weight. Energy expenditure is cumulative, including both low-intensity activities of daily life, such as stair climbing and housecleaning, and more vigorous exercise like swimming and cycling. Someone in a largely sedentary occupation can achieve the exercise goal by engaging in a moderate-intensity activity (such as walking at 4 miles per hour) for a total of 60 minutes every day, or engaging in a high-intensity activity (such as jogging at

good health and preventing disease according to the American College of Sports Medicine. In 1995 the Centers for Disease Control and Prevention and the American College of Sports Medicine issued a revised joint recommendation that everyone should try to engage in a minimum of 30 minutes of physical activity on most days—ideally, every day. This 30-minute total did not have to consist solely of what has traditionally been considered exercise (walking, swimming, cycling, etc.) (Figure 3-5). It could involve a series of short bouts of physical activity that collectively accumulate to a total of at least 30 minutes of moderate-intensity physical exercise and that may include more intermittent activities such as walking up or down stairs, doing lawn work or gardening, and cleaning the house. (See the Activity Pyramid in Figure 3-6).

This recommendation relative to the quantity and quality of exercise was substantially less formal than what had been recommended in the past. Research had indicated that many health benefits could be achieved by engaging in moderate-intensity physical activities not typically associated with formal exercise. The total amount of activity appeared to be more critical

PHYSICAL ACTIVITY PYRAMID

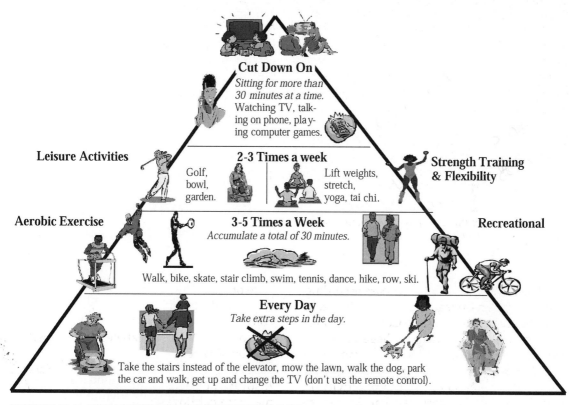

Cut Down On
Sitting for more than 30 minutes at a time. Watching TV, talking on phone, playing computer games.

Leisure Activities

2-3 Times a week
Golf, bowl, garden.   Lift weights, stretch, yoga, tai chi.

Strength Training & Flexibility

Aerobic Exercise

3-5 Times a Week
Accumulate a total of 30 minutes.

Recreational

Walk, bike, skate, stair climb, swim, tennis, dance, hike, row, ski.

Every Day
Take extra steps in the day.

Take the stairs instead of the elevator, mow the lawn, walk the dog, park the car and walk, get up and change the TV (don't use the remote control).

FIGURE 3-6. THE PHYSICAL ACTIVITY PYRAMID.
Exercises or activities are divided into four groups and are put on different level of the Physical Activity Pyramid.
From http://www.islandcounty.net/health/CHAB/phyactpyr.pdf

6 miles per hour), for 20 to 30 minutes, 4 to 7 days per week.

It has been estimated that the majority of Americans do not meet this minimum standard for daily physical activity. Thus it is recommended that everyone make an effort to gradually incorporate physical activity into their daily routine, eventually increasing to a minimum total of 60 minutes on a consistent basis.

It must be pointed out that the recommendations from the American College of Sports Medicine were made with the idea of reducing risks for chronic diseases, while the recommendations from the Institute of Medicine were primarily referring to avoiding weight gain.

In 2007, the American College of Sports Medicine (ACSM) and the American Heart Association (AHA) provided new recommendations that all healthy adults under the age of 65 do either moderately intense aerobic exercise 30 minutes a day, a minimum of five days a week; or vigorously intense aerobic exercise

20 minutes a day, a minimum of 3 days a week. Either of these approaches should also include 8 to 10 strength-training exercises, 8 to 12 repetitions of each exercise twice a week. Moderate-intensity physical activity means working hard enough to raise your heart rate and break a sweat, yet still being able to carry on a conversation. The 30-minute recommendation is for the average healthy adult to maintain health and reduce the risk for chronic disease.

The most recent guidelines for exercise come from the 2008 Physical Activity Guidelines for Americans published by the Centers for Disease Control. Fit List 3-4 summarizes those guidelines.

FIT LIST 3-4

For Important Health Benefits

Adults need at least:

2 hours and 30 minutes (150 minutes) of moderate-intensity aerobic activity (i.e., brisk walking) every week **and** muscle-strengthening activities on 2 or more days a week that work all major muscle groups (legs, hips, back, abdomen, chest, shoulders, and arms).

OR

1 hour and 15 minutes (75 minutes) of vigorous-intensity aerobic activity (i.e., jogging or running) every week **and** muscle-strengthening activities on 2 or more days a week that work all major muscle groups (legs, hips, back, abdomen, chest, shoulders, and arms).

OR

An equivalent mix of moderate- and vigorous-intensity aerobic activity **and** muscle-strengthening activities on 2 or more days a week that work all major muscle groups (legs, hips, back, abdomen, chest, shoulders, and arms).

WHERE DO YOU BEGIN?

Just as you are never too sedentary to begin a fitness program, you are also never too old. It is wise to start a fitness program early in life, but all of us can benefit from exercise no matter when we begin. Long-term success in staying with an exercise program undoubtedly has some basis in your underlying motivation for beginning such a program in the first place.

PRECAUTIONS IN BEGINNING A FITNESS PROGRAM

For most high school and college students, chances are that overall health is pretty good. In the normal healthy individual, there is virtually no reason to expect that participation in any type of fitness activity will pose a threat to health or well-being. Generally, exercise is considered a safe activity for most individuals. Nevertheless, it is always a good idea to assess your medical history by identifying any pre-existing medical conditions that should be considered before beginning an exercise program. For nontraditional students, this is especially true for anyone over 35 years of age. If your medical history identifies any health-related problem, it is advisable to consult appropriate medical personnel before engaging in any type of activity. Lab Activity 3-1 will help you assess your current medical history and may indicate a reason for you to seek additional medical advice.

Paying attention to the principles and guidelines of fitness as detailed earlier in this chapter can markedly reduce your chances of suffering injuries associated with exercise. Many of the injuries that occur with exercise can be eliminated by an awareness of the way you exercise, by "listening" to what your body is telling you through aches and pains.

READY TO BEGIN?

At this point you have been given the basic guidelines and considerations for beginning a fitness program. The chapters that follow will provide you with knowledge about and understanding of the various aspects of fitness. The chapters are designed to show the importance of fitness's essential ingredients, and they will explain how you can assess, develop, and maintain fitness. Finally, the rest of this text will demonstrate how to plan, develop, and implement a personalized fitness program based on your individual interests Fit List 3-5 provides a checklist for beginning a physical activity program. Lab Activity 3-2 will help you begin planning your physical activity program.

FIT LIST 3-5

Points to Consider When Starting a Physical Activity Program

Assess fitness level

- Poor, fair, average, good, excellent
- Begin at a lower intensity with lower cardio fitness and higher intensities with greater cardio fitness
- Determine your health or medical history

Determine fitness goal(s)

- Improve health
- Increase strength
- Improve flexibility
- Increase fat loss
- Improve cardiovascular performance
- Improve sport performance

Time constraints

- Time of day
- Times per day
- Days available

Exercise preferences

- Type of activity

Equipment availability

SUMMARY

- The type of physical activity that you choose to engage in should be fun and enjoyable.
- The basic considerations of any training and conditioning program should include the following principles: overload, progression, consistency, diminishing returns, reversibility, specificity, individuality, and safety.
- The three basic elements of any training and conditioning program are the warm-up routine, the workout or conditioning activity, and the cool-down period.
- As a precaution, before you begin an exercise program, you should complete a medical history questionnaire to identify any problems.

SUGGESTED READINGS

American College of Sports Medicine. 1998. ACSM position stand on the recommended quantity and quality of exercise for developing and maintaining cardiorespiratory and muscular fitness and flexibility in adults. *Medicine and Science in Sports and Exercise* 30(6):975–991.

American College of Sports Medicine. 2009. *ACSM's resource manual: For guidelines for exercise testing and prescription.* Baltimore: Lippincott, Williams & Wilkins.

American College of Sports Medicine. 2003. *ACSM fitness book.* 2nd ed. Champaign, IL: Human Kinetics.

Bouchard, C., R. Shepard, and T. Stephens. 1994. *Physical activity, fitness and health.* Champaign, IL: Human Kinetics.

Dupont, G., W. Moalla, and C. Guinhouya. 2004. Passive versus active recovery during high-intensity intermittent exercises. *Medicine and Science in Sports and Exercise* 36(2):302–8.

Faccioni, A. 2007. Dynamic warm up routines for sports. *Coaching Update* 22(2):16–17; 28.

Gray, S., and M. Nimmo. 2001. Effects of active, passive or no warm-up on metabolism and performance during high-intensity exercise. *Journal of Sports Sciences* 19(9):693–700.

Halas, J., and G. Gannon. 2005. Principles of physical fitness development: Implications for fitness assessment. *Physical and Health Education Journal* 71(4):4.

Halvorson, R. 2009. Dynamic warm-ups reduce sports injuries. *IDEA Fitness Journal* 6(4):14.

Haskell, W., I. Lee, and R. Pate. 2007. Physical activity and public health: Updated recommendations for adults from the American College of Sports Medicine and the American Heart Association. *Medicine and Science in Sports and Exercise* 39(8):1423–34.

Herman, S., Derek, T. 2008. Four-week dynamic stretching warm-up intervention elicits longer term performance benefits, *Journal of Strength and Conditioning Research* 22(4):1286.

Heyward, V. 2010. *Advanced fitness assessment and exercise prescription.* Champaign, IL: Human Kinetics.

Howley, E., D. Franks, and W. Westcott. 2007. *Health fitness instructor's handbook.* Champaign, IL: Human Kinetics.

Mannie, K. 2004. Dynamic warm-up/flexibility. *Coach and Athletic Director* 73(6):8–10.

Mannie, K. 2004. Overloading without overtraining. *Coach and Athletic Director* 74(4):9–12.

Molkin, M. 2004. Warming up, cooling down and stretching: Preparing for a workout and recovering afterward deserve a lot more attention than many believe. *Fitness Management* 20(2):30–32.

Nelson, M., W. Rejeski, and S. Blair. 2007. Physical activity and public health in older adults: Recommendations from the American College of Sports Medicine and the American Heart Association. *Medicine and Science in Sports and Exercise* 39(8):1435–45.

Pate, R. et al. 1995. Physical activity and public health: A recommendation from the Centers for Disease Control and Prevention and the American College of Sports Medicine. *Journal of the American Medical Association* 273(5):402–7.

Swain, D. 2006. Moderate- or vigorous-intensity exercise: What should we prescribe? *ACSM's Health and Fitness Journal* 10(5):7–11.

US Department of Health and Human Services. 2008. *Physical activity guidelines for Americans.* Washington DC.

Weil, A. 2007. *Healthy aging: A lifelong guide to your well-being.* New York, Anchor.

Young, S. 2010. From static stretching to dynamic exercises: Changing the warm-up paradigm. *Strategies* 24(1):13.

SUGGESTED WEB SITES

Aerobics and Fitness Association of America

AFAA, the world's largest fitness educator, links members, consumers, corporate subscribers, and allied professionals throughout the world with a revolutionary group of dynamic fitness services. Whether you're looking for aerobics certification, a personal trainer, or just some fitness facts, this is the place to be.
www.afaa.com

American Alliance for Health, Physical Education, Recreation and Dance

This site is sponsored by the national organization of physical education, health, and fitness professionals.
www.aahperd.org

The American College of Sports Medicine

ACSM is a professional society providing basic and applied exercise science conferences, meetings, and workshops.
www.acsm.org/

American Fitness Professionals and Associates

Provides a list of fitness and nutrition certifications as well as a list of providers of continuing education and resources.
www.afpafitness.com

International Dance Exercise Association

The IDEA supports the world's leading health and fitness professionals with credible information, education, career development, and leadership.
www.ideafit.com

Internet's Fitness Resource

The primary purpose of this site is the dissemination of information on exercise and nutrition. IFR offers a comprehensive listing of fitness related sites as well as the Fitness Instructor FAQ, the Fitness Plan, guest editorials, fitness classifications and more.
www.netsweat.com

International Health, Racquet, and Sportsclub Association

This organization promotes fitness through education and sport club membership.
www.ihrsa.org

National Academy of Sports Medicine

This site addresses fitness, sports performance, and sports medicine, and provides live, online, and home-study courses.
www.nasm.org

National Association for Health and Fitness

This not-for-profit organization exists to improve the quality of life of every individual in the United States through the promotion of physical fitness and healthy lifestyles and by fostering and supporting councils for physical activity, health, and sports.
www.physicalfitness.org

National Center on Physical Activity and Disability

The NCPAD encourages persons with disabilities to participate in regular physical activity to promote healthy lifestyles and prevent secondary conditions.
www.ncpad.org

National Institute for Fitness and Sport

This nonprofit organization is committed to enhancing human health, physical fitness, and athletic performance through research, education, and service.
www.nifs.org

www.fitness.com

Fitness.com includes everything about fitness: chat, discussion board, links and shopping.
www.fitness.com/

Centers for Disease Control and Prevention

This site discusses all aspects of physical activity and provides recommendations for everyone of all ages.
http://www.cdc.gov/physicalactivity/everyone/guidelines/adults.htm

Medical History Questionnaire

Name _____   Section _____   Date _____

PURPOSE   To determine whether your past medical history warrants further medical evaluation before beginning an exercise program.

PROCEDURE   Check the appropriate column below if you think you have or if you have ever been told you had any of the conditions listed below.

	Yes	No
Coronary heart disease	____	____
Chest pain (during rest or during exercise)	____	____
Pain in your shoulder and jaw	____	____
Irregular heartbeats	____	____
High blood pressure	____	____
Shortness of breath	____	____
Family history of heart disease	____	____
Rheumatic fever	____	____
High cholesterol levels	____	____
Respiratory problems	____	____
Chronic cough	____	____
Diabetes	____	____
Sickle cell anemia	____	____
Dizziness or loss of consciousness	____	____
Seizures or convulsions	____	____
Severe headaches	____	____
Obesity	____	____
Arthritis	____	____
Serious bone, joint, or muscle injury	____	____
Low back pain	____	____
Do you smoke cigarettes?	____	____
Are you using any prescription drugs?	____	____
Do you have any physical problems that are of concern to you?	____	____

If you have checked the yes column for any of the conditions listed, it is recommended that you consult your physician before engaging in a physical activity program.

The American College of Sports Medicine* and the American Medical Association have established the following guidelines and recommendations for medical evaluation before engaging in a physical activity program.

1. Any individual less than 35 years of age who has (1) no previous history of cardiovascular disease, (2) no known primary risk factors, and (3) undergone a medical evaluation within the past 2 years may generally begin a physical activity program without additional medical evaluation or clearance.
2. Any individual less than 35 years of age who exhibits (1) evidence of coronary heart disease or (2) a significant combination of risk factors should be examined and cleared medically before engaging in a physical activity program.
3. For all individuals over 35 years of age, medical evaluation and clearance are recommended before any major increase in physical activity levels.

*American College of Sports Medicine: *Guidelines for exercise testing and prescription*, Philadelphia, 1991, Lea & Febiger.

Planning for a Physical Activity Program

_____   _____   _____
Name   Section   Date

PURPOSE   To determine whether you have addressed the necessary considerations for beginning a physical activity program.

PROCEDURE   In the space provided, indicate your best response.

1. Based on your responses in Lab Activity 1–1, list the goals you wish to accomplish by engaging in a physical activity program. _____
   _____
   _____
   _____
   _____
   _____

2. What are the components of fitness that you want to concentrate on to accomplish these goals? (muscular strength, flexibility, cardiorespiratory endurance, etc.) _____
   _____
   _____
   _____

3. What are the physical activities that you most enjoy participating in that you think will be the most effective in accomplishing these goals? _____
   _____
   _____

4. When do you think will be the best time during the day for you to work out? _____
   _____

5. How many days a week do you plan to engage in physical activity? _____
   _____

6. Do you plan to work out on your own, or will you choose a workout partner? List the people with whom you might like to work out._____
   _____

7. How long do you think your warm-up, workout/activity, cool-down will take? _____
   _____

8. What will your warm-up activity consist of? _____
_____
_____
_____

9. Briefly describe what you plan to do during your workout. (Specific exercises and instruction relative to the various health-related components of fitness will be covered in subsequent chapters.)_____
_____
_____
_____

10. What will your cool-down activity consist of?_____
_____
_____
_____

11. What things can you do to make your physical activity program safe and reduce the possibility of injury? _____
_____
_____
_____

Developing **Cardiorespiratory** Fitness

Objectives

After completing this chapter, you should be able to do the following:

- Relate the importance of cardiorespiratory endurance to overall fitness and health.
- Contrast aerobic and anaerobic activity.
- Explain how maximum aerobic capacity determines your level of cardiorespiratory endurance.
- Describe the principles of continuous, interval, and fartlek training and the potential of each technique for improving cardiorespiratory endurance.
- Analyze specific aerobic activities that can be used to improve cardiorespiratory endurance.
- Identify methods for assessment of cardiorespiratory endurance.

WHY IS CARDIORESPIRATORY FITNESS IMPORTANT FOR YOU?

Of all the components of physical fitness listed in Chapter 1, none is more important than cardiorespiratory endurance, also referred to as cardiovascular endurance. Cardiorespiratory endurance is the ability to perform whole-body activities and continue movement for extended periods without undue fatigue. We rely on the cardiorespiratory system to transport and supply the oxygen needed by the various tissues within our bodies. It is the basic life-support system of the body. Without oxygen, the cells within the human body cannot function, and ultimately death occurs.

Everyone needs some degree of cardiorespiratory endurance to carry out normal daily activities. If you are engaged in exercise, the cardiorespiratory system must work harder to

KEY TERMS	
aerobic activity	*slow-twitch muscle*
anaerobic activity	*fibers*
stroke volume	*FIT principle*
cardiac output	*continuous training*
aerobic capacity	*target heart rate*
maximum aerobic	*rating of perceived*
capacity	*exertion*
fast-twitch muscle	*interval training*
fibers	*fartlek*
heart rate reserve and	
Karvonen equation	

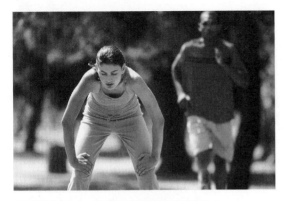

FIGURE 4-1. CHALLENGING THE CARDIORESPIRATORY SYSTEM.
Engaging in exercise forces the cardiorespiratory system to become more efficient at supplying needed oxygen and thus improves fitness.

deliver enough oxygen to sustain that activity. Thus as the cardiorespiratory system becomes more efficient at supplying the needed oxygen, your level of cardiorespiratory fitness improves and you are likely to be more resistant to fatigue (Figure 4-1).

For older individuals such as nontraditional college students, the health benefits of improving cardiorespiratory endurance may be more important than the fitness benefits.

Engaging in regular exercise will also improve your cardiovascular health and can greatly reduce your chance of heart disease. If you have low levels of cardiorespiratory endurance, your risk of developing heart disease is higher than normal.

WHAT IS THE DIFFERENCE BETWEEN AEROBIC VERSUS ANAEROBIC ACTIVITIES?

Without oxygen, the body is incapable of producing energy for an extended period of time. Muscles must generate energy to move. Three energy-generating systems function in

muscle tissue to produce a chemical compound called *adenosine triphosphate (ATP)*, which is the ultimate usable form of energy for muscular activity. They are the ATP, glycolytic, and oxidative systems. During sudden outbursts of activity in intensive, short-term exercise, ATP can be rapidly metabolized to meet energy needs. However, after a few seconds of intensive exercise, the small stores of ATP are used up. The body then turns to stored glycogen as an energy source. Glycogen is broken down to supply glucose, which is then metabolized within the muscle cells to generate ATP for muscle contractions without the need for oxygen. This breakdown also produces a byproduct called lactic acid or *lactate*, which seeps out of the muscle cells into the blood to be used elsewhere. This energy system is referred to as *anaerobic metabolism.* As exercise continues, the body has to rely on a more complex form of carbohydrate and fat metabolism to generate ATP. This second energy system requires oxygen and is therefore referred to as *aerobic metabolism.* The aerobic system burns the lactate using oxygen, thus removing it and creating far more ATP than the anaerobic system. Normally it takes about 20 minutes to clear the lactate from the system. Training to improve endurance helps an individual get rid of the lactic acid before it can build to the point where it causes muscle fatigue.

In most activities both aerobic and anaerobic systems function simultaneously. The degree to which the major energy systems are involved is determined by the intensity and duration of the activity. If the intensity of the activity is such that sufficient oxygen can be supplied to meet the demands of working tissues, the activity is considered to be **aerobic.** Conversely, if the activity is of high enough intensity or the duration is such that insufficient oxygen is available to meet energy demands, the activity becomes **anaerobic.**

Table 4-1 provides a comparison summary between aerobic and anaerobic activities.

TABLE 4-1
COMPARISON OF AEROBIC VERSUS ANAEROBIC ACTIVITIES

	Mode	Relative Intensity	Performance	Frequency	Duration
Aerobic Activities	Continuous, long-duration, sustained activities	Less intense	60% to 85% of maximum range	At least 3 but no more than 6 times per week	20 to 60 minutes
Anaerobic Activities	Explosive, short-duration, burst-type activities	More intense	85% to 100% range	3 to 4 days per week	10 seconds to 2 minutes

HOW DOES EXERCISE AFFECT THE FUNCTION OF THE HEART?

The capacity of the cardiorespiratory system to carry oxygen throughout the body depends on the coordinated function of four components: (1) the heart, (2) the blood vessels, (3) the blood, and (4) the lungs. Improvement of cardiorespiratory endurance through exercise occurs because of an increase in the capability of each of these four components in providing necessary oxygen to the working tissues. A basic discussion of what occurs in the heart in response to training and exercise should make it easier

aerobic activity: an activity in which the intensity of the activity is low enough that the cardiovascular system can supply enough oxygen to continue the activity for long periods

anaerobic activity: an activity in which the intensity is so great that the demand for oxygen is greater than the body's ability to deliver oxygen

for you to understand why the training techniques discussed later are effective in improving cardiorespiratory endurance.

The heart is the main pumping mechanism and circulates oxygenated blood throughout the body to the various tissues. The heart receives oxygen-poor blood from the venous system and then pumps the blood through the pulmonary vessels to the lungs, where carbon dioxide is exchanged for oxygen. The oxygen-rich blood then returns to the heart, from which it exits through the aorta to the arterial system and is circulated throughout the body, supplying oxygen to the tissues (Figure 4-2).

As you begin to exercise, your muscles use the oxygen at a much higher rate, and thus your heart must pump more oxygenated blood to meet this increased demand. Like any other muscle, the heart will adapt to the increased demands placed on it over a period of time. The heart is capable of adapting to this increased demand through three mechanisms, as listed below.

1. *Increased heart rate.* As the intensity of the exercise increases, the heart rate also increases, reaching a plateau at a given level after about 2 to 3 minutes. At rest, the heart beats about 70 times per minute. The maximal

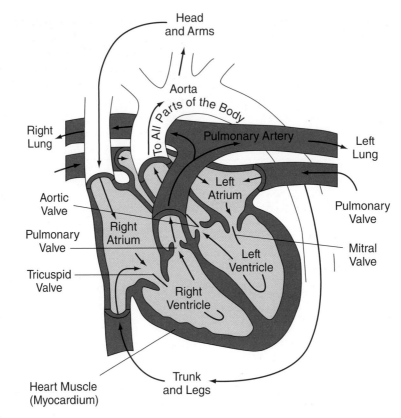

Head
and Arms

Aorta

To All Parts of the Body

Right
Lung

Pulmonary Artery

Left
Lung

Aortic
Valve

Left
Atrium

Pulmonary
Valve

Pulmonary
Valve

Right
Atrium

Mitral
Valve

Tricuspid
Valve

Left
Ventricle

Right
Ventricle

Heart Muscle
(Myocardium)

Trunk
and Legs

FIGURE 4-2.
Anatomy of the Heart and Blood Flow.

heart rate is different in everybody, but it can be estimated by subtracting the person's age (in years) from 220.

2. *Increased stroke volume.* The volume of blood being pumped out of the heart with each beat is called the **stroke volume.** At rest, the heart pumps out approximately 70 ml of blood per beat. During acute exercise, stroke volume increases. Stroke volume can continue to increase only to a point (about 110 ml/beat) at which there is simply not enough time between beats for the heart to fill up. The long term effects of exercise produce an increase in maximum stroke volume during exercise, particularly in individuals who are sedentary.

3. *Increased cardiac output.* **Cardiac output** indicates how much blood the heart is capable of pumping in exactly 1 minute. It is determined by heart rate (the rate of pumping) and stroke volume (the quantity of blood ejected with each heartbeat). Cardiac output is the primary determinant of the maximal rate at which oxygen can be

stroke volume: the volume of blood being pumped out of the heart with each beat

cardiac output: indicates how much blood the heart is capable of pumping in exactly 1 minute

used. Approximately 5 liters (L) of blood are pumped through the heart during each minute at rest. During exercise, cardiac output increases to approximately four times that experienced during rest (about 20L) in the normal individual and may increase as much as six times in the elite endurance athlete (about 30L). As your level of fitness improves, the heart becomes more efficient because it is capable of pumping more blood with each stroke and thus heart rate during exercise will be lower.

WHAT DETERMINES HOW EFFICIENTLY THE BODY IS USING OXYGEN?

The greatest rate at which oxygen can be taken in and used during exercise is referred to as **aerobic capacity,** or as your **maximum aerobic capacity.** Maximum aerobic capacity is measured in a laboratory to determine how much oxygen can be used during 1 minute of maximal exercise. It is most often presented in terms of the volume of oxygen used relative to body weight per unit of time (ml/kg/min). Normal maximum aerobic capacity for most men and women ages 15 to 25 years would fall in the range of 38 to 46 ml/kg/min. However, a world-class male marathon runner may have

a maximum aerobic capacity in the 70 to 80 ml/kg/min range, and a female marathoner may have a 60 to 70 ml/kg/min range.

The performance of any activity requires a certain rate of oxygen utilization that is about the same for everybody. Generally, the greater the rate or intensity of the activity, the greater the oxygen demands. Each person has his or her own maximal rate of oxygen utilization, and his or her ability to perform an activity is closely related to the amount of oxygen required by that activity.

The maximal rate at which oxygen can be used is largely a genetically determined characteristic. Each person's maximal aerobic capacity falls within a given range. The more active you are, the higher the existing maximum aerobic capacity will be within that range. The less active you are, the lower your maximum aerobic capacity will be in that range. Thus, by engaging in a training program, it is possible to increase your aerobic capacity to its highest limit within your range.

The range of maximal aerobic capacity that you inherit is determined in large part by the types of muscle fibers that you have. **Fast-twitch muscle fibers** (FT), or fast-contracting fibers, are not as dependent on the presence of oxygen for contraction and tend to tire very rapidly. Fast-twitch fibers are responsible for speed or power activities such as sprinting or weight lifting. **Slow-twitch muscle fibers** (ST) are slow-contracting fibers that require large amounts of oxygen for contraction and are more resistant to fatigue. Slow-twitch fibers are more useful in long-term, endurance activities such as marathon running or cross-country skiing. If you have a greater percentage of slow-twitch muscle fibers than fast-twitch

aerobic capacity: the greatest rate at which oxygen can be taken in and used during exercise

maximum aerobic capacity: measured in a laboratory to determine how much oxygen can be used during 1 minute of maximal exercise

fast-twitch muscle fibers: a type of muscle fiber used for speed or power activities such as sprinting or weight lifting

slow-twitch muscle fibers: a type of muscle fiber that is resistant to fatigue and is more useful in long-term endurance activities

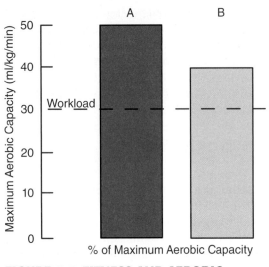

FIGURE 4-3. FITNESS AND AEROBIC CAPACITY.

Individual A should be able to work longer than can individual B as a result of lower use of maximum aerobic capacity.

fibers throughout your body, you will be able to use oxygen more efficiently and thus your maximum aerobic capacity will be higher. It appears that different forms of training can to some extent selectively hypertrophy one type of fiber more than the others.

Fatigue is closely related to the percentage of maximum aerobic capacity that a particular activity demands. It should be apparent that the greater the percentage of maximal aerobic capacity required during an activity, the shorter the time the activity may be performed. Fatigue partly occurs when insufficient oxygen is supplied to muscles. For example, Figure 4-3 compares two people, A and B. A has a maximum aerobic capacity of 50 ml/kg/min, whereas B has a maximum aerobic capacity of only 40 ml/kg/min. If A and B are exercising at the same intensity, then A is working at a much lower percentage of maximum aerobic capacity than is B. Consequently, A should be able to sustain his or her activity over a much longer period. Everyday activities such as walking up stairs or running to catch a bus may be

adversely affected if your ability to use oxygen efficiently is impaired. Thus improvement of cardiorespiratory endurance should be an essential component of any fitness program.

HOW DO YOU KNOW WHAT YOUR AEROBIC CAPACITY IS?

The most accurate technique for measuring aerobic capacity is done in a laboratory. It involves exercising a person on a treadmill or bicycle ergometer at a specific intensity and then monitoring heart rate and collecting samples of expired air using somewhat expensive and sophisticated equipment. Obviously, this is a somewhat impractical technique for the typical person. Therefore, what we most often do is monitor the heart rate as a means of estimating a percentage of maximum aerobic capacity.

Monitoring heart rate is an indirect method of estimating oxygen uptake. In general, heart rate and oxygen uptake have a linear relationship, although at very low intensities as well as at high intensities this linear relationship breaks down (Figure 4-4). The greater the intensity of the exercise, the higher the heart rate. Because of this existing relationship, it should be apparent that the rate of oxygen utilization can be estimated by measuring the heart rate. The Lab Activities at the end of this chapter, which all monitor heart rates, are a means of estimating maximum aerobic capacity.

THE FIT PRINCIPLE

The **FIT principle** is a basic philosophy of what is necessary to gain a training effect from an exercise program. FIT is an acronym that

> **FIT principle:** An approach to exercise that takes into consideration frequency, intensity, and time of an activity.

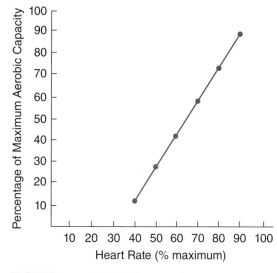

FIGURE 4-4. MAXIMAL HEART RATE AND MAXIMUM AEROBIC CAPACITY.
Maximal heart rate is achieved at about the same time as maximum aerobic capacity.

stands for Frequency, Intensity, and Time, all of which are factors that can be altered or modified within the context of a fitness program. The FIT principle is most often applied to training techniques for improving cardiorespiratory endurance and less frequently to techniques of resistance training.

WHAT TRAINING TECHNIQUES CAN BE USED TO IMPROVE CARDIORESPIRATORY ENDURANCE?

Several methods can be used to improve cardiorespiratory endurance, including (1) continuous or sustained training, (2) interval training, and (3) fartlek. The amount of improvement possible is largely determined by initial levels of cardiorespiratory endurance. The lower your endurance at the start, the more you will improve. Regardless of the training technique

used for the improvement of cardiorespiratory endurance, one principal goal remains the same. You are trying to increase the ability of the cardiorespiratory system to supply a sufficient amount of oxygen to working muscles. Without oxygen, the body is incapable of producing energy for an extended period.

CONTINUOUS TRAINING

Continuous training is a technique that uses exercises performed at the same level of intensity for long periods. The type of activity used in continuous training must be aerobic. Aerobic activities are any type that use large amounts of oxygen, elevate the heart rate, and maintain it at that level for an extended time. Aerobic activities generally involve repetitive, whole body, large-muscle movements performed over an extended time. Examples of aerobic activities are found in Fit List 4-1. The advantage of these aerobic activities as opposed to more intermittent activities, such as racquetball, squash, basketball, or tennis, is that it is easy to regulate the intensity of aerobic activities by either speeding up or slowing down the pace. Because we already know that the given intensity of the workload elicits a given heart rate, these aerobic activities allow us to maintain heart rate at a specified or

FIT LIST 4-1

Examples of Aerobic Fitness Activities

- Walking
- Jogging
- Running
- Swimming
- Cycling
- Stepping
- Aerobic dance exercise
- In-line skating
- Cross-country skiing
- Rowing

target level. Intermittent activities involve variable speeds and intensities that cause the heart rate to fluctuate considerably. Although these intermittent activities will improve cardiorespiratory endurance, they are much more difficult to monitor in terms of intensity. It is important to point out that any type of activity, from gardening to aerobic exercise, can improve fitness and reduce the risks for developing several chronic diseases. Again, the fact that you enjoy a specific type of activity should be an important factor in your selection of one. If the FIT Principle is applied to continuous training, we need to look at three variables:

- Frequency of activity
- Intensity of activity
- Time or duration of activity

▶ Frequency of Activity

To see at least minimal improvement in cardiorespiratory endurance, it is necessary for a previously sedentary or unfit individual to engage in no fewer than 3 sessions per week. A person who is fit should engage in 5 sessions of moderate-intensity activity per week. An individual who is very fit should engage in at least 3 sessions of vigorous-intensity activity each week. In addition it is also recommended that everyone do 8-10 strength-training exercises (8-12 repetitions of each) twice each week. A competitive athlete should be prepared to train as often as six times per week. Everyone should take off at least 1 day per week to give damaged tissues a chance to repair themselves.

▶ Intensity of Activity

The intensity of the exercise is also a critical factor, even though recommendations regarding training intensities vary. This is particularly true in the early stages of training, when the body is forced to make a lot of adjustments to increased

continuous training: a technique that uses exercises performed at the same level of intensity for long periods

workload demands. Activity intensity can be classified as either low-intensity, moderate-intensity, or vigorous-intensity. In low-intensity activities, the individual is not sweating and there will not be noticeable changes in the breathing pattern. Moderate-intensity activity means working hard enough to raise your heart rate and break a sweat, yet still being able to carry on a conversation. In vigorous-intensity activities heavy sweating occurs in 3-5 minutes, breathing is rapid and deep, and you can only talk in short phrases.

Determining Exercise Intensity by Monitoring Heart Rate. There are several sites at which heart rate is easily measured. The most accurate site for measuring the pulse rate is the radial artery (located on the thumb side of the wrist joint). By placing your index and middle fingers on the thumb side of the wrist, you should be able to locate a strong pulse (Figure 4-5, *A*). Do not use your thumb to monitor pulse rate. Each pulse represents one heartbeat. You should count the number of beats that occur in 30 seconds and then multiply that number by 2 to give you an accurate heart rate. Heart rate should be monitored within 15 seconds after stopping exercise.

A heart rate monitor can also be used to monitor heart rate during exercise. A number of different heart rate monitors are available at all price ranges. Figure 4-5 *C* provides an example of a typical heart rate monitor.

The objective of aerobic exercise is to elevate your heart rate to a specified target rate and maintain it at that level during your entire workout. Because heart rate is directly related to the intensity of the exercise as well as to the rate of oxygen use, it becomes a relatively simple process to identify a specific workload (pace) that will make the heart rate plateau at the desired level. By monitoring heart rate, we know whether the pace is too fast or too slow to get the heart rate into a target range. If for whatever reason you cannot increase your pace while walking or jogging, you can increase the intensity of the activity by walking or jogging up an incline.

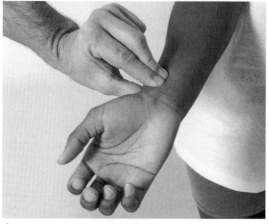

A

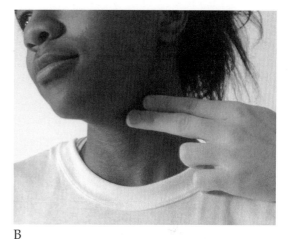

B

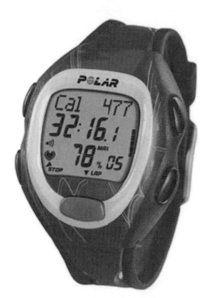

C

FIGURE 4-5. MEASURING PULSE RATE.
Measuring pulse rate at A, Radial artery and B, Carotid artery. C, Heart rate monitor. (Courtesy Polar Electro, Inc., Lake Success, NY.)

Heart rate can be increased or decreased by speeding up or slowing down your pace. It has already been indicated that heart rate increases proportionately with the intensity of the workload and will plateau after 2 to 3 minutes of activity. Thus you should be actively engaged in the workout for 2 to 3 minutes before measuring your pulse.

Several formulas allow you to easily identify a training **target heart rate.** To calculate a specific target heart rate, you must first determine your maximal heart rate. Exact determination of maximal heart rate (HR) involves exercising an individual at a maximal level and monitoring the HR using an electrocardiogram. This is a difficult process outside of a laboratory. However, an approximate estimate of maximum HR for individuals of both genders is that maximum HR is thought to be about 220 beats per minute. However, maximum HR is related to age, and, as you get older, your maximum HR decreases. Thus a relatively simple estimate of maximum HR in adults would be $HR_{max} = 220 - Age$. For a 20-year-old individual, maximum heart rate would be about 200 beats per minute $(220 - 20 = 200)$. **Heart rate reserve** is used to determine exercise heart rates. Heart rate reserve (HRR) is the

target heart rate: a specific heart rate to be achieved and maintained during exercise

heart rate reserve:

$$HRR = HR_{max} - HR_{rest}$$

TABLE 4-2
CALCULATING HEART RATES

Formula	Example (for a 20-year-old with a resting) heart rate of 70 beats per minute)
Maximal heart rate = 220 − Age	220 − 20 = 200 beats per minute
Heart rate reserve = maximal heart rate − resting heart rate	200 − 70 = 130
Lower limit of target heart rate range = (Heart Rate Reserve × 70%) + resting heart rate	(130 × 0.7) + 70 = 161
Upper limit of target heart rate range = (Heart Rate Reserve × 79%) + resting heart rate	(130 × 0.79) + 70 = 173

difference between resting heart rate (HR_{rest})* and maximum heart rate (HR_{max}).

$$HRR = HR_{max} - HR_{rest}$$

The greater the difference, the larger your heart rate reserve and the greater your range of potential training heart rate intensities. The **Karvonen equation** is used to calculate exercise heart rate at a given percentage of training intensity. To use the Karvonen equation you need to know your HR_{max} and HR_{rest}.

Exercise HR = % of target intensity ($HR_{max} - HR_{rest}$) + HR_{rest}.

When using estimated HR_{max} or/and HR_{rest}, the values are always predictions. So in a 20-year-old with a resting heart rate of 70 beats per minute the heart rate reserve is 130 (200 − 70 = 130). For moderate-intensity activity, the heart works in a range between the lower limit and an upper limit. The lower limit is calculated by taking 70 percent of the heart rate reserve and adding the resting heart rate, which would be 161 beats per minute ((130 × 0.7) + 70 = 161).

The upper limit is calculated by taking 79 percent of the heart rate reserve and adding

the resting heart rate ((130 × 0.79) + 70 = 173. (See Table 4-2.)

Lab Activity 4-1 will help you calculate a Target Heart Rate.

The American College of Sports Medicine recommends that young healthy individuals train either at moderate-intensity (70 to 79% of maximum heart rate) or vigorous-intensity (greater than 80% of maximum heart rate) levels to improve cardiorespiratory endurance and reduce the risk for chronic disease. Individuals who are less fit, who have led a previously sedentary lifestyle, are overweight, have a history or risk factors for heart disease, as well as the elderly, and anyone with arthritis and those of us with special instructions from a physician should initially engage in low-intensity workouts. For those individuals, the important thing is for them to become active and that if they are persistent they should gradually be able to increase the intensity of the activity.

Karvonen equation:

Exercise HR = % of target intensity ($HR_{max} - HR_{rest}$) + HR_{rest}.

*True resting heart rate should be monitored with the subject lying down.

TABLE 4-3
RATING PERCEIVED EXERTION

15-Grade Scale		10-Grade Scale	
6		0	Nothing
7	Very, very light	0.5	Very, very weak (just noticeable)
8		1	Very weak
9	Very light	2	Weak (light)
10		3	Moderate
11	Fairly light	4	Somewhat strong
12		5	Strong (heavy)
13	Somewhat hard	6	
14		7	Very strong
15	Hard	8	
16		9	
17	Very hard	10	Very, very strong (almost maximum)
18			
19	Very, very hard		Maximum
20			

The original scale (6–20) on the left and the newer 10-point category scale with ratio properties on the right. From Borg, GA. 1982. Psychological bases of perceived exertion. *Medicine and Science in Sports and Exercise*; 14: 377–387.

Determining Exercise Intensity Through Rating of Perceived Exertion (RPE). **Rating of perceived exertion** (RPE) can be used in addition to monitoring heart rate to indicate exercise intensity. During exercise, individuals are asked to rate on a numerical scale from 6 to 20 exactly how they feel relative to their level of exertion (Table 4-3). More intense exercise that requires a higher level of oxygen consumption and energy expenditure is directly related to higher subjective ratings of perceived exertion. Over a period of time, individuals can be taught to exercise at a specific RPE that relates directly to more objective measures of exercise intensity.

►**Time or Duration of Activity**

For a sedentary or unfit individual beginning a fitness program to improve cardiorespiratory endurance it is recommended to engage in no less than 20 minutes of exercise with the heart rate at recommend training intensities. But if that is too difficult it is okay for the person to slow down and take a break whenever necessary. Initially they should just try and finish the 20–minute session. For a healthy, fit individual to maintain health and reduce the risk for chronic disease, it is recommended to engage in either 30 minutes of moderate-intensity activity 5 days a week or 20 minutes of vigorous-intensity activity 3 days a week. Combinations of moderate- and vigorous-intensity physical activity can be

rating of perceived exertion: a technique used to subjectively rate exercise intensity on a numerical scale

TABLE 4-4
GUIDELINES FOR CONTINUOUS TRAINING

Training Level	Frequency (Sessions per Week)	% Maximum Heart Rate	RPI	Time	Physical Signs
Low-intensity (Beginner)	3	55–69%	6–9	20 minutes	No sweating. No noticeable change in breathing.
Moderate-intensity (Fit)	5	70–79%	10–15	30 minutes	Heart rate increases; break a sweat in 10 min; able to carry on a conversation.
Vigorous-intensity (Very Fit)	3	>80%	16–20	20 minutes	Heavy sweating in 3 to 5 mins; rapid and deep breathing; can only talk in short phrases.

used to meet the guidelines. It has been shown that moderate-intensity physical activity can be accumulated throughout the day in 10-minute bouts, which can be just as effective as exercising for 30 minutes straight. It should be added that to lose weight or maintain weight loss, 60 to 90 minutes of physical activity may be necessary.

▶ Guidelines for Continuous Training

In summary, when using the continuous training method, the activity selected must be aerobic and should be enjoyable. To see minimal improvement in cardiorespiratory endurance, training must be done for 20 to 30 minutes, three to five times per week with the heart rate elevated to an intensity of no less than 55 percent of its maximal rate. As mentioned in Chapter 3, each training program should be designed to meet individual needs and abilities. The principle of overload states that you must stress the system if you are to see improvement and progress from one level to another. Everyone

should begin slowly with the idea that he or she will progress as quickly as possible at his or her own rate. If you are able to perform an activity at a given level without undue stress and it seems that you are not being "challenged" at that particular level, you may progress to the next level. Remember, however, that beginning at a level that is too high will probably produce various musculoskeletal injuries that often cause setbacks in a training program.

All training programs are based on monitoring heart rate during some type of aerobic activity. Heart rate can be increased or decreased by altering the pace. The guidelines in Table 4-4 can be applied to low-intensity, moderate-intensity, or vigorous-intensity activities.

INTERVAL TRAINING

Unlike continuous training, **interval training** involves activities that are more intermittent.

TABLE 4-5
RECOMMENDED INTERVAL TRAINING WORKOUTS

Level	Intensity during Training Period	Intensity during Recovery Period
Beginner	70%–75% of MHR	55%–60% of MHR
Intermediate	75%–85% of MHR	60%–65% of MHR
Advanced	85%–95% of MHR	60%–65% of MHR

Interval training consists of alternating periods of relatively intense work with periods of active recovery. It permits you to perform much more work at a more intense workload over a longer period than you could if you were working continuously. It is most desirable in continuous training to work at an intensity of about 60 to 85 percent of maximal heart rate. Obviously, sustaining activity at a relatively high intensity over a 20-minute period would be extremely difficult. The advantage of interval training is that it allows work at this 85 percent or higher level for a short period, followed by an active period of recovery during which you may be working at 60 percent of maximal heart rate. Thus the intensity of the workout and its duration can be greater than with continuous training.

Most sports are anaerobic, involving short bursts of intense activity followed by a type of active recovery period (football, basketball, soccer, and tennis all qualify). Training with the interval technique allows you to be more sport-specific during the workout. With interval training you can apply the overload principle by making the training period much more intense. Several important factors should be considered in interval training. The *training period* is the amount of time that continuous activity is actually being performed, and the *recovery period* is the time between training periods. A *set* is a group of combined training and recovery periods, and a *repetition* is the number of training/recovery periods per set. *Training time* or *distance* refers to the rate or distance of the training period. The *training/recovery ratio* indicates a time ratio for training versus recovery. (Table 4-5 provides specific recommendations for an interval training workout.)

An example of interval training would be a soccer player running sprints. An interval workout would involve running ten 120-yard sprints in under 20 seconds, with a 1-minute recovery period (walking) between each sprint. During this training session the soccer player's heart rate would probably increase to 85 to 95 percent of maximal level during the sprint and should probably fall to the 60 to 65 percent level during the recovery period.

Inactive or sedentary individuals should exercise some caution when using interval training as a method for improving cardiorespiratory endurance. The intensity levels attained during the active periods may be too high for the inactive individual.

FARTLEK TRAINING

Fartlek is a training technique, a type of cross-country running, that originated in Sweden.

interval training: alternating periods of relatively intense work with periods of active recovery

fartlek: a type of workout that involves jogging at varying speeds over varying terrain

Fartlek literally means "speed play." It is similar to interval training in that you must run for a specified period; however, specific pace and speed are not identified. The course for a fartlek workout should be some type of varied terrain including some level running, some uphill and downhill running, and some running around obstacles such as trees or rocks. The object is to put surges into a running workout, varying the length of the surges according to individual purposes. One big advantage of fartlek training is that because the pace and terrain are always changing, the training session is less regimented and allows for an effective alternative in the training routine. When you really think about it, most people who jog or walk are really engaging in a fartlek-type workout.

Again, if fartlek training is going to improve cardiorespiratory endurance, it must elevate the heart rate to at least minimal training levels (60 to 85 percent). Fartlek may best be used as an off-season conditioning activity or as a change-of-pace activity to counteract the boredom of a training program that uses the same activity day after day.

GOOD AEROBIC ACTIVITIES FOR IMPROVING CARDIO-RESPIRATORY ENDURANCE

WALKING

If walking is your primary form of exercise, you're part of a large club that has become the fitness phenomenon of the new millenium. More than 60 million Americans now walk for exercise, making it the number one participation sport in the country (Figure 4-6).

People walk for fitness for several reasons. It is, after all, an activity that can be pursued at almost any time, anywhere, with anyone, at no cost. Besides being fun, walking can expend a lot of energy. A walking regimen can be started

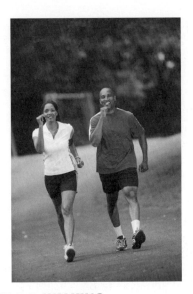

FIGURE 4-6. WALKING.
Walking is the most popular aerobic activity.

easily at any age and can be worked into almost anybody's daily schedule. Although some techniques are better than others, walking demands little skill or practice. Walking is an action that is low impact, which means that the chances of injury to the joints of the lower extremities are much lower than jogging or running. It does require a pair of comfortable shoes, but no other specialized clothing or equipment is really necessary. As long as you're in relatively good health, the activity presents few, if any, health hazards. As with any program involving your health, just check with your physician before you begin.

Walking's greatest value as a fitness activity is that you can just go out and walk. Like other physical activities, technique becomes a factor in developing a more effective program. In walking, the development of proper technique involves correct stride, arm swing, posture, and a steady pace. Although it's fun to experiment with techniques, it's by no means mandatory in walking. You know how to put one foot in front of the other, and there's no reason to complicate a simple activity.

RUNNING

For decades now, running has been viewed by the American public as an important fitness activity. Within the last 20 years, millions of people have taken to the streets and now run or jog on a regular basis. And the running phenomenon doesn't seem to be restricted to any one segment of the population. Young children, college students, office personnel, laborers, elderly persons, people of all backgrounds and both sexes regularly put on their running shoes and go for a run (Figure 4-7).

Although many people run to control their weight and attain a healthful physical appearance, other people run for the other physiological benefits a running program offers. Many people report that running (or jogging) is relaxing and alleviates stress, tension, and depression. They express feelings of greater self-worth and enthusiasm toward life after a run. This euphoric feeling has been called a "runner's high," and most people agree that

this is both a psychological and a physiological phenomenon.

As is the case with walking, the only equipment required is a pair of running shoes and some shorts. Running offers the advantages of low cost, flexibility of time, year-round availability, and a relatively high level of benefit in return for time and effort.

However, there are some disadvantages to running. Because the feet and legs are subjected to repetitive pounding on the running surface, overuse injuries are very likely. Most of these injuries involve the muscles, tendons, ligaments, and occasionally bones of the lower extremities. Proper running and training techniques and properly fitted running shoes can reduce the number of injuries associated with running.

SWIMMING

Like running, swimming is an excellent method of developing cardiorespiratory fitness (Figure 4-8). The physiological benefits of swimming are similar to those of running; however, several differences should be addressed. The first difference is that not only must the energy of the arms and legs be used

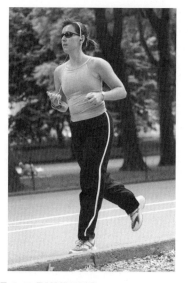

FIGURE 4-7. RUNNING.
Running is an excellent activity for improving cardiorespiratory endurance.

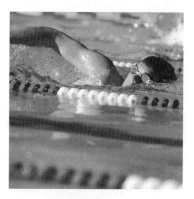

FIGURE 4-8. SWIMMING.
Swimming is a good activity for improving cardiovascular endurance.

to propel the body through the water, but some energy must also be expended to keep the body afloat. For these reasons, it has been estimated that the amount of energy required to swim a given distance is approximately four times as great as running an equal distance. Energy expenditure and heart rates vary with the type of stroke. For both trained and highly skilled swimmers swimming at any given speed, the breaststroke seems to require the greatest amount of energy, then the backstroke, and last the front crawl. Monitoring heart rate is difficult in swimmers.

Swimming also eliminates many of the stresses and strains on the weight-bearing joints that are commonly experienced in running. Although the shoulder joint undergoes a significant amount of overuse-type stress, the ankle and knee joints are spared the trauma of the foot repeatedly banging into a hard surface.

A swimsuit and perhaps a pair of goggles for persons whose eyes are irritated by chlorine are all that is necessary to begin a swimming program. For many, the biggest drawback of using a swimming program for cardiorespiratory conditioning is the unavailability of a swimming pool.

AEROBIC EXERCISE

In today's terminology, the word *aerobics* is primarily used to refer specifically to aerobic exercise, which may well be the country's largest, most widespread, organized fitness endeavor. Aerobics is a combination of choreographed fitness routines set to music. In other words, it is movement to music that contributes to physical fitness by improving cardiorespiratory endurance, strength, flexibility, and muscular endurance.

As a rapidly developing participation sport, aerobics is undergoing an evolutionary process. Different styles of aerobics have been advocated over the last few years.

▶Floor Aerobics

Floor aerobics can be divided into low-impact and high-impact (Figure 4-9). In low-impact aerobics, the impact to the lower extremities is reduced by eliminating excessive jumping and by keeping one leg slightly bent and in constant contact with the floor throughout the conditioning phase of the workout. Traveling movements rather than stationary steps are used, with an emphasis on maintaining proper body alignment at all times. In high-impact aerobics, the conditioning component consists of running, jumping, and hopping movements set to music. High-impact aerobics can produce musculoskeletal injuries as a result of the repetitive pounding of the lower extremities against a hard surface. Fit List 4-2 provides a list of some common movements used in floor aerobics.

▶Step Aerobics

Step aerobics offers a great cardio workout without the need for extensive space or

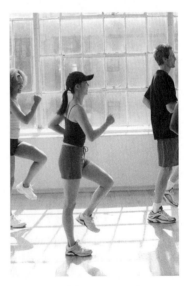

FIGURE 4-9. FLOOR AEROBICS.
Floor aerobics can either be high- or low-impact.

FIT LIST 4-2

Floor Aerobic Movements

Jazz Stretch This is a stretch, so reach as high as possible, but don't strain. Feet apart, jazz hands on hips. L arm reaches overhead. Palm of hand facing forward with fingers stretched. R hand on hip. L knee slightly bent (isolation). Repeat on other side.

Attitude Lift Keep your torso tall while you lift your legs and arms. Turn out from the hip keeping your pelvis neutral. Bend your knee slightly to get the maximum benefit. Feet together. Arms at side. Body supported on L leg, knee slightly bent. R leg lifts up and is turned out, slightly bent. L arm extended forward. R arm extended out to the side.

Diagonal Toe Touch Arm and leg reach out to the diagonal. Make sure you are reaching rather than swinging your arms. Bring feet together. Arms at side. Face L diagonal. Touch R foot to forward diagonal. Extend R arm to forward diagonal. L arm on L hip. Repeat on other side.

Flick Kick Bring feet together. Arms at side. Body supported on L leg, knee slightly bent. Kick R foot forward. Keep leg low and point toe. L arm extends forward. Bring feet together, arms at side. R arm extends to the side. Back to arms at side. Repeat in opposite direction.

Heel Hop Keep your torso tall. Flex your heels R and L. Heels touch out directly in front of your body. Make a controlled stopping point with your arms. Bring feet together. Body supported on L leg, R foot flexed. L arm extended overhead. R arm extended out to the diagonal. Arms at side. Feet come together.

Knee Lift Lift your knees and squeeze your glutes. Keep your abdominals tight and your torso tall. Bring feet together. Raise R knee. R arm extended out to side, L arm extended forward. Repeat on opposite side.

Pendulum Lift Movement flows with the music as legs lift side to side. Push your leg out to the side and pull your leg back towards your body. Body supported on L leg, R leg lifts out to the side. L arm extends forward. R arm extends out to the side. Reverse direction.

Lunges Arms swing naturally. Use your legs. Shift your body weight from one side to another. Lean to R. R knee turned out, knee bent over toe. Lean to L. L knee turned out, knee bent over toe.

Plies Work your quads and squeeze your glutes. Arms at sides, elbows slightly bent. Heels together, toes turned out. R foot steps out, toes and knees turned out. Knees bent over toes. Bring L foot back to starting position. Heels together. Reverse direction.

Jazz Square Take four steps making a square on the floor. Arms swing naturally. Keep your body forward at all times. Use those legs! Bring feet together. R foot crosses over L (counts 1–2). L foot steps back (counts 3–4). R foot steps to the side (counts 5–6). L foot steps front (counts 7–8). Return to starting position. Bring feet together.

Chasse Toes and knees face forward. Chasse means one foot chases the other. Count 1 and 2 and 3 and 4. Land toe, ball, heel. Then repeat going the opposite direction. You're traveling with this step, so look out for your neighbor! Step out R. Bring L foot to R foot. Step out R. Bring feet together. Bring L foot to R foot. Bring feet together.

Grapevine The foot pattern is step, cross, step and lift. Then reverse the direction. You are traveling with this step, so watch where you are going! Step out R. Arms swing overhead. L foot crosses behind R foot. Step out R. Arms swing down.

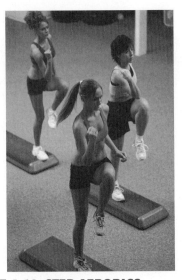

FIGURE 4-10. STEP AEROBICS.
*Step aerobics uses a stepping platform
4 to 10 inches high.*

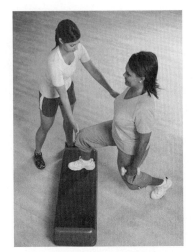

FIGURE 4-11. CIRCUIT AEROBICS.
*Circuit aerobics uses resistance equipment (dumb-
bells) combined with advanced aerobic exercise.*

equipment (Figure 4-10). The only equipment needed is an aerobic stepping platform 4 to 10 inches high sitting on a flat surface. Stepping onto the platform increases the intensity of the workout. Risers can be added to the initial step as the fitness level increases. In step aerobics, your workout travels vertically rather than horizontally. Steps up onto and down off of the platform are combined with arm movements to increase large-muscle movements. Routines are arranged so that students step up and down to the music. Posture is important in stepping—keep the head up and shoulders back and don't lean forward from the waist. The feet should be centered on the platform and they should meet it wholly, heel to ball of foot unless moving fast or doing lunges. When stepping down, let the toe hit the ground first, then the ball of foot, then the heel. Step down close to the step platform rather than stretching away from it. The knee should consistently bend to 60 degrees. Qualified instructors should be able to quickly correct

faulty techniques. Fit List 4-3 provides a list of common movements used in step aerobics.

▶ Circuit Aerobics

Circuit aerobics combines the use of resistance equipment with an advanced aerobic exercise class (Figure 4-11). Holding light hand weights or wearing banded wrist weights is a common practice in various forms of aerobic exercise. Addition of these light weights increases energy expenditure during activity. Approximately 30 minutes is devoted to aerobic dance and 30 minutes to resistance training at various stations. Fit List 4-4 provides a list of exercises using weights that can be used with either floor or step aerobics.

▶ Water Aerobics

Like any other form of aerobic exercise, water aerobics can provide a challenging cardio workout (Figure 4-12). However exercising in water takes advantage of the bouyancy of the body, thus supporting body weight and reducing the risk of muscle or joint injury. Water

FIT LIST 4-3

Step Aerobics Common Movements

Basic can be done with the R or L foot leading. Step up with one foot and then down (different instructors may use different arm movements with this move).

Diagonal or Corner to Corner The side of your body is facing the step. Rather than going over the top to the other side, go over at a diagonal so you end up on the other side at the opposite end of the step.

Hamstring Curl Step with one foot and bring the opposite heel toward your rear until there is tension in the hamstring muscle. (Can be done with the right or left leg leading.)

Hip Lift or Glute Lift Step with one foot and lift the opposite leg back. This is a small movement that works the glutes. The abdominals should remain tight so the lower back isn't stressed. Once the leg is lifted, try to squeeze the glutes before lowering the leg. This move can be done with the right or left leg leading.

Kicks Step with one foot and kick the opposite leg. (Can be done with the right or left leg leading.)

Knee Lift Step with one foot and lift the opposite knee. (Can be done with the right or left leg leading.)

Lunge From the top of the step, lean forward and touch your toe on the floor behind you. Your weight should be slightly forward, not on the foot that is touching the floor. Do NOT press your heels down in this move, just touch the toe and return the foot to the step platform. Repeat with the opposite leg.

Over the Top The side of your body is toward the step. Bring one foot onto the step followed by the other foot. The first foot steps down on the opposite side of the step followed by the second foot.

Side Lifts Step with one foot and lift the opposite leg to the side. You don't need to lift very high, just lift the leg straight up to the side and squeeze the muscle when you feel tension. This move can be done with the right or left leg leading.

Straddle Down From the top of the step, one leg steps down on one side, the other leg steps down on the other (so you are "straddling" the step). Each leg then returns to the top of the step. A wide variety of arm movements can be used with this leg pattern.

Turn Step Like the Alternating V-Step except as you bring both legs down, the side of your body is facing the step rather than the front of your body.

V-Step can be done with the R or L foot leading. Take the feet wide on the step and then close together on the floor (arm patterns will vary).

Repeaters Any alternating step pattern where the weight bearing phase of the movement (such as knee lifts, hip lifts, etc.) can be repeated (usually 3 times).

aerobics is ideal for individuals with joint problems, back pain, obese individuals, pregnant women, or people who get overheated easily. The water also provides resistance to movement in any direction, which helps strengthen muscles. Though aquatic activities in general expend more energy than many land-based activities performed at the same

FIT LIST 4-4

Circuit Aerobics Exercises

Arm Circles Arms are overhead or shoulder level. Circle the arms clockwise down toward the body and then back to the starting point.

Bicep Curls Elbows should be at the side of the trunk with the palms of the hand facing upward. Bring the hands toward the chest by flexing the elbow and return them to the side of the trunk.

Alternating Bicep Curls Same as the movement above, but only flex/extend one arm at a time.

Double Side Out Fists should be under the chin at chest level with the palms facing downward. Extend both arms out to the side keeping the elbows at shoulder height. Return the arms to their starting position. (This can also be done by alternating the R and L arm).

Frontal Pull With arms at shoulder level, pull the arms in toward the body (so fists rest on thighs), then return them to shoulder level.

Frontal Raise Begin with fists on each thigh. Raise the arms to shoulder level and return to the thigh.

Hammer Curls Similar to bicep curls except the palms are facing each other rather than facing upward. This movement can also be done by alternating arm movements.

Lateral Raise Fists should be together with palms touching the thighs. Lift the arms outwards and upwards with the palms facing down. Elbows should be leading this movement and should be slightly bent. Lift until the arms are slightly below shoulder level and then return them to the thigh.

Low Row With arms in front of the body, pull the elbows in toward the waist until the hands are next to the waist and then return the arms to the front of the body.

Overhead Press Fists are resting on the shoulders with the palms facing each other. Extend the arms up over the head, keeping the elbows close to the ears. Lower the arms back to the shoulders. This can be down with both arms at the same time or by alternating arms.

Overhead Pull With arms above the head, pull the arms in toward the thighs and then return them overhead.

Pec Press Elbows are shoulder height and bent. Hands are in a fist with palms facing forward. Press the arms together until the palms (and fists) are facing each other in front of your face. Return the arms to their starting position.

Shoulder Punch With hands at shoulder level, punch one arm and then return to shoulder level.

Slice Similar to the double side out except one arm goes up and the other goes down. This is usually done with a side lift move. The leg that lifts to the side corresponds to the arm which is down (the opposite arm goes up).

Tricep Kickbacks Arms should be at your side with the elbows slightly bent and behind the shoulders. Your hands are next to your trunk with your palms facing the body. Extend the elbow back and then return to your starting position. This movement can be done by pressing both arms back at the same time or alternating back and forth.

Upright Row Fists should be together next to your thighs. Bring the arms up toward your chin (keeping the fists close together and next to the body). Return the arms to their starting position.

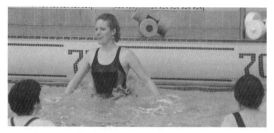

FIGURE 4-12. WATER AEROBICS.
Water aerobics allows exercise against resistance in non-weight bearing.

pace due to the increased resistance of water, the speed with which movements can be performed is greatly reduced. Fit List 4-5 provides a sample water aerobics workout.

►Kickboxing Aerobics

A kickboxing aerobics class is a high-impact cardiovascular workout that blends elements of boxing, martial arts and traditional aerobics into a 30- to 60-minute exercise routine (Figure 4-13). Typical routines include a series of repetitive punches, hand strikes, kicks, and other self-defense moves, interspersed with a bouncing "base" move, to music. Even though one is thrusting through the air rather than working against resistance it qualifies as a total body workout because it uses several muscle groups and is intensely aerobic. It has become extremely popular in both health clubs and in home exercise videos. Fit List 4-6 provides a list of common kickboxing aerobics movements.

FIT LIST 4-5

Sample Water Aerobics Workout

- Begin in shallow water. The water level should be between the rib cage and the underarm.
- Jog around the pool and do kicks, jumping jacks, strides, and knee lifts to warm up the body for 6 to 8 minutes.
- Lightly stretch the quadriceps, calf muscles, hip flexors, and hamstrings.
- Perform the moves listed in the second bullet point at a higher intensity for 8 to 10 minutes. Make the movements long and exaggerated.
- Execute a tuck jump. Start in a standing position, then keep the knees and ankles together as you pull the knees into the chest. Return to a standing position. Move the arms in a circular motion at the side of the body; the arms lengthen as the knees lift, and bend at the elbow as the legs straighten.
- Perform a frog jump. Begin with the toes, knees, and thighs slightly turned out. The arms are bent in a diamond shape, with the fists close to the chest. Push the arms down to the hips while lifting the legs up and into a diamond shape. The knees point to each side at the top of the jump and mimic frog legs. Return to the starting position.
- Execute a scissors jump. Start in a standing position. As you jump, one leg moves straight forward and the other moves directly behind the body. Alternate front and back. The arms move in opposition to the legs.
- Begin in a standing position for a heel lift. While keeping the knees and heels close together, jump and lift the heels toward the buttocks. The heels should not lift higher than knee height. The arms are extended away from the body at shoulder height, slightly rounded at the elbows. As you lift the legs, pull the arms down to the hips.
- Kick the legs and jog for 2 to 3 minutes.
- Stretch the quadriceps, hamstrings, hip flexors, and calves deeply.

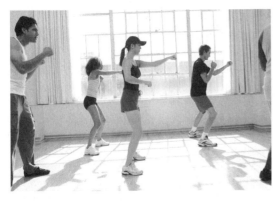

FIGURE 4-13. KICKBOXING AEROBICS.
Kickboxing aerobics blends traditional aerobics with boxing and martial arts.

CYCLING

Cycling is another aerobic activity that is excellent for improving cardiorespiratory endurance (Figure 4-14). People of all ages enjoy it, primarily because of the ease with which anyone can learn to ride without formal training. Like running and swimming, cycling produces some very desirable physiological responses in terms of strength, endurance, and weight control.

Bicycles come in thousands of different makes and models, with countless numbers of available accessories and options. The cost of purchasing an inexpensive bicycle is not much more than that of buying a pair of good running shoes for the average person.

Perhaps the biggest problem with cycling is locating a safe place to ride. No matter how safety conscious you are on the bicycle, there is always a danger posed by traffic. For this reason, stationary exercise bikes, or ergometers, have become popular. The stationary bike allows you to gain all the cardiovascular benefits of cycling without having to worry about dealing with traffic safety. Additionally, you can exercise in privacy, regardless of outdoor conditions, and read, watch TV, or listen to music at the same time.

SPINNING

Spinning is an exercise technique that is basically aerobic exercise performed on stationary

FIT LIST 4-6

Kickboxing Aerobics Movements

Squat Bending the knees separately or together using any depth, or stance.

Leg Extension Kicking either leg forward, diagonally, sideways, or backward while keeping the knee straight, bent, or in motion.

Lower Leg Extension or Curl Kicking the lower leg forward or back.

Toe Raises Lifting or standing up on the toes.

Trunk Tilt or Twist Tilting the trunk forward (as in kicking, crunches, or toe touches) or to either side, or twisting the torso in a rotary motion while punching.

Straight or Bent Arm Extension Punching or swinging the arm straight out, up, down, back, diagonally, or sideways, in any direction, with the elbow bent, straight, or in motion.

Forearm Extension or Flexion Straightening the forearm out in a chopping motion or curling it in.

Knee Raises Kicking with the knee or lifting it as in a leg raise.

Punches Jab, round house, power punch, uppercut, left hook, elbow thrusts, forearm smash.

Kicks Front kick with front leg, front kick with back leg, side kick to either side, round house kick, various knee kicks.

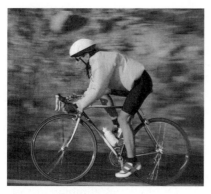

FIGURE 4-14. CYCLING.
Cycling can be enjoyed by people of all ages.

exercise bikes (Figure 4-15). It is being recommended as a great workout with no impact, thus minimizing chances of injury. Spinning usually involves a 40- to 45-minute workout. It is good for all levels in any class because you can get a very intense workout or a low-level workout in the same class depending on your fitness level and how hard you want to work. The workout is done to music, with the class instructor acting as a coach to work you through the routine. At this point spinning classes are found primarily in health clubs and

spinning clubs. Videos are widely available to the consumer.

IN-LINE SKATING

In-line skating, also called rollerblading, is another fitness and recreational activity that has quickly gained popularity throughout the United States (Figure 4-16). However, contrary to popular belief, skating is not a new activity. In-line skating is essentially "high-tech" roller-skating. A pair of Rollerblades looks like ice skates that have had the blade replaced with a series of four to six small wheels. These wheels are made for gliding on hard, smooth surfaces. In-line skaters are capable of attaining speeds approaching 25 miles per hour. For this reason, pads must be worn to protect elbows, knees, and hands. It is also recommended that protective headgear, such as a cycling helmet, be worn to minimize the likelihood of injury.

The motions used with in-line skating are similar to those used in ice skating—pushing

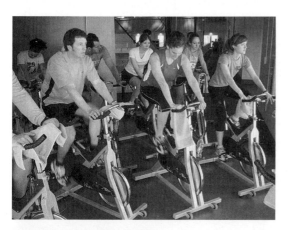

FIGURE 4-15. SPINNING.
Spinning is performed in a group class on stationary exercise bicycles.

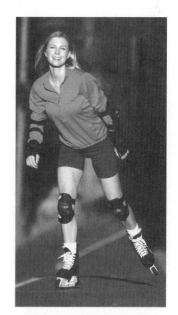

FIGURE 4-16. ROLLERBLADING.
Rollerblading is popular on college campuses.

with the legs from side to side and using a side-to-side swinging motion of the arms for balance. In-line skating uses gross movements of both the arms and the legs, making it an excellent aerobic activity.

HIKING OR BACKPACKING

Hiking or backpacking is a simple way to add a little variety to a fitness or exercise routine (Figure 4-17). It is a great way to get outdoors and improve your endurance at the same time. Unlike some of the other activities discussed in this chapter, it is important that you plan ahead and take some simple safety precautions to ensure an enjoyable experience. Hiking and backpacking demand that you be prepared physically, so you should select a trail that matches your conditioning, the amount of time you have, and the type of terrain you enjoy. Initially, you should start with moderate hikes and gradually increase your endurance by progressively selecting more difficult trails. It is essential to pack the right gear (lightweight) for changing weather, dress in layers of fabric that insulates well and dries rapidly, and make sure your hiking boots fit properly to avoid developing blisters and sore spots.

Always know where you are and where you are going by having a compass, a map, or a hiking guidebook. You should avoid hiking alone. If you must go by yourself, it is wise to pick more popular trails so that there are other hikers around. You must know how to take care of yourself should an emergency arise.

ROCK CLIMBING

Rock climbing is becoming an increasingly popular sport. Outdoor rock climbing in mountainous, sometimes remote, terrain is not only challenging but can also be extremely dangerous if the individual is not properly trained or experienced. Knowledge of climbing techniques and the use of essential pieces of gear and equipment are crucial to avoid serious and potentially fatal injury. Normally, climbers use gear and safety equipment specifically designed for the purpose. Flexibility, strength, endurance, and mental control, as well as balance and agility, are required to cope with difficult, dangerous physical challenges. Indoor climbing is an increasingly popular variation of rock climbing performed on artificially manufactured structures that attempt to mimic the experience of real rock climbing but in a more controlled environment (Figure 4-18). Walls are

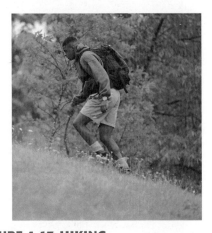

FIGURE 4-17. HIKING.
Hiking or backpacking can be a relaxing activity that can also improve cardiorespiratory endurance.

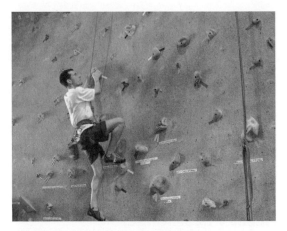

FIGURE 4-18. ROCK CLIMBING.
Climbing walls simulate outdoor rock climbing.

constructed using different sized resin hand-holds placed at varying angles and distances. The handholds can be moved to make the climb more or less difficult depending on the skill of the climber. Because environmental conditions including the climbing surface and proper use of equipment can be more controlled, indoor climbing is a safer alternative introduction to the sport.

WHAT IS YOUR LEVEL OF CARDIO-RESPIRATORY ENDURANCE?

How fit is your cardiorespiratory system? Several tests have been developed to evaluate fitness levels. Most of these tests are based on the idea that cardiorespiratory endurance capacity is best indicated by the maximum aerobic capacity of the working tissues to use oxygen. We know from an earlier discussion that maximum aerobic capacity can be predicted or estimated by measuring heart rates at varying workloads. You can use Lab Activities 4-2 and 4-3 as tests to determine your specific levels of cardiorespiratory endurance. Remember that each of these activities is based largely on one or both of the following factors: (1) the motivation of the person, and (2) the minimal level of cardiovascular endurance.

SUMMARY

- Cardiorespiratory endurance involves the coordinated function of the heart, lungs, blood, and blood vessels to supply sufficient amounts of oxygen to the working tissues.
- The best indicator of how efficiently the cardiorespiratory system functions is aerobic capacity, or the maximal rate at which oxygen can be used by the tissues.
- Heart rate is directly related to the rate of oxygen consumption. It is therefore possible to predict the intensity of the exercise in terms of a rate of oxygen use by monitoring heart rate.
- Aerobic exercise involves an activity in which the level of intensity and duration is low enough to provide a sufficient amount of oxygen to supply the demands of the working tissues.
- In anaerobic exercise the intensity of the activity is so high that oxygen is being used more quickly than it can be supplied; thus an oxygen debt is incurred that must be repaid before working tissue can return to its normal resting state.
- Continuous training for improving cardiorespiratory endurance involves selecting an activity that is aerobic in nature and training at least three times per week for a period of no less than 20–30 minutes with the heart rate elevated to 55 to 85 percent of maximal rate.
- Interval training involves alternating periods of relatively intense work followed by periods of active recovery. Interval training allows performance of more work at a relatively higher workload than does continuous training.
- Fartlek makes use of jogging or running over varying types of terrain at changing speeds.
- Walking, running, swimming, aerobic exercise, cycling, in-line skating, hiking and backpacking, and rock climbing are all excellent activities for improving cardiorespiratory endurance.

SUGGESTED READINGS

American College of Sports Medicine. 1998. American College of Sports Medicine position stand: The recommended quantity and quality of exercise for developing and maintaining cardiorespiratory and muscular fitness, and flexibility in healthy adults. *Medicine and Science in Sports and Exercise.* Jun; 30(6):975–91.

American College of Sports Medicine. 2005. *Guidelines for exercise testing and prescription.* Philadelphia: Lippincott Williams, and Wilkins.

Baun, M. 2007. *Fantastic water workouts.* Champaign, IL: Human Kinetics.

Bishop, J. 2007. *Fitness through aerobics,* Upper Saddle River, NJ:Benjamin Cummings.

Borg, G. A. 1982. Psychophysical basis of perceived exertion. *Medicine and Science in Sports and Exercise* 14:377.

Bracko, M. 2007. Advantages of interval training. *ACSM's Health & Fitness Journal* 11(5):31.

Colwin, C. M. 2002. *Breakthrough swimming.* Champaign, IL: Human Kinetics.

Cook, G. 2008. *Gym survival guide: Your road map to fearless fitness.* New York: Sterling Publishing.

Crouter, S.E., C. Albright, and D. R. Bassett Jr. 2004. Accuracy of Polar S410 heart rate monitor to estimate energy cost of exercise. *Medicine and Science in Sports and Exercise* 36(8):1433–1439.

Decker, J., ed. 2002. *Walking games and activities.* Champaign, IL: Human Kinetics.

Dreyer, D., and K. Dreyer. 2005. *Chi walking: The five mindful steps for lifelong health and energy.* New York: Simon and Schuster.

Fenton, M. 2008. *The complete guide to walking, new and revised: For health, weight loss, and fitness (Walking Magazine).* New York: Lyons Press.

Fleck, S. J. and W. J. Kraemer. 2004. Integrating other fitness components. In *Designing resistance training programs,* 3rd ed., edited by S. J. Fleck, 129–47, 325–61. Champaign, IL: Human Kinetics.

Furia, E. 2010. *The big book of bicycling: Everything you need to know to get started, train, and race.* Emmaus, PA: Rodale.

Glidewell, S. 2004. *Inline skating.* Minneapolis: Lerner Publishing Group.

Greene, L., and R. Pate. 2004. *Training for young distance runners.* Champaign, IL: Human Kinetics.

Grier, T. D., L. K. Lloyd, J. L. Walker, and T. D. Murray. 2002. Metabolic cost of aerobic dance bench stepping at varying cadences and bench heights. *Journal of Strength and Conditioning Research* 16(2):242–49.

Haskell, W., Lee, I., and R. Pate. 2007. Physical activity and public health. Updated recommendation for adults from the American College of Sports Medicine and the American Heart Association. *Circulation* 2007; 116; DOI:10.1161/circulationaha.107.185649.

Haywood, K. M., and N. Getchell. 2001. Development of cardiorespiratory endurance. In *Learning activities for life span motor development,* 3rd ed., edited by K. M. Haywood, 181–86, 212–23. Champaign, IL: Human Kinetics.

Hewitt, B. 2005. *Bicycling Magazine's mountain biking skills: Skills and techniques to master any terrain.* New York: Rodale Press.

Hewitt, B. 2005. *Bicycling Magazine's new cyclists handbook.* New York: Rodale Press.

Hewitt, B. 2005. *Bicycling Magazine's training techniques for cyclists: Greater power, faster speed, longer endurance, better skills.* Emmaus, PA: Rodale Press Inc.

Iknoian, T. 2005. *Fitness walking.* Champaign, IL: Human Kinetics.

Jackson, A. S., J. B. Kampert, and C. E. Barlow. 2004. Longitudinal changes in cardiorespiratory fitness: Measurement error or true change? *Medicine and Science in Sports and Exercise* 36(7):1175–80.

Katz, J. 2003. *Your water workout: No impact aerobic and strength training from yoga, pilates, tai chi and more.* New York: Broadway Books.

Kemsley, W. 2005. *The backpacker and hikers handbook: The ultimate guide.* Guilford, CT: Globe Pequot Press.

Kubukeli, Z. N., T. D. Noakes, and S. C. Dennis. 2002. Training techniques to improve endurance exercise performances. *Sports Medicine* 32(8):489–509.

Lagally, K. M., R. J. Robertson, K. I. Gallagher, R. Gearhart, and F. L. Goss. 2002. Ratings of perceived exertion during low- and high-intensity resistance exercise by young adults. *Perceptual and Motor Skills* 94(3 Part I): 723–31.

Larsen, G. E., et al. 2002. Prediction of maximum oxygen consumption from walking, jogging, or running. *Research Quarterly for Exercise and Sport* 73(1):66–72.

Laughlin, T. 2001. *Swimming made easy: The total immersion way for any swimmer to achieve fluency, ease, and speed in any stroke.* Swimwear Inc. New Paltz, NY.

Lepretre, P. M., J. P. Koralsztein, and V. L. Billat. 2004. Effect of exercise intensity on relationship between VO2max and cardiac output. *Medicine and Science in Sports and Exercise* 36(8):1357–63.

Long, J. 2005. *How to rock climb.* Guilford, CT: Globe Pequot Press.

Luebben, C. 2004. *Rock climbing: Mastering basic skills.* Seattle, WA: Mountaineers Books.

MacNeill, I. *The beginning runner's handbook: The proven 13-week walk/run program.* Vancouver: Douglas & McIntyre Publishing Group.

Marshall, P., J. Somerville, and F. Rosato. 2002. *Walking and jogging for health and wellness.* Belmont, CA: Wadsworth.

Mazzeo, K. 2006. *Fitness through aerobics and step training.* Belmont, CA: Wadsworth.

Murphy, M., and S. Blair. 2009. Accumulated versus continuous exercise for health benefit. *Sports Medicine* 39(1):29.

Ordas, T., and T. Rochford. 2005. Kickboxing fitness : A guide for fitness professionals from the American Council on Exercise. Monterry, CA: Coaches Choice.

Powers, S., and E. Howley. 2008. *Exercise physiology: Theory and application to fitness and performance.* New York: McGraw-Hill.

Robergs, R., and S. Keteyian. 2002. *Fundamentals of exercise physiology: For fitness, performance, and health.* New York: McGraw-Hill.

Sandrock, M. 2001. Fartlek training: Mixing it up. In *Running tough,* edited by M. Sandrock. Champaign, IL: Human Kinetics.

Sharkey, B. J., ed. 2002. *Fitness and health.* 5th ed. Champaign, IL: Human Kinetics.

Sidman, C. L., C. B. Corbin, and G. Le Masurer. 2004. Promoting physical activity among sedentary women using pedometers. *Research Quarterly for Exercise and Sport* 75(2):122–29.

Swain, D. P., and B. C. Leutholtz. 2002. Exercise prescription for cardiorespiratory fitness. In *Exercise prescription: A case study approach to the ACSM guidelines,* edited by D. P. Swain and B. C. Leutholtz, 29–42. Champaign, IL: Human Kinetics.

Swain, D. P., J. A. Parrott, and A. R. Bennett. 2004. Validation of new method for estimating VO2max based on VO2reserve. *Medicine and Science in Sports and Exercise* 36(8):1421–26.

Talbert, D. 2002. *Bicycling for fun and fitness.* Santa Barbara, CA. Daniel & Daniel.

Wallack, R., Saxton, K. 2011. *The complete book of barefoot running: Learn the scientifically proven technique for improving your stride and reducing injuries.* Beverly, MA: Fair Winds Press.

Wendel, G., A. Schuit, and R. De Niet. 2004. Factors of the physical environment associated with walking and bicycling. *Medicine and Science in Sports and Exercise* 36(4):725–30.

Yeager, S. 2010. *Ride your way lean: The ultimate plan for burning fat and getting fit on a bike.* Emmaus, PA: Rodale Books.

SUGGESTED WEB SITES

Active.com

This site provides information to active individuals who are selecting a variety of fitness events to participate in.
www.active.com

Bicycling Life

This online journal discusses issues, editorials, bicycling how-to's, solutions for little problems, adjustments, repairs, and practical cycling.
www.bicyclinglife.com

BikeRide

This site allows cyclists to find bicycling events that are taking place all over America.
www.bikeride.com

Cooper Institute for Aerobics Research

This nonprofit research and education organization is dedicated to preventive medicine and research.
www.cooperinst.org

International Inline Skating Association

The IISA is a nonprofit trade association that represents the 29 million people who are regular inline skaters. The IISA conducts educational and safety programs about inline skating and promotes the benefits and pleasures of inline skating for sport, recreation, fitness, and vitality.
www.iisa.org

Road Runners Club of America

The RRCA maintains an extensive list of programs for its clubs and individual members.
www.rrca.org

Rollerblade

This site provides several resources for in-line skaters. Tips for beginners, skate maintenance videos and instruction, information on places to skate, assistance in finding a certified instructor, and industry history are some of the resources available. In addition, there is a plethora of information on skating for fitness, with a calorie-burning chart, healthy recipes, a 10-week workout program, and information on the fitness benefits of skating.
www.rollerblade.com

Runners Web

The Runners Web is designed for runners and triathletes. It contains a variety of running and triathlon (and some cycling) information.
www.runnersweb.com/running.html

Runner's World Online

This site presents a beginner's program, marathon training, health, and fitness.
www.runnersworld.com

Swimmersworld.com

This site features competitive swimming news and information.
www.swimmersworld.com

Walking for Fitness

This site includes the best new content, relevant links, how-to's, forums, and answers to just about any question concerning walking.
http://walking.about.com/mbody.htm

WebAerobics

WebAerobics, Inc., offers aerobics enthusiasts a destination on the Internet where they can find information about aerobics.
www.webaerobics.com

Name   Section   Date

PURPOSE   To calculate a target heart rate range.

EQUIPMENT   Clock or watch

PROCEDURE   Count resting heart rate during a 1-minute period. Then perform the following calculations.

220
−   _____ age
=   _____ maximum heart rate
        - resting heart rate
=   _____ heart rate reserve
×   _.60_ intensity (60%)
=   _____
+   _____ resting heart rate
=   _____ lower limit of THR range

220
−   _____ age
=   _____ maximum heart rate
        - resting heart rate
=   _____ heart rate reserve
×   _.85_ intensity (85%)
=   _____
+   _____ resting heart rate
=   _____ upper limit of THR range

Target Heart Rate Range = _____ bpm to _____ bpm
                        Lower Limit   Upper Limit

Name   Section   Date

PURPOSE   To determine relative fitness.

PROCEDURE

1. Walk 1 mile as fast as you can. Stretch for 5 to 10 minutes before and after. Wear good walking shoes and loose-fitting clothes. Maintain a steady pace.
2. Record your time. Do this to the nearest second. Most people walk between 3.0 and 6.0 miles per hour, so it should take 10 to 20 minutes to walk the mile.
3. Record your heart rate immediately at the end of the mile. (It begins to slow almost immediately after you stop walking.) Count your pulse for 15 seconds and multiply by 4, then record this number. This gives you your heart rate per minute after your test walk.

FIND YOUR FITNESS LEVEL

The information in the following charts pertains to both the nontreadmill walker and the treadmill walker.

Turn to the appropriate Rockport Fitness Walking Test™ charts according to your age and sex. These show the established fitness norms from the American Heart Association.

Using your Relative Fitness Level chart, find your time in minutes and your heart rate per minute. Follow these lines until they meet, and mark this point on the chart. This point is designed to tell you how fit you are compared to other individuals of your same age and sex. For example, if your mark falls in the "above average" section of the chart, you are in better shape than the average person in your category.

The charts are based on weights of 170 lb for men and 125 lb for women. If you weigh substantially less, your relative cardiovascular fitness level will be slightly underestimated. Conversely, if you weigh substantially more, your relative cardiovascular fitness level will be slightly overestimated.

HOW TO DETERMINE YOUR 20-WEEK WALKING PROGRAM

EXERCISE PROGRAM CHARTS

Using the exercise program chart, find your time in minutes and your heart rate per minute. Follow these lines until they meet, and mark this point on your chart. Note the color area you fall into and turn to the exercise program, starting on p. 105, corresponding to that color.

You can improve your aerobic capacity and promote lifelong health with the walking program outlined here. Your designated program is designed specifically for your current fitness level.

From The Rockport Company, 1993.

At the end of the 20-week period, retake the Rockport Fitness Walking Test™ to determine your new fitness level and exercise program.

On each program there are columns labeled "pace" and "heart rate." Pace is only an approximation. Your walking speed should be determined by the pace that keeps your heart rate at the percentage of maximum listed. For your percentage of maximum heart rate, use the chart provided.

THE WALKING TEST

1. Find a measured track or measure out a mile, using your car's odometer, on a flat uninterrupted road.
2. Walk 1 mile as fast as you can, maintaining a steady pace.
3. Upon completion, record your time to the nearest second.
4. Continue walking, but slow down the pace. Count your pulse beginning with zero for 15 seconds and multiply the number of beats by four; record this number in the space provided. This gives you your heart rate per minute after your test walk. Note: Your heart rate begins to slow almost immediately after you stop walking, so continue moving while you take your pulse.
5. Cool down. Remember to repeat the stretching exercises once you've cooled down.

Resting heart rate _____

Heart rate at the end of the mile _____

Time to walk the mile _____

Helpful items needed for test: loose-fitting clothes, comfortable walking shoes (we recommend Rockports!), and a watch with a second hand.

The Rockport Fitness Walking Test

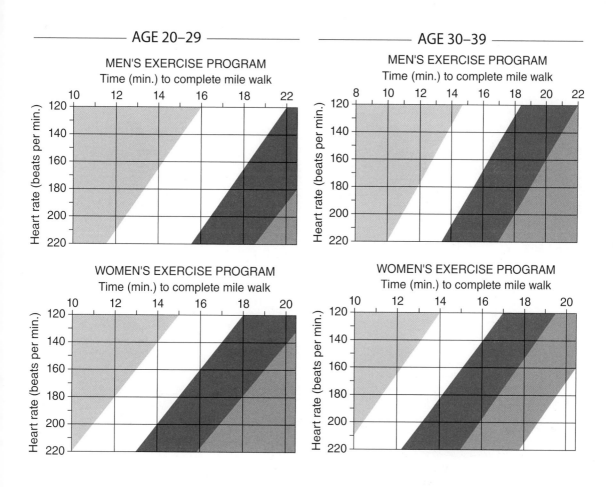

The Rockport Fitness Walking Test

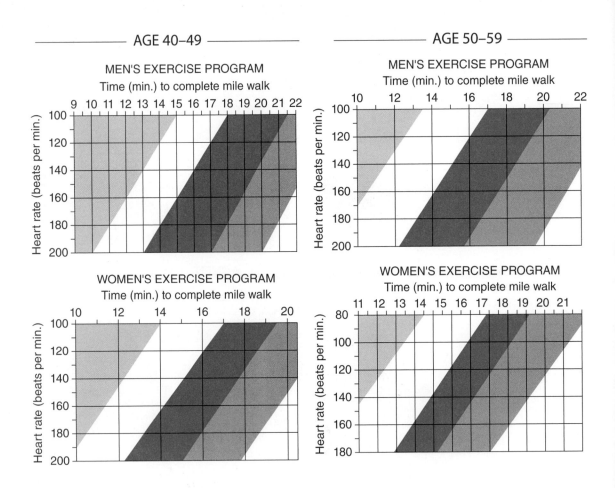

AGE 40–49

MEN'S EXERCISE PROGRAM
Time (min.) to complete mile walk

WOMEN'S EXERCISE PROGRAM
Time (min.) to complete mile walk

AGE 50–59

MEN'S EXERCISE PROGRAM
Time (min.) to complete mile walk

WOMEN'S EXERCISE PROGRAM
Time (min.) to complete mile walk

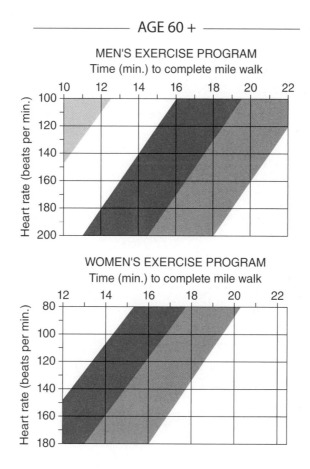

AGE 60 +

MEN'S EXERCISE PROGRAM
Time (min.) to complete mile walk

WOMEN'S EXERCISE PROGRAM
Time (min.) to complete mile walk

The Rockport Fitness Walking Test

% OF MAXIMUM HEART RATE CHART (10-SECOND COUNT)			
Age	60%	70%	80%
20–29	19–20	22–23	25–27
30–39	18–19	21–22	24–25
40–49	17–18	20–21	23–24
50–59	16–17	19–20	21–23
60+	14–16	16–18	19–21

Week	1–2	3–4	5	6	7–8	9	10	11	12–13	14	15–16	17–18	19–20
WARM-UP/COOL-DOWN (stretches before and after walk in min.)	5–7	5–7	5–7	5–7	5–7	5–7	5–7	5–7	5–7	5–7	5–7	5–7	5–7
MILEAGE	1.0	1.25	1.5	1.5	1.75	2.0	2.0	2.0	2.25	2.5	2.5	2.75	3
PACE (mph)	3.0	3.0	3.0	3.5	3.5	3.5	3.75	3.75	3.75	3.75	4.0	4.0	4
HEART RATE (% of max)	60	60	60	60–70	60–70	60–70	60–70	70	70	70	70	70–80	70
FREQUENCY (times per week)	5	5	5	5	5	5	5	5	5	5	5	5	5

Week	1–2	3–4	5–6	7	8–9	10–12	13	14	15–16	17–18	19–20
WARM-UP/COOL-DOWN (stretches before and after walk in min.)	5–7	5–7	5–7	5–7	5–7	5–7	5–7	5–7	5–7	5–7	5–7
MILEAGE	1.5	1.75	2.0	2.0	2.25	2.5	2.75	2.75	3.0	3.25	3.5
PACE (mph)	3.0	3.0	3.0	3.5	3.5	3.5	3.5	4.0	4.0	4.0	4.0
HEART RATE (% of max)	60–70	60–70	60–70	70	70	70	70	70–80	70–80	70–80	70–80
FREQUENCY (times per week)	5	5	5	5	5	5	5	5	5	5	5

The Rockport Fitness Walking Test

Week	1	2	3–4	5	6–8	9–10	11–12	13–14	15	16–17	18–20	Maintenance
WARM-UP/COOL-DOWN (stretches before and after walk in min.)	5–7	5–7	5–7	5–7	5–7	5–7	5–7	5–7	5–7	5–7	5–7	5–7
MILEAGE	2.0	2.25	2.5	2.75	2.75	3.0	3.0	3.25	3.5	3.5	4.0	4.0
PACE (mph)	3.0	3.0	3.0	3.0	3.5	3.5	4.0	4.0	4.0	4.5	4.5	4.5
HEART RATE (% of max)	70	70	70	70	70	70	70–80	70–80	70–80	70–80	70–80	70–80
FREQUENCY (times per week)	5	5	5	5	5	5	5	5	5	5	5	3–5

Week	1	2	3–4	5	6	7	8	9–10	11–14	15–20	Maintenance
WARM-UP/COOL-DOWN (stretches before and after walk in min.)	5–7	5–7	5–7	5–7	5–7	5–7	5–7	5–7	5–7	5–7	5–7
MILEAGE	2.5	2.75	3.0	3.25	3.25	3.5	3.75	4.0	4.0	4.0	4.0
PACE (mph)	3.5	3.5	3.5	3.5	4.0	4.0	4.0	4.0	4.5	4.5	4.5
HEART RATE (% of max)	70	70	70	70	70–80	70–80	70–80	70–80	70–80	70–80	70–80
FREQUENCY (times per week)	5	5	5	5	5	5	5	5	5	5	3–5

Week	1	2	3	4	5	6	7–20	Maintenance
WARM-UP/COOL-DOWN (stretches before and after walk in min.)	5–7	5–7	5–7	5–7	5–7	5–7	5–7	5–7
MILEAGE	3.0	3.25	3.5	3.5	3.75	4.0	4.0	4.0
PACE (mph)	4.0	4.0	4.0	4.5	4.5	4.5	4.5	4.5
HEART RATE (% of max)	70	70	70	70–80	70–80	70–80	70–80	70–80
FREQUENCY (times per week)	5	5	5	5	5	5	5	3–5

Name   Section   Date

PURPOSE   To determine the level of cardiorespiratory endurance of college students during a 12-minute running or walking activity.

EQUIPMENT   1. Measured running course, preferably a track
2. Stopwatch

PROCEDURE   During a 12-minute period the subject attempts to cover as much distance as possible by either running or walking.

TREATMENT OF DATA   1. Distance covered should be rounded off to the nearest 1/8 mile.
2. Consult Table 4-6. Locate the distance covered for either men or women under the appropriate age classification, and determine the level of fitness.

Sample Worksheet for Cooper's 12-Minute Walking/Running Test		Example
1. Measure distance covered, and round off to nearest ⅛ mile	_____	1. 1.50
2. Locate this distance in appropriate "Age" column	_____	2. Age 20
3. Determine fitness level	_____	3. Good

Continued

TABLE 4-6
12-MINUTE WALKING/RUNNING TEST DISTANCE [MILES] COVERED IN 12 MINUTES

Fitness Category		Age (Years)					
		13–19	20–29	30–39	40–49	50–59	60+
I. Very poor	(men)	<1.30*	<1.22	<1.18	<1.14	<1.03	<.87
	(women)	<1.0	<.96	<.94	<.88	<.84	<.78
II. Poor	(men)	1.30–1.37	1.22–1.31	1.18–1.30	1.14–1.24	1.03–1.16	.87–1.02
	(women)	1.00–1.18	.96–1.11	.95–1.05	.88–.98	0.84–.93	.78–.86
III. Fair	(men)	1.38–1.56	1.32–1.49	1.31–1.45	1.25–1.39	1.17–1.30	1.03–1.20
	(women)	1.19–1.29	1.12–1.22	1.06–1.18	.99–1.11	.94–1.05	.87–.98
IV. Good	(men)	1.57–1.72	1.50–1.64	1.46–1.56	1.40–1.53	1.31–1.44	1.21–1.32
	(women)	1.30–1.43	1.23–1.34	1.19–1.29	1.12–1.24	1.06–1.18	.99–1.09
V. Excellent	(men)	1.73–1.86	1.65–1.76	1.57–1.69	1.54–1.65	1.45–1.58	1.33–1.55
	(women)	1.44–1.51	1.35–1.45	1.30–1.39	1.25–1.34	1.19–1.30	1.10–1.18
VI. Superior	(men)	>1.87	>1.77	>1.70	>1.66	>1.59	>1.56
	(women)	>1.52	>1.46	>1.40	>1.35	>1.31	>1.19

Monitoring heart rate is an indirect method of estimating oxygen consumption. In general, heart rate and oxygen consumption have a direct relationship; the longer the intensity of the exercise, the higher the heart rate. Because of these existing relationships, it should become apparent that the rate of oxygen consumption can be estimated by taking the heart rate.

From Cooper K. H. 1982. *The aerobics program for total wellbeing,* New York: Bantam Books. Reprinted with permission of the publisher, Bantam Books, New York.
*< Means "less than"; > means "more than."

5

Improving Muscular **Strength,** Endurance, and Power

Objectives

After completing this chapter, you should be able to do the following:

- Define strength, endurance, and power and indicate their relevance to health and skill of performance.
- Discuss factors that determine levels of muscular strength.
- Explain the physiological changes that occur which increase strength.
- Explain why core stabilization exercises should be a part of all strength-training programs.
- Demonstrate proper techniques for using progressive resistance exercise to develop strength and muscular endurance in specific muscle groups.
- Discuss isometric and circuit training exercises as techniques for improving muscle strength.
- Explain how functional strengthening exercises and plyometrics can be incorporated into strength training programs.
- Demonstrate various calisthenic exercises that can be used for increasing muscular strength and endurance.

WHY IS MUSCULAR STRENGTH IMPORTANT FOR EVERYONE?

The development of **muscular strength** is an essential component of fitness for any-one involved in a physical activity pro-gram. By definition, strength is the ability of a muscle to generate maximum force against some heavy resistance. The development of

muscular strength: the ability of a muscle to generate force against some resistance

KEY TERMS

muscular strength	*core stabilization*
muscular endurance	*training*
power	*progressive resistance*
concentric	*exercise*
contraction	*isometric exercise*
eccentric	*isokinetic exercise*
contraction	*circuit training*
hypertrophy	*functional strength*
atrophy	*training*
motor unit	*plyometric exercise*
myofilaments	*calisthenic exercise*

muscular strength may be considered as both a health-related and a performance-related component of physical fitness. Maintenance of at least a normal level of strength in a given muscle or muscle group is important for normal healthy living. Muscle weakness or imbalance can result in abnormal movement or gait and can impair normal functional movement. Muscle weakness can also produce poor posture, which can affect appearance. One of the most common health ailments in the United States is lower back pain. In most cases lower back pain is related to lack of muscular fitness, especially lack of muscular strength in the abdominals and loss of flexibility of the hamstrings. (See Chapter 9 for more discussion of lower back pain.) Thus strength training may play a critical role not only in fitness programs but also in injury prevention and rehabilitation.

HOW ARE STRENGTH AND MUSCULAR ENDURANCE RELATED?

Muscular strength is closely associated with **muscular endurance.** Muscular endurance is the ability to perform repetitive muscular contractions against some resistance for an extended period of time. As we will see later, as muscular strength increases, there tends to be a corresponding increase in endurance. For example, suppose a person can lift a given weight 25 times. If that person's muscular strength increases by 10 percent through weight training, it is very likely that his or her maximal number of repetitions also would be increased because it is easier for the person to lift the weight. For most people, developing muscular endurance is more important than developing muscular strength because muscular endurance is probably more critical in carrying out the everyday activities of living. It is important for anyone beginning a physical activity program to understand the need to develop muscular endurance prior to engaging in an aggressive fitness program. This

becomes increasingly true with age. However, muscular strength is essential for anyone involved in certain types of competition.

WHY IS MUSCULAR POWER IMPORTANT IN SPORT ACTIVITIES?

Most movements in sports are explosive and must include elements of both strength and speed if they are to be effective. If a large amount of force is generated quickly, the movement can be referred to as a **power** movement. Without the ability to generate power, your performance capabilities will be limited. It is difficult to hit a softball, drive a golf ball, or kick a soccer ball without generating power.

TYPES OF SKELETAL MUSCLE CONTRACTION

Skeletal muscle is capable of three different types of contraction: (1) an isometric contraction, (2) a **concentric,** or positive, **contraction,** and (3) an **eccentric,** or negative, **contraction.** An isometric contraction occurs when the muscle contracts to produce tension but there is no

muscular endurance: the ability to perform repetitive muscular contractions against some resistance for an extended period of time

power: a large amount of force that is generated quickly

concentric contraction: a contraction where the muscle shortens when contracting

eccentric contraction: a contraction where the muscle lengthens when contracting

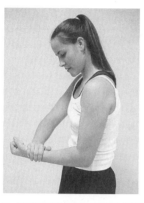

FIGURE 5-1. ISOMETRIC EXERCISE.
In isometric exercise the force is exerted against some immovable resistance and the length of the muscle does not change.

change in length of the muscle (Figure 5-1). Considerable force can be generated against some immovable resistance, even though no movement occurs. In a concentric contraction, the muscle shortens in length while tension is developed to overcome or move some resistance. In an eccentric contraction, the resistance is greater than the muscular force being produced, and the muscle lengthens while producing tension. For example, when lifting a bookbag in your hand, the biceps muscle in the upper arm is shortening as it contracts, which is a concentric contraction. As you lower the bookbag, the biceps muscle is still contracting but now it is lengthening. This is an eccentric contraction. Concentric and eccentric contractions must occur to allow most movements.

FAST-TWITCH VERSUS SLOW-TWITCH FIBERS

As mentioned in Chapter 4, all fibers in a particular muscle unit are either slow-twitch or fast-twitch fibers. Each has distinctive contractile as well as metabolic capabilities. Within a particular muscle, both types of fibers exist, and the ratio in an individual muscle varies with each person. Those muscles that function

primarily to maintain posture against the pull of gravity require more endurance and have a higher percentage of slow-twitch fibers. Muscles that produce powerful, explosive, and strength movements tend to have a much greater percentage of fast-twitch fibers.

Because this ratio is genetically determined, it may play a large role in determining ability for a given sport activity. For example, sprinters and weight lifters have a large percentage of fast-twitch fibers in relation to slow-twitch ones. One study has shown that sprinters may have as many as 95 percent fast-twitch fibers in certain muscles. Conversely, marathon runners generally have a higher percentage of slow-twitch fibers. The question of whether fiber types can change as a result of training has not been completely resolved. However, both types of fibers can improve their metabolic capabilities through specific strength and endurance training.

WHAT FACTORS INFLUENCE HOW MUCH STRENGTH YOU HAVE?

SIZE OF THE MUSCLE

Muscular strength is proportional to the size of a muscle as determined by the cross-sectional diameter of the muscle fibers. The greater the cross-sectional diameter or the bigger a particular muscle, the stronger it is, thus the more force it is capable of generating. The size of a muscle tends to increase in cross-sectional diameter with weight training. This increase in muscle size is referred to as **hypertrophy.** Conversely, a decrease in the size of a muscle is referred to as **atrophy.** Significant muscle

hypertrophy: an increase in muscle size in response to training

atrophy: a decrease in muscle size caused by inactivity

hypertrophy depends on the presence of an anabolic steroidal hormone called *testosterone*. Testosterone is primarily a male hormone. Males tend to gain muscle bulk due to the presence of this hormone.

Strength is a function of the number and diameter of muscle fibers composing a given muscle. The number of fibers is an inherited characteristic; a person who inherits a large number of muscle fibers has the potential to hypertrophy to a much greater degree than does someone with relatively few fibers. However, anyone can increase strength through exercise.

NEUROMUSCULAR EFFICIENCY

Traditionally, the thinking among experts has been that change in the size of the muscle (hypertrophy) is primarily responsible for increases in strength. However in large part, increases in strength are caused by neural adaptations. Strength is directly related to the efficiency of the neuromuscular system and the function of the **motor unit** in producing muscular force. Initial increases in strength during a weight-training program can be attributed primarily to increased neuromuscular efficiency in both males and females. In females, strength gains occur primarily as a result of increased neuromuscular efficiency rather than inceases in the size of a muscle. For a muscle to contract, an impulse must be transmitted from the nervous system to the muscle. Each muscle fiber is innervated by a specific motor unit. By overloading a particular muscle, as in weight training, the muscle is forced to work efficiently. Efficiency is achieved by getting more motor units to fire, causing a stronger contraction of the muscle.

motor unit: a group of muscle fibers innervated by a single motor nerve

BIOMECHANICAL FACTORS

Strength in a given muscle is determined not only by the physical properties of the muscle but also by biomechanical factors. Bones along with muscles and their tendons form a system of levers and pulleys that collectively generate force that can move an external object. The position of attachment of a particular muscle tendon on the bone will largely determine how much force this muscle is capable of generating.

AGE AND GENDER

The ability to generate muscular force is also related to age. Both males and females seem to be able to increase strength throughout puberty and adolescence, reaching a peak around 20 to 25 years of age. After that, this ability begins to level off and in some cases decline. It has been shown that after about age 25 a person generally loses an average of 1 percent of her or his maximal remaining strength each year. Thus at age 65 a person would have only about 60 percent of the strength he or she had at age 25.

A critical difference between men and women regarding strength developing is the ratio of strength to body weight. The reduced strength/body weight ratio in females is the result of a higher percentage of body fat. The strength/body weight ratio may be significantly improved through weight training by decreasing the percent body fat while increasing lean weight. Strength-training programs for females should follow the same guildelines as those for men.

LEVEL OF PHYSICAL ACTIVITY

Loss in muscle strength is definitely related to individual levels of physical activity. Those people who are more active, or perhaps those who continue to strength train, considerably reduce this tendency toward declining muscle strength. In addition, exercise may have an effect in slowing the decrease in cardiorespiratory endurance and flexibility, as well as in slowing increases in body fat that tend to occur with aging. Therefore strength maintenance is important for all individuals regardless of age or the level of competition if total wellness and health are an ultimate goal.

OVERTRAINING

Overtraining can have a negative effect on the development of muscular strength. The statement "if you abuse it, you will lose it" is applicable here. Overtraining can result in psychological breakdown ("staleness") or physiological breakdown, which may involve musculoskeletal injury, fatigue, or sickness. Engaging in proper and efficient resistance training, eating a proper diet, and getting appropriate rest can all minimize the potential negative effects of overtraining.

REVERSIBILITY

Gains in muscular strength resulting from resistance training are reversible. Individuals who interrupt or stop resistance training altogether will see gradual decreases in strength gains over time. "If you don't use it, you'll lose it."

WHAT PHYSIOLOGICAL CHANGES OCCUR TO CAUSE INCREASED STRENGTH?

There is no question that weight training to improve muscular strength results in increased size, or hypertrophy, of a muscle. What causes a muscle to hypertrophy? Over the years, several theories have been proposed to explain this increase in muscle size; most of these have been discounted.

The primary explanation for this hypertrophy is best attributed to an increase in the size and number of small contractile protein filaments within the muscle, called **myofilaments.** Increases in both size and number of the myofilaments as a result of strength training cause the individual muscle fibers to increase in cross-sectional diameter. This increase is particularly found in males, although females will also see some increase in muscle size. More research is needed to further clarify and determine the specific causes of muscle hypertrophy. In addition to muscle hypertrophy, there are a number of other physiological adaptations to resistance training. Health Link 5-1 identifies them.

> **myofilaments:** small protein structures that are the contractile elements in a muscle fiber

HEALTH LINK 5-1

Adaptations to Resistance Training

- The strength of noncontractile structures such as tendons and ligaments is increased.
- The mineral content of bone is increased, making the bone stronger and more resistant to fracture.
- Aerobic capacity may be improved when resistance training is done at a high enough intensity to increase heart rate to the 60 to 85 percent range.
- The levels of several enzymes important to aerobic and anaerobic metabolism increase.

www.nsca-lift.org

OVERLOAD

For a muscle to improve in strength, it must be forced to work at a higher than accustomed level. In other words, the muscle must be *overloaded*. Without overload the muscle will be able to *maintain* strength as long as training is continued against a level of resistance to which the muscle is accustomed. However, *no additional* strength gains will be realized. This maintenance of existing levels of muscular strength may be more important in weight-training programs that emphasize muscular endurance rather than strength gains. It is certainly true that many individuals can benefit more in terms of overall health by concentrating on improving muscular endurance. However, to most effectively build muscular strength, weight training requires a consistent, increasing effort against

progressively increasing resistance. Progressive resistance exercise is based primarily on the principles of overload and progression. However, the principle of overload applies to all eight training techniques that produce improvement of muscular strength over a period of time. Table 5-1 summarizes the eight techniques for improving muscular strength.

WHAT ARE THE TECHNIQUES OF RESISTANCE TRAINING?

If you were to go into a weight room or gym and ask 10 different people what weight-lifting technique they thought was the most effective for improving muscular strength, you would likely get 10 different responses. The key is to figure

TABLE 5-1
TECHNIQUES OF IMPROVING MUSCULAR STRENGTH

Technique	Action	Equipment/Activity
Core stabilization	Provides a stable base on which prime movers in the extremities function	Uses stability balls, weighted balls, etc., to strengthen the lumbo-pelvic-hip complex
Progressive resistive exercise	Force develops while the muscle shortens or lengthens	Free weights, Free Motion, Cybex, Eagle, Body Master
Isometric exercise	Force develops while muscle length remains constant	Any immovable resistance
Circuit training	Used as a combination of isometric, PRE, or isokinetic exercises organized into a series of stations	May use any of the equipment listed above, Calisthenics
Functional strength training	Uses concentric, eccentric, and isometric contractions in multiple planes to improve strength and neuromuscular control	Functional movements
Calisthenics	Uses body weight to provide resistance	No special equipment required
Plyometric exercise	Uses a rapid eccentric stretch of the muscle to facilitate an explosive concentric contraction	Hops, bounds, and depth jumping

out which technique will best allow you to achieve the goals you have established for yourself. There are a number of different techniques of resistance training for strength improvement, including **core stabilization training, progressive resistance exercise, isokinetic exercise, circuit training, functional strength training, plyometric exercise, and calisthenic exercise.**

CORE STABILIZATION TRAINING

A dynamic **core stabilization training** program should be an important component of all comprehensive strengthening programs. The core is defined as the lumbo-pelvic-hip complex. The core is where the centre of gravity is located and where all movement begins. There are 29 muscles in the lumbar spine, the abdomen, and around the hip and plevis that have their attachment to the lumbo-pelvic-hip complex. (See Figure 5-5 on page 128)

A core stabilization program will improve dynamic postural control, ensure appropriate muscular balance and joint movement around the lumbo-pelvic-hip complex, allow for the development of functional strength, and improve neuromuscular efficiency throughout the entire body.

Many individuals work on developing the strength, power, neuromuscular control, and muscular endurance in specific muscles that enable them to perform functional activities. However, relatively few individuals have developed the muscles required for stabilization of the spine. The body's stabilization system

has to be functioning optimally to effectively utilize the strength, power, neuromuscular control, and muscular endurance that they have developed in their prime movers. If the extremity muscles are strong and the core is weak, then there will not be enough force to produce efficient movements. A weak core is a fundamental problem of inefficient movements that lead to injury.

A core stabilization training program is designed to help an individual gain strength,

core stabilization training: a technique for increasing the ability and efficiency of the muscles of the hip, lower back, pelvis, and abdomen, and for providing stability and a base of support for movement of the extremities

progressive resistance exercise: a technique that gradually strengthens muscles through a muscle contraction that overcomes some fixed resistance

isometric exercise: an exercise in which the muscle contracts against resistance but does not change in length

isokinetic exercise: an exercise in which the speed of movement is constant regardless of the strength of a contraction

circuit training: a series of exercise stations that consist of various combinations of weight training, flexibility, calisthenics, and brief aerobic exercises

functional strength training: uses integrated exercises designed to improve functional movement patterns for increasing strength and neuromuscular control by using eccentric, concentric, or isometric contractions in three planes of motion simultaneously

plyometric exercise: a technique of exercise that involves a rapid eccentric (lengthening) stretch of a muscle, followed immediately by a rapid concentric contraction of that muscle for the purpose of producing a forceful explosive movement

calisthenic exercises: exercises done using body weight as resistance

neuromuscluar control, power, and muscle endurance of the lumbo-pelvic-hip complex. A comprehensive core stabilization training program should be systematic, progressive, and functional. When designing a functional core stabilization training program, you should select the appropriate exercises to elicit a maxi-

mal training response. The execises must be safe but challenging, stress multiple planes, incorporate a variety of resistance equipment (physioball, weighted ball, dumbbells, tubing, etc.), be derived from fundamental movement skills, and be activity specific. Figure 5-2 shows examples of exercises that may be used

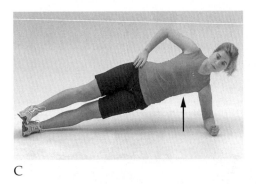

A

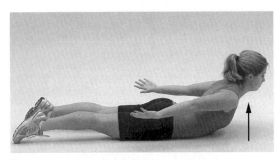

B

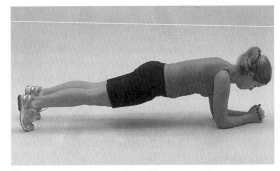

C

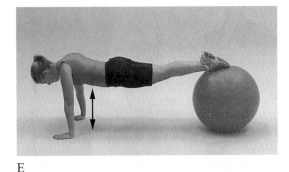

D

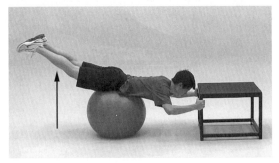

E

F

FIGURE 5-2. CORE STABILIZATION EXERCISES.
A, *Bridging.* **B,** *Prone cobra.* **C,** *Sidelying isolated abdominal.* **D,** *Human arrow.* **E,** *Stability ball push-up.*
F, *Hip-ups on stability ball.*

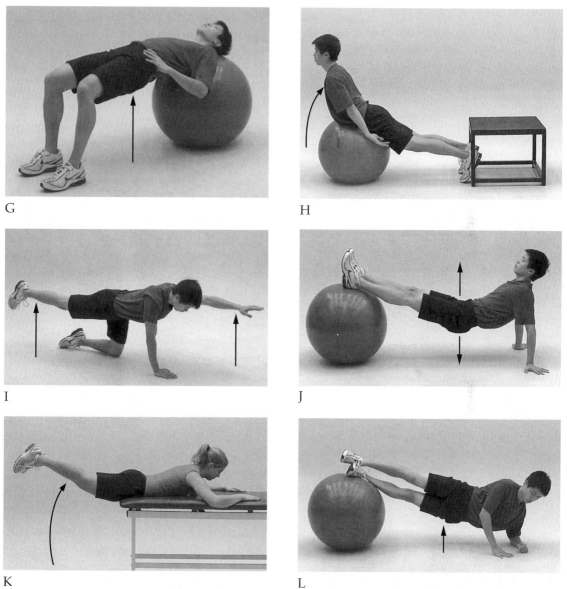

FIGURE 5-2. (cont.). CORE STABILIZATION EXERCISES.
G, *Bridging on stability ball,* **H,** *Prone cobra on stability ball,* **I,** *Alternating opposite leg-arm,*
J, *Pikeups on stability ball,* **K,** *Prone hip extension on table* **L,** *Side plank on stability ball.*

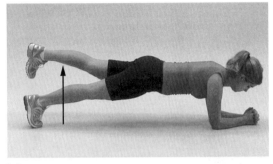

M

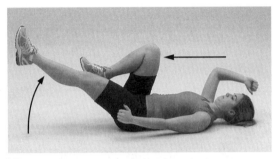

N

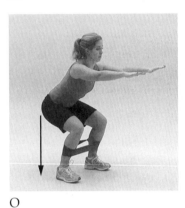

O

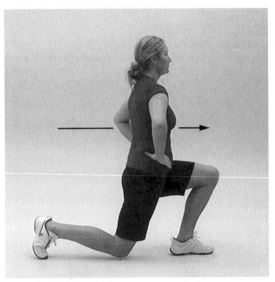

P

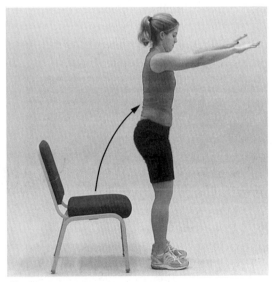

Q

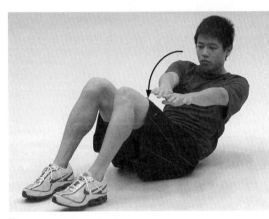

R

FIGURE 5-2. (cont.). CORE STABILIZATION EXERCISES.
M, *Human arrow with single leg extension,* **N,** *Dying bug,* **O,** *Squats with Theraband.* **P,** *Lunges,* **Q,** *Sit to stand with abdominal bracing.* **R,** *Three-point crunches.*

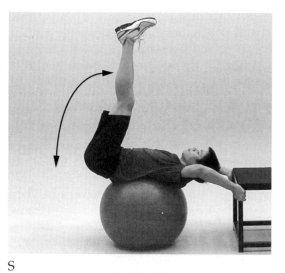

S

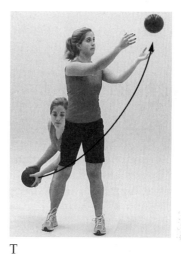

T

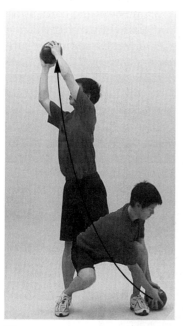

U

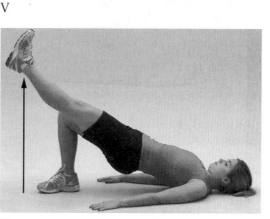

V

W

FIGURE 5-2. (cont.). CORE STABILIZATION EXERCISES.
*S, Straight-leg raises on stability ball. **T,** Weighted ball double-arm rotation toss. **U,** Weighted ball toss with rotation. **V,** Stability ball diagonal rotations. **W,** Bridge with single-leg extension.*

to improve core stability. You should start with execises in which you can maintain stability and optimal neuromuscular control.

PROGRESSIVE RESISTANCE EXERCISE

Progressive resistance exercise is perhaps the most commonly used and most popular technique for improving muscular strength. Progressive resistance exercise training uses exercises that strengthen muscles through a contraction that overcomes some fixed resistance, such as with dumbbells, barbells, or various weight machines. Progressive resistance exercise uses isotonic contractions, in which force is generated while the muscle is changing in length.

▶ Isotonic Contractions

Isotonic contractions may be either concentric or eccentric. Suppose you are going to perform a biceps curl (see Figure 5-14, page 134). To lift the weight from the starting position, the biceps muscle must contract and shorten in length (concentric or positive contraction). If the biceps muscle does not remain contracted when the weight is being lowered, gravity would cause

this weight to simply fall back to the starting position. Thus to control the weight as it is being lowered, the biceps muscle must continue to contract while at the same time gradually lengthening (eccentric or negative contraction).

▶ Exercise Machines versus Free Weights

Various types of exercise equipment can be used with progressive resistive exercise, including free weights (barbells and dumbbells) or exercise machines such as Universal, Cybex, Tough Stuff, Icarian Fitness, King Fitness, Body Solid, Pro-Elite, Life Fitness, Nautilus, BodyCraft, Yukon, Flex, Cam-Bar, GymPros, Nugym, Body Works, DP, Soloflex, Eagle, Free Motion Fitness, and Body Master, to name a few (Figure 5-3, *A*). Dumbbells and barbells require the use of iron plates of varying weights that can be easily changed by adding or subtracting equal amounts of weight to both sides of the bar. The exercise machines have a stack of weights that is lifted through a series of levers or pulleys. The stack of weights slides up and down on a pair of bars that restrict the movement to only one plane (Figure 5-3, *B*). Weight can be increased or decreased simply

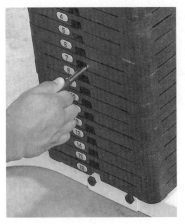

A   B

FIGURE 5-3. ISOTONIC EXERCISE EQUIPMENT.
A, Most exercise equipment is isotonic. B, Resistance may be easily altered by changing the key in the stack of weights.

by changing the position of a weight key. Machines are useful in isolating a weak muscle or muscle group, such as the hamstrings versus the quadriceps or internal shoulder rotators versus external shoulder rotators.

Both the free weights and the machines have advantages and disadvantages. The machines are relatively safe to use in comparison with free weights. For example, if you are doing a bench press with free weights, it is essential to have someone "spot" you (help you lift the weights back onto the support racks if you don't have enough strength to complete the lift). If you don't, you may end up dropping the weight on your chest. A spotter has three functions: to protect the lifter from injury, to make recommendations on proper lifting technique, and to motivate the lifter. See Safe Tip 5-1 for proper spotting techniques.

With the exercise machines, you can easily and safely drop the weight without fear of injury. It is also a simple process to increase or decrease the weight with the exercise machines by moving a single weight key, although changes can generally be made only in increments of 10 or 15 pounds. With free weights, iron plates must be added or removed from each side of the barbell.

Persons who have strength-trained using both free weights and the exercise machines realize the difference in the amount of weight that can be lifted. Unlike the machines, free weights have no restricted motion and can thus move in many different directions, depending on the forces applied. Also, with free weights, an element of muscular control on the part of the lifter is required to prevent the weight from moving in any direction other than vertically, helping to improve balance and neuromuscular coordination of the lifter. This control will usually decrease the amount of weight that can be lifted. Regardless of which type of equipment is used, the same principles of isotonic training may be applied.

SAFE TIP 5-1

Proper spotting techniques

- Make sure the lifter uses the proper grip.
- Check to see that the lifter is in a safe, stable position.
- Make sure the lifter moves through a complete range of motion at the appropriate speed.
- Make sure the lifter inhales and exhales during the lift.
- When spotting dumbbell exercises, spot as close to the dumbbells as possible above the elbow joint.
- Make sure the lifter understands how to get out of the way of missed attempts, particularly with overhead techniques.
- Stand behind the lifter.
- If heavy weights exceed the limits of your ability to control the weight, use a second spotter.
- Communicate with the lifter to know how many reps are to be done, whether a liftoff is needed, and how much help the lifter wants in completing a rep.
- Always be in a position to protect both the lifter and yourself from injury.

▶ Using both Concentric and Eccentric Contractions

In progressive resistance exercise, it is essential to incorporate both concentric and eccentric contractions. It is possible to generate greater amounts of force against resistance with an eccentric contraction than with a concentric contraction. Eccentric contractions are more resistant to fatigue than are concentric contractions. The mechanical efficiency of eccentric exercise may be several times higher than that of concentric exercise. Research has clearly demonstrated that the muscle should be overloaded and fatigued both concentrically and eccentrically for the greatest strength improvement to occur.

When training specifically for the development of muscular strength, the concentric or positive portion of the exercise should require 1 to 2 seconds, while the eccentric or negative portion of the lift should require 2 to 4 seconds. The ratio of negative to positive should be approximately two to one. Physiologically, the muscle will fatigue much more rapidly concentrically than eccentrically. For many years the importance of using both positive and negative contractions in strength training programs has been stressed, regardless of which brand of equipment is being used.

▶ Accomodating Resistance

It has been argued that a disadvantage of any type of isotonic exercise is that the force required to move the resistance is constantly changing throughout the range of movement. One manufacturer attempted to alleviate this problem of changing force capabilities by using a cam in its pulley system (Figure 5-4). The cam was individually designed for each piece of equipment so that the resistance is variable throughout the movement. This change in

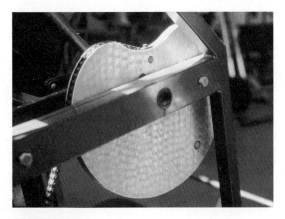

FIGURE 5-4.
A cam has been used in an attempt to equalize resistance throughout the full range of motion.

resistance at different points in the range has been labeled *accommodating resistance* or variable resistance. Whether this design does what it claims to do is debatable. It must be remembered that in real-life situations it does not matter whether the resistance is changing. What is important is that you develop enough strength to move objects from one place to another. The amount of strength necessary for each person largely depends on his or her lifestyle and occupation.

▶ Progressive Resistance Exercise Techniques

Perhaps the most confusing aspect of progressive resistance exercise is the terminology used to describe specific programs. Fit List 5-1, which identifies specific terms with their operational definitions, may provide some clarification.

FIT LIST 5-1

Progressive Resistance Exercise Terminology	
Repetition	Number of times you repeat a specific movement
Repetition maximum	Number of maximum repetitions at a given weight
One repetition maximum*	The absolute maximum weight you can lift in an exercise only one time
Set	A particular number of repetitions
Intensity	The amount of weight or resistance lifted
Recovery	The rest interval between sets
Frequency	The number of times an exercise is done in a week's period

*It should be emphasized that a one repetition maximum test can potentially cause unnecessary injury and is therefore not recommended.

There are probably as many fallacies and misconceptions associated with resistance training as with any other component of fitness. It seems that everyone has his or her own ideas about the best techniques for increasing muscular strength. A considerable amount of research has been done in the area of resistance training to determine optimal techniques in terms of (1) the intensity or the amount of weight to be used, (2) the number of repetitions, (3) the number of sets, (4) the recovery period, and (5) the frequency of training. The FIT principle as described in Chapter 4 can also be applied to progressive resistance exercise.

There is no such thing as an optimal strength-training program. Achieving total agreement on a program of resistance training that includes specific recommendations relative to repetitions, sets, intensity, and frequency is impossible. However, the following general recommendations will provide you with an effective resistance training program.

Selecting a Starting Weight. For any given exercise, the amount of weight selected should be sufficient to allow 6 to 8 repetitions maximum (RM) in each of the 3 sets with a recovery period of 60 to 90 seconds between sets. Initial selection of a starting weight may require some trial and error to achieve this 6 to 8 RM range. If at least 3 sets of 6 repetitions cannot be completed, the weight is too heavy and should be reduced. If it is possible to do more than 3 sets of eight repetitions, the weight is too light and should be increased. Health Link 5-2 summarizes this technique.

Progression. Progression to heavier weights is determined by the ability to perform at least 8 repetitions maximum in each of 3 sets. When progressing weight, an increase of about 10 percent of the current weight being lifted should still allow at least 6 RM in each of 3 sets.

Frequency. A particular muscle or muscle group should be exercised consistently every other day. Thus the frequency of weight training should be at least three times per week but no more than four times per week. It is common for serious weight trainers to lift every day; however, they exercise different muscle groups on successive days. For example, they may work upper-body muscles on Monday, Wednesday, and Friday and lower-body muscles on Tuesday, Thursday, and Saturday (Figure 5-5).

It is important to realize that there are many effective techniques and training regimens that weight lifters and body builders can use. One may decide from looking at the size of a muscle or seeing the amount of weight these people are able to lift that they are doing something right even though their training regimens may not always follow the recommendations of researchers.

HEALTH LINK 5-2

Progressive Resistance Exercises

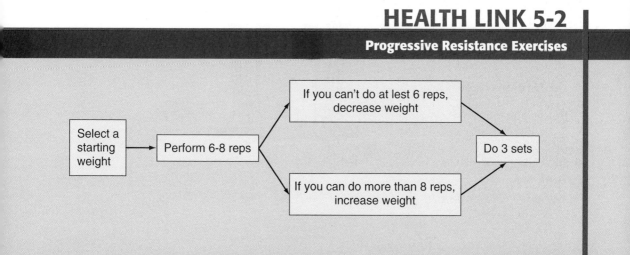

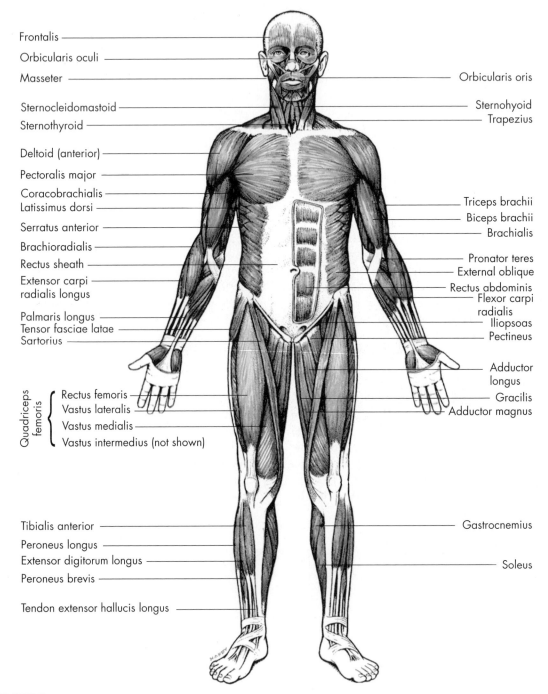

Frontalis
Orbicularis oculi
Masseter
Sternocleidomastoid
Sternothyroid
Deltoid (anterior)
Pectoralis major
Coracobrachialis
Latissimus dorsi
Serratus anterior
Brachioradialis
Rectus sheath
Extensor carpi radialis longus
Palmaris longus
Tensor fasciae latae
Sartorius

Quadriceps femoris
{
Rectus femoris
Vastus lateralis
Vastus medialis
Vastus intermedius (not shown)
}

Tibialis anterior
Peroneus longus
Extensor digitorum longus
Peroneus brevis
Tendon extensor hallucis longus

Orbicularis oris
Sternohyoid
Trapezius
Triceps brachii
Biceps brachii
Brachialis
Pronator teres
External oblique
Rectus abdominis
Flexor carpi radialis
Iliopsoas
Pectineus
Adductor longus
Gracilis
Adductor magnus
Gastrocnemius
Soleus

FIGURE 5-5.

A, Superficial muscles of the human body, anterior view from anatomical position.

Chapter 5

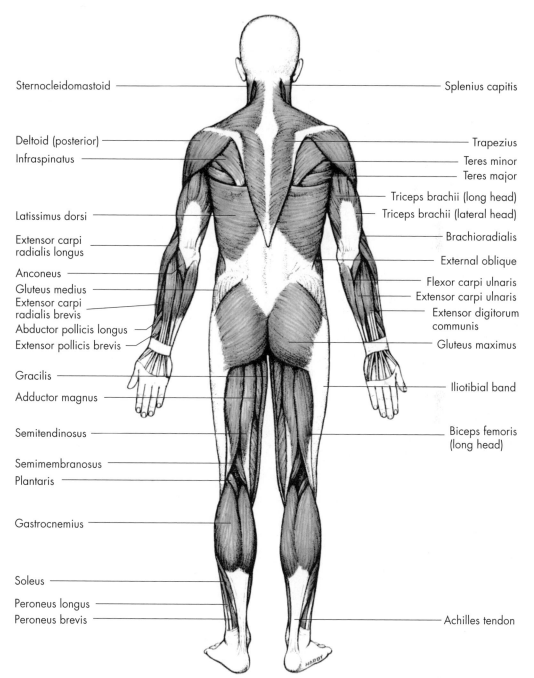

FIGURE 5-5. (cont.)

B, Superficial muscles of the human body, posterior view.

From Thompson CW and Floyd RT: *Manual of Structural Kinesiology*, ed. 15, New York: McGraw-Hill, 2004.

Regardless of specific techniques used, to improve strength the muscle must be overloaded in a progressive manner. This is the basis of progressive resistance exercise. The amount of weight used and the number of repetitions performed must be sufficient to make the muscle work at a higher intensity than it is used to. This is the single most critical factor in any strength-training program. It is also essential to design the strength-training program to meet the specific needs of a person, whether he or she is a competitive athlete or an individual interested in improving total-body health and fitness.

▶ Should You Exercise Differently to Improve Muscular Endurance?

Muscular endurance was defined as the ability to perform repeated muscle contractions against resistance for an extended period of time. Most weight-training experts believe that muscular strength and muscular endurance are closely related. As one improves, there is a tendency for the other to improve also. It is generally accepted that when weight training for strength, heavier weights with a lower number of repetitions should be used. Conversely, endurance training uses relatively lighter weights with a greater number of repetitions.

It has been suggested that endurance training should consist of three sets of 10 to 15 repetitions, using the same criteria for weight selection progression and frequency as recommended for progressive resistive exercise. Thus suggested training regimens for both muscular strength and endurance are similar in terms of sets and numbers of repetitions. Persons who have great strength levels tend to also exhibit greater muscular endurance when asked to perform repeated contractions against resistance.

▶ Specific Progressive Resistance Exercises

To say that a *person* is strong is probably incorrect. We should instead refer to a specific muscle, muscle group, or movement as being strong because increases in strength occur only in muscles that are regularly subjected to overload. Because muscle contractions result in joint movement, the goal of weight training should be to increase strength in every movement possible about a given joint. Exercises must be designed to place stress on those groups of muscles collectively to produce a specific joint movement.

For this reason our approach to specific strength-training exercises deviates from the traditional approach. The following illustrations are organized to show exercises for all motions about a particular joint rather than for each specific muscle. These exercises are demonstrated using free weights (barbells, dumbbells, weights, and some machine weights). Any of the exercises described may be applied to various commercial exercise machines such as Universal or Nautilus. Positions may differ slightly when different pieces of equipment are used. However, the joint motions that affect the various muscles indicated are still the same.

Figures 5-6 to 5-28 describe exercises for strength improvement of shoulder, hip, knee, and ankle joint movements. Figure 5-5 shows the anatomic location of the muscles that are referred to with specific exercises. Complete the worksheets in Table 5-2 to assess your progress in strength increases while doing the following exercises. Safe Tip 5-2 provides guidelines and precautions to be used in resistance training.

ISOMETRIC EXERCISE

An isometric exercise involves a muscle contraction in which the length of the muscle remains constant while tension develops toward a maximal force against an immovable resistance (see Figure 5-1, page 115). To develop strength, the muscle should generate a maximal force for 10 seconds at a time, and this contraction should be repeated 5 to 10 times per day.

Isometric exercises are capable of increasing muscular strength; unfortunately, strength gains in a particular muscle will occur only in the position in which resistance is applied. At other positions in the range of motion, the strength curve drops off dramatically because

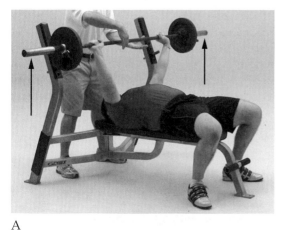

A

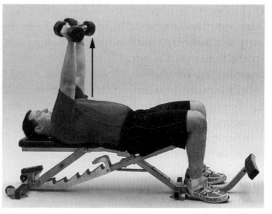

B

FIGURE 5-6. BENCH PRESS.
A, Barbell (with spotter). B, Dumbbells.
Joints affected: shoulder, elbow.
Movement: pushing away.
Position: supine, feet flat on bench or floor, back flat on bench.
Primary muscles: pectoralis major, triceps.

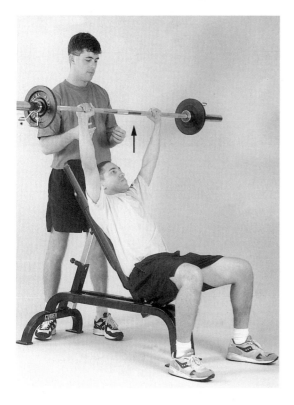

FIGURE 5-7. INCLINE PRESS.
Joints affected: shoulder, elbow.
Movement: pushing upward and away.
Position: supine at an inclined angle, feet flat on floor, back flat against bench.
Primary muscles: pectoralis major, triceps.

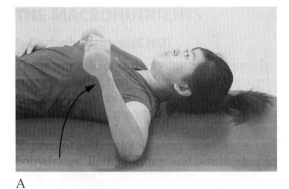

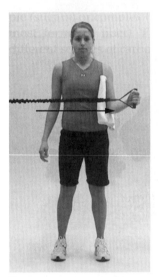

A

B

FIGURE 5-8. SHOULDER LATERAL ROTATION.
(A) Lying using dumbbell
(B) Standing using tubing
Joints affected: shoulder.
Movement: external rotation.
Position: supine, shoulder at 90-degree angle and elbow flexed at 90-degree angle.
Primary muscles: infraspinatus, teres minor.

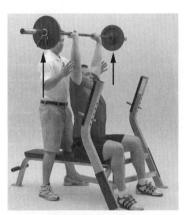

FIGURE 5-9. MILITARY PRESS.
Joints affected: shoulder, elbow. Movement: pressing the weight overhead.
Position: sitting, back straight.
Primary muscles: deltoid, trapezius, triceps.

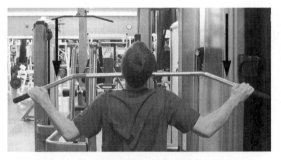

FIGURE 5-10. LAT PULL-DOWNS.
Joints affected: shoulder, elbow.
Movement: pulling the bar down in front of the head.
Position: kneeling, back straight, head up.
Primary muscles: latissimus dorsi, biceps.

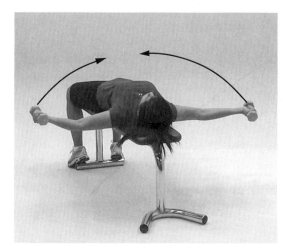

FIGURE 5-11. FLYS.
Joint affected: shoulder.
*Movement: horizontal flexion. Bring arms
together over head.*
*Position: lying on back, feet flat on floor, back flat
on bench.*
Primary muscles: deltoid, pectoralis major.

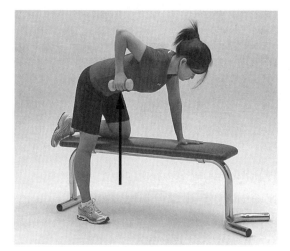

FIGURE 5-12. BENT-OVER ROWS.
Joint affected: shoulder.
Movement: adduction of scapula.
Position: standing, bent over at waist.
Primary muscles: trapezius, rhomboids.

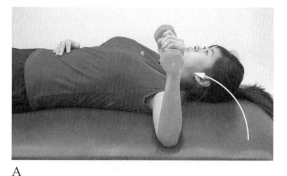

A

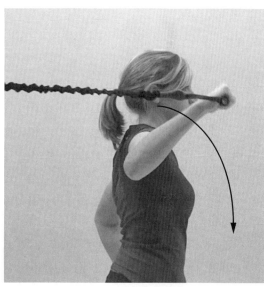

B

**FIGURE 5-13. SHOULDER MEDIAL
ROTATION.**
(A) Lying using dumbbell
(B) Standing using tubing
Joint affected: shoulder.
Movement: internal rotation.
Lifting weight off the floor.
*Position: supine, shoulder abducted and
elbow flexed.*
Primary muscles: subscapularis.

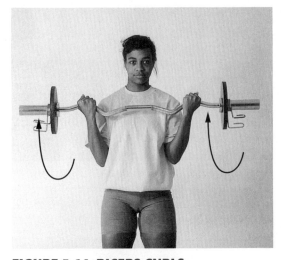

FIGURE 5-14. BICEPS CURLS.
Joint affected: elbow.
Movement: elbow flexion. Curling the weight up to the shoulder.
Position: standing feet front and back rather than side to side, back straight, arms extended.
Primary muscles: biceps.

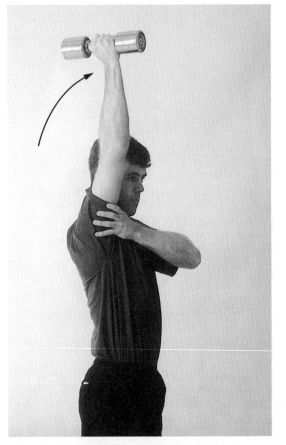

FIGURE 5-15. TRICEPS EXTENSIONS.
Joint affected: elbow.
Movement: elbow extension. Pressing weight toward ceiling.
Position: standing, elbows pointing directly forward beside ears.
Primary muscles: triceps.

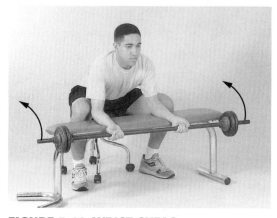

FIGURE 5-16. WRIST CURLS.
Joint affected: wrist.
Movement: wrist flexion. Curling weight upward.
Position: seated, forearms on table, palms up.
Primary muscles: long flexors of forearm.

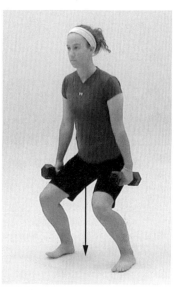

FIGURE 5-18. SQUAT.
Joint affected: hips and knees.
Movement: hip flexion and knee extension.
Position: standing, feet shoulder width apart, back straight, a dumbbell in each hand, bend knees to lower to either 3/4 or 1/2 squat position then stand up.
Muscles: hip extensors, quadriceps.

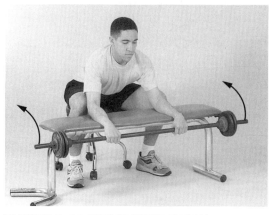

FIGURE 5-17. WRIST EXTENSIONS.
Joint affected: wrist.
Movement: extension. Curling weight upward.
Position: seated, forearms on table, palms down.
Primary muscles: long extensors of forearm.

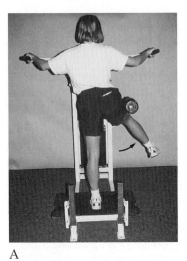

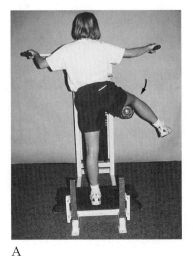

A

A

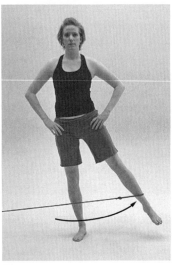

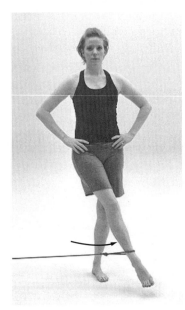

B

FIGURE 5-19. HIP ABDUCTION.
*A, On machine. **B**, Using tubing.*
Joint affected: hip.
Movement: hip abduction. Lifting leg up.
Position: standing, leg under resistance arm.
Primary muscles: hip abductors.

B

FIGURE 5-20. HIP ADDUCTION.
*A, On machine. **B**, Using tubing.*
Joint affected: hip.
Movement: hip adduction. Pulling leg toward midline of body.
Position: standing leg on top of resistance arm.
Primary muscles: hip adductors.

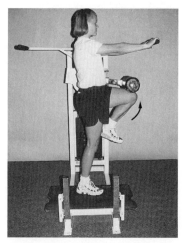

A

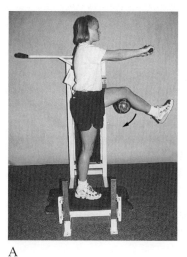

A

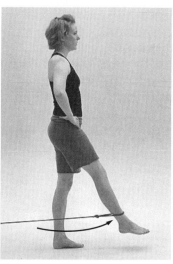

B

FIGURE 5-21. HIP FLEXION.
A, Bent knee on machine. B, Straight leg using tubing.
Joint affected: hip.
Movement: hip flexion. Lifting knee up.
Position: Standing, knee flexed, Knee under resistance arm.
Primary muscles: iliopsoas.

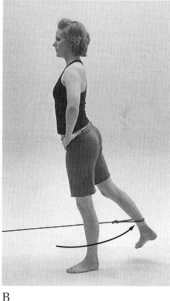

B

FIGURE 5-22. HIP EXTENSIONS.
A, On machine. B, Standing with tubing.
Joint affected: hip.
Movement: hip extension. Pulling leg downward.
Position: Standing, knee extended, resistance arm under thigh.
Primary muscles: gluteus maximus, hamstrings.

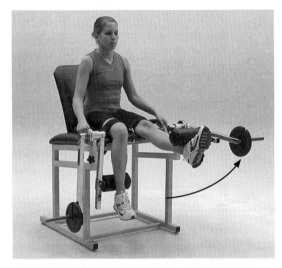

FIGURE 5-23. QUADRICEPS EXTENSIONS.
Joint affected: knee.
Movement: extension. Straightening knee.
Position: sitting, on knee machine.
Primary muscles: quadriceps group.

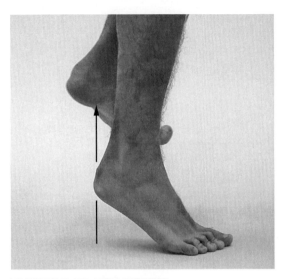

FIGURE 5-25. TOE RAISES.
Joint affected: ankle.
Movement: plantar flexion. Pressing up on toes.
Position: standing and lifting body weight.
Primary muscles: gastrocnemius, soleus.

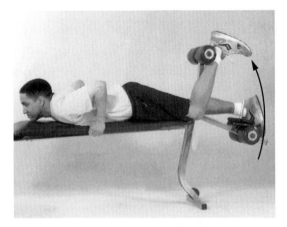

FIGURE 5-24. HAMSTRING CURLS.
Joint affected: knee.
Movement: flexion. Bending knee and lifting the weight up.
Position: prone, on knee machine.
Primary muscles: hamstring group.

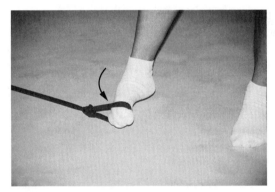

FIGURE 5-26. ANKLE INVERSION.
Joint affected: ankle.
Movement: inversion. Turning the sole of the foot up and in.
Position: sitting, resistance tubing around forefoot.
Primary muscles: anterior tibialis.

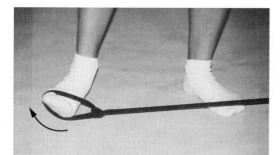

FIGURE 5-27. ANKLE EVERSION.
Joint affected: ankle.
Movement: eversion. Turning the sole of the foot up and out.
Position: sitting, resistance tubing around forefoot.
Primary muscles: peroneals.

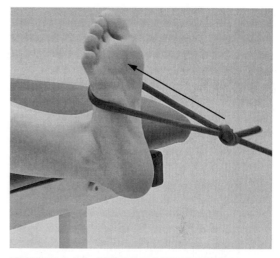

FIGURE 5-28. ANKLE DORSIFLEXION.
Joint affected: ankle.
Movement: dorsiflexion. Pulling the toes upward.
Position: sitting, resistance tubing around forefoot.
Primary muscles: dorsiflexors in shin.

TABLE 5-2
STRENGTH TRAINING WORKSHEET I: UPPER-BODY EXERCISES

Exercise	Reps	Sets	Date/Weight														
Shoulder lateral rotation	6–8	3															
Bench press	6–8	3															
Incline press	6–8	3															
Military press	6–8	3															
Lateral pull-downs	6–8	3															
Flys	6–8	3															
Reverse flys	6–8	3															
Shoulder medial rotation	6–8	3															
Biceps curls	6–8	3															
Triceps curls	6–8	3															
Wrist curls	6–8	3															
Wrist extensions	6–8	3															

Exercise	Reps	Sets	Date/Weight													
Squat	6–8	3														
Hip abduction	6–8	3														
Hip adduction	6–8	3														
Bent-knee leg lifts	6–8	3														
Hip extension	6–8	3														
Quadriceps extensions	6–8	3														
Hamstring curls	6–8	3														
Toe raises	6–8	3														
Ankle inversion	6–8	3														
Ankle eversion	6–8	3														
Ankle dorsiflexion	6–8	3														

SAFE TIP 5-2

Guidelines and Precautions in Resistance Training

The following guidelines can improve your effectiveness and your safety during strength training:

- Do appropriate warm-up activities before beginning workout.
- Use proper lifting techniques as recommended on the following pages. Improper lifting techniques can result in injury.
- To ensure balanced development, exercise all muscle groups.
- Avoid doing one-repetition maximum lifts. This can result in muscle strains, especially if you are not properly warmed up.
- Always have a spotter if you are lifting free weights.
- Before using a machine (e.g., Cybex), make sure you understand how to use it properly.
- Progress gradually and within your own individual limits.
- Always train throughout a full range of motion.
- Use both concentric and eccentric contractions.
- Try to exercise the larger muscle groups first, and alternate exercises to allow previously exercised muscle groups a chance to recover.
- Do not hold your breath during a lift.
- Do not overtrain. Overtraining may result in injury.
- If you have questions about weight training, seek out an expert who can give you specific, correct advice.
- Do not try to show off; always work within your own limits.

of a lack of motor activity at those angles, and there is no corresponding increase in strength.

Another major disadvantage of these isometric, "sit at your desk" exercises is that they tend to produce a spike in blood pressure that can result in potentially life-threatening cardiovascular accidents. This sharp increase in blood pressure results from holding your breath and increasing pressure within the chest cavity. Consequently, the heart experiences a significant increase in blood pressure. This has been referred to as the *Valsalva effect*. To avoid or minimize this effect, it is recommended that breathing be done during the maximal contraction.

Isometric exercises certainly have a place in a fitness program. There are instances in which an isometric contraction can greatly enhance a particular movement. A common use for isometric exercises would be for injury rehabilitation or reconditioning. A number of conditions or ailments resulting either from trauma or from overuse must be treated with strengthening exercises. Unfortunately, these problems may be aggravated with full range-of-motion strengthening exercises. It may be more desirable to make use of isometric exercises until the injury has healed to the point that full-range activities can be performed.

CIRCUIT TRAINING

Circuit training uses a series of exercise stations consisting of various combinations of weight training, flexibility, calisthenics, and brief aerobic exercises. Circuits may be designed to accomplish many different training goals. With circuit training, you move rapidly from one station to the next and perform whatever exercise is to be done at that station within a specified time period. A typical circuit would consist of eight to twelve stations, and the entire circuit would be repeated three times.

Circuit training is definitely an effective technique for improving strength and flexibility. Certainly, if the pace or the time interval between stations is rapid and if the workload is maintained at a high level of intensity with heart rates at or above target training levels, the cardiorespiratory system may benefit from this circuit. It should be and most often is used as a technique for developing and improving muscular strength and endurance. Figure 5-29 provides an example of a simple circuit training setup that can be easily completed by healthy college students.

FUNCTIONAL STRENGTH TRAINING

Functional strength training is a rapidly evolving technique of improving not only muscular strength but also neuromuscular control. The strength-training techniques discussed to this point have traditionally focused on isolated, single-plane exercises used to elicit muscle hypertrophy in a specific muscle. These exercises have a very low neuromuscular demand because they are performed primarily with the rest of the body artificially stabilized on stable pieces

▶ Station 1: Push-ups (30 repetitions)
▶ Station 2: Hamstring (low back stretching)
▶ Station 3: Bent-knee sit-ups (25 repetitions)
▶ Station 4: Bench press (10 repetitions at 75% maximal weight)
▶ Station 5: Rope skipping (100 repetitions)
▶ Station 6: Knee extensions (15 repetitions at 80% maximal weight)
▶ Station 7: Shoulder adduction (15 repetitions)
▶ Station 8: Knee flexions (15 repetitions at 80% maximal weight)

Allow 60 seconds to complete each station, and repeat the entire circuit three times in succession.

FIGURE 5-29. EXAMPLE OF CIRCUIT TRAINING SETUP.

of equipment. The central nervous system controls the ability to integrate the proprioceptive function of a number of individual muscles that must act simultaneously to produce a specific movement pattern that occurs in three planes of motion. If the body is designed to move in three planes of motion, then isolated training does little to improve functional ability. When strength training using isolated, single-plane, artificially stabilized exercises, the entire body is not being prepared to deal with the imposed demands of normal daily activities (walking up and down stairs, getting groceries out of the trunk, etc.).

Earlier in this chapter it was stated that muscles are capable of three different types of contraction: concentric, eccentric, and isometric. During functional movements, some muscles are contracting concentrically (shortening) to produce movement, others contracting eccentrically (lengthening) to allow movement to occur, and still other muscles contracting isometrically to create a stable base on which the functional movement occurs.

Since all muscles involved in a movement function either eccentrically, concentrically, or isometrically in three planes of motion simultaneously, functional strength training uses integratred exercises designed to improve functional movement patterns in terms of both increased strength and improved neuromuscular control. When using functional strengthening exercises, individuals not only develop functional strength and neuromuscular control, but also high levels of core stabilization strength and flexibility. Figures 5-30 and 5-31 provide examples of functional strengthening exercises.

PLYOMETRIC EXERCISE

Plyometric exercise is a technique of exercise that involves a rapid eccentric (lengthening) stretch of a muscle, followed immediately by a rapid concentric contraction of that muscle for the purpose of producing a forceful explosive movement over a short period of time.

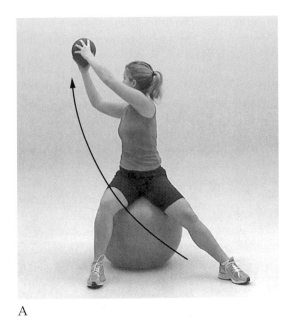

A

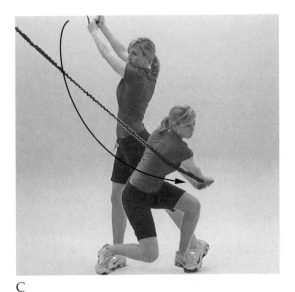

C

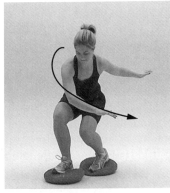

B

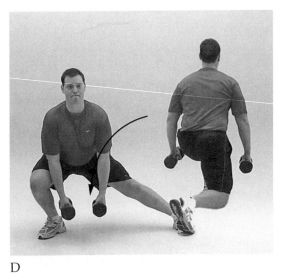

D

FIGURE 5-30. FUNCTIONAL STRENGTHENING EXERCISES.

*Functional strengthening exercises use simultaneous movements (concentric, eccentric, and isometric contractions) in three planes on either stable or unstable surfaces. **A,** Stability ball diagonal rotations with weighted ball. **B,** Tandem stance on DynaDisc with trunk rotation. **C,** Standing diagonal rotations with cable or tubing reistance. **D,** Weight-resisted multiplanar lunges.*

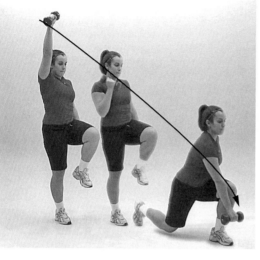

E

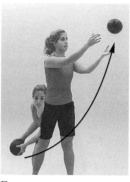

F

**FIGURE 5-30. (cont.). FUNCTIONAL
STRENGTHENING EXERCISES.**
*E, Front lunge balance to one-arm press.
F, Weighted-ball double arm rotation toss
from squat.*

Essentially, plyometric exercises are used to de-velop muscular power. Plyometric exercises in-volve hops, bounds, and depth jumping for the lower extremities. and the use of medicine balls and other types of weighted equipment for the upper extremities. Depth jumping is an ex-ample of a plyometric exercise in which an in-dividual jumps to the ground from a specified height and then quickly jumps again as soon as ground contact is made. (see Figure 5-32.)

The greater the stretch put on the muscle from its resting length immediately before the concentric contraction, the greater the resistance the muscle can overcome. Plyomet-rics emphasize the speed of the stretch phase. The rate of stretch is more critical than the magnitude of the stretch. An advantage to using plyometric exercise is that it can help de-velop eccentric control in dynamic move-ments. Plyometrics tend to place a great deal of stress on the musculoskeletal system. The learning and perfection of specific jumping skills and other plyometric exercises must be technically correct and specific to one's age, ac-tivity, and physical and skill development. Plyometric exercises often cause muscle sore-ness in individuals who are not used to doing

them. Therefore, they should be considered as a more advanced technique of strength train-ing, and only individuals who have experience in weight training should use them.

Recommendations for plyometric exercise vary. However, performing 3 sets of approxi-mately 15 repetitions is a good place to start.

CALISTHENIC STRENGTHENING EXERCISES

Until recently the thought of doing calisthenic exercises probably conjured up the image of a hard-nosed Marine drill instructor leading a group of recruits through a boring, regimented exercise session. But add music and bright-colored exercise clothing and change the name to aerobic exercise, aerobic dance, or tae bo and you have a multimillion-dollar industry that has swept a large segment of the Ameri-can population into exercise fanaticism. This new fascination with aerobic exercise has shown that calisthenic exercise can be enjoy-able without being excessively regimented.

We have already discussed weight training for the development of muscular strength.

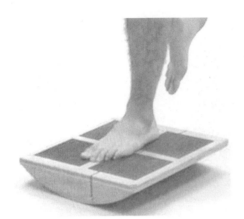

A

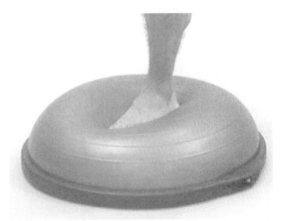

B

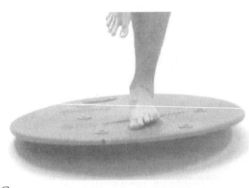

C

FIGURE 5-31. FUNCTIONAL STRENGTH-TRAINING EXERCISES TO ENHANCE STRENGTHENING NEUROMUSCULAR CONTROL FOR THE ANKLE ON DIFFERENT PIECES OF EQUIPMENT.

A, Rocker board. B, Bosu balance trainer.
C, Biomechanical Ankle Platform (BAPS) board.
D, DynaDisc.

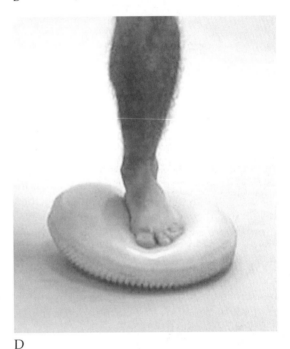

D

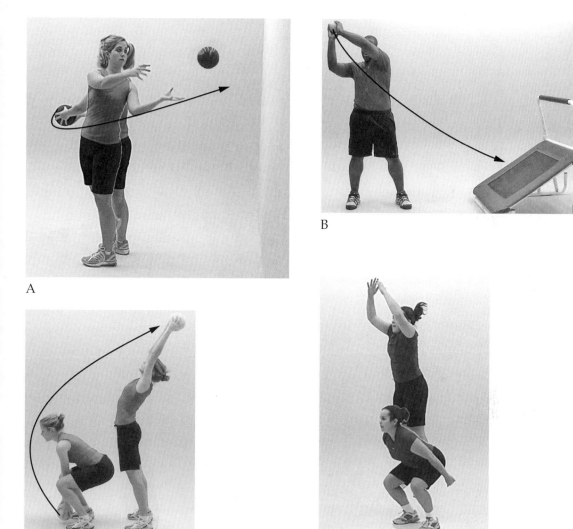

FIGURE 5-32. PLYOMETRIC EXERCISES.

*A, Weighted ball double arm rotation toss. **B,** Plyback two-arm toss with rotation. **C,** Weighted ball squat to stand extension. **D,** Squat jumps.*

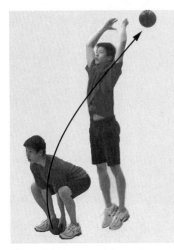

E

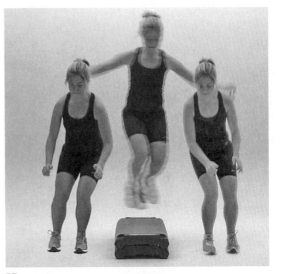

H

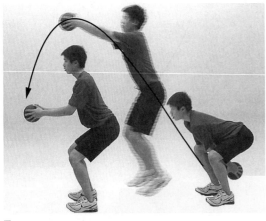

F

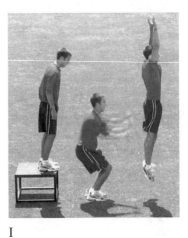

I

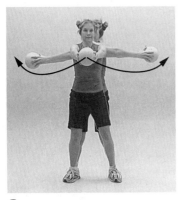

G

FIGURE 5-32. (cont.) PLYOMETRIC EXERCISES.

E, Overhead weighted ball throw. F, Weighted ball forward jump from squat. G, Weighted ball standing rotations. H, Double leg lateral hop overs. I, Depth jump to vertical jump.

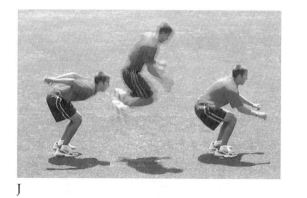

J

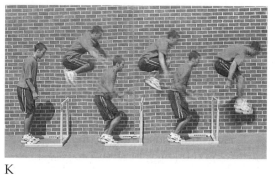

K

FIGURE 5-32. (cont.) PLYOMETRIC EXERCISES.
J, Repeat two-leg standing long jump. K, Three-hurdle jumps.

Calisthenic exercises, if done properly, can improve muscular strength and endurance, flexibility, and cardiorespiratory endurance. However, they are best suited as a supplemental activity to other previously discussed techniques rather than as a substitute for resistance-training exercises.

▶ Muscle Strength and Endurance

Calisthenics can help to increase muscular strength, tone, and endurance by using the weight of the body and its extremities as resistance. For example, chinning exercises (see Figure 5-41) use the weight of the body to resist the biceps and brachialis muscles in elbow flexion. The primary advantage of calisthenics over training with weights is that you do not need any expensive equipment or machines to provide resistance. Most of these exercises can be accomplished without the use of any equipment.

▶ Flexibility

Calisthenic exercises can also help to improve flexibility as long as each exercise is done through a full range of motion. The weight of a body part can assist in passively stretching a muscle to its greatest length. However, caution must be used when doing

calisthenic exercise to improve flexibility. The repetitive, bouncing nature of many of these exercises causes a muscle to be stretched ballistically, which can predispose a muscle to injury, particularly in an untrained person. Through calisthenic exercises, the muscle should be progressively stretched during the set of exercises. Do not neglect a warm-up that includes flexibility exercises before engaging in calisthenics.

▶ Cardiorespiratory Endurance

There is some question as to whether calisthenic exercises can increase resting heart rate significantly. However, if exercise is of sufficient intensity, frequency, and duration, cardiorespiratory endurance can be improved. Anyone who has gone through a 20- to 30-minute aerobics class will agree that heart rate is elevated to training levels. Calisthenic exercises should be done at a quick pace and without much rest between sets for optimal improvement of cardiorespiratory endurance.

▶ Specific Exercises

The exercises illustrated in Figures 5-33 to 5-42 are recommended because they work on specific muscle groups and with a specific

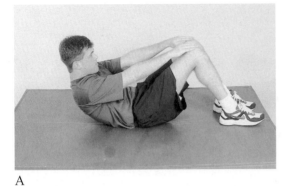

A

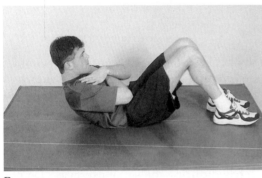

B

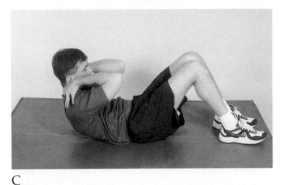

C

FIGURE 5-33. SIT-UPS.

A, Beginning; B, Intermediate, C, Advanced.
Joints affected: spinal vertebral joints.
Movement: trunk flexion.
Instructions: Lying on back, hands either on chest or behind back, knees flexed to 90-degree angle, feet on floor, curl trunk and head to approximately 45-degree angle.
Primary muscles: rectus abdominis.
Caution: *It has been suggested by some experts on low back pain that sit-up exercises done with both bent and straight legs should be avoided due to the high compressive loads on the low back and spine. This is particularly true in individuals with existing low back pain. (McGill, 2001) While this view is not universally accepted, if sit-ups, crunches, or even straight leg raises cause increased low back pain, they should be avoided.*

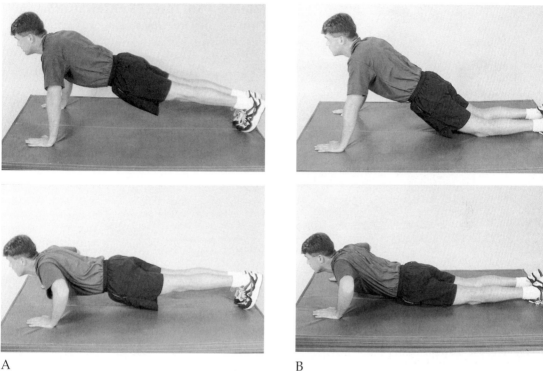

A

B

FIGURE 5-34. PUSH-UPS.

A, Push-ups. *B,* Modified push-ups.

Purpose: strengthening.

Muscles: triceps, pectoralis major.

Repetitions: beginner 10; intermediate 20; advanced 30.

Instructions: Keep the upper trunk and legs extended in a straight line. Touch floor with chest.

Caution: Avoid hyperextending the back, especially in modified push-ups.

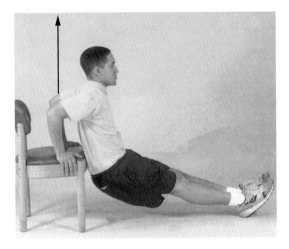

FIGURE 5-35. TRICEPS EXTENSIONS.
Purpose: strengthening and range of motion at shoulder joint.
Muscles: triceps, trapezius.
Repetitions: beginner 7; intermediate 12; advanced 18.
Instructions: Begin with arms extended and body straight. Lower buttocks until they touch the ground, then press back up.

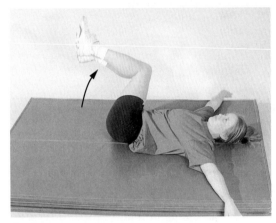

A

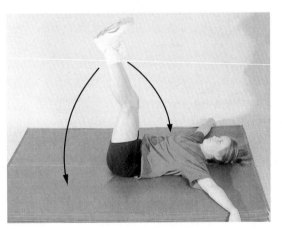

B

FIGURE 5-36. TRUNK ROTATION.
A, Beginner; B, Advanced.
Muscles: internal and external obliques.
Repetitions: beginner 10 each direction; intermediate 15 each direction; advanced 20 each direction.
Instructions: Rotate trunk from side to side until knees touch the floor, keeping knees slightly bent.
Caution: *This exercise should be done only by those who already have strong abdominals.*

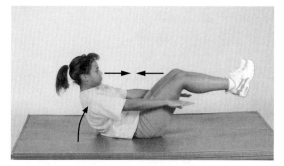

FIGURE 5-37. SITTING TUCKS.

Purpose: strengthen abdominals and stretch low back.

Muscles: rectus abdominis, erector muscles in low back.

Repetitions: beginner 10; intermediate 20; advanced 30.

Instructions: Keep legs and upper back off the ground and pull knees to chest.

Caution: It has been suggested by some experts on low back pain that sit-up type exercises done with both bent and straight legs should be avoided due to the high compressive loads on the low back and spine. This is particularly true in individuals with existing low back pain. (McGill, 2001) While this view is not universally accepted, if sitting tucks cause increased low back pain, they should be avoided.

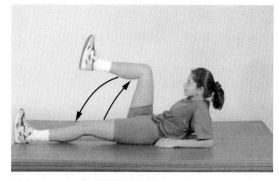

FIGURE 5-38. BICYCLE.

Purpose: strengthen hip flexors and stretch lower back.

Muscles: iliopsoas.

Repetitions: beginner 10 each side; intermediate 20 each side; advanced 30 each side.

Instructions: Alternately flex and extend legs as if you were pedaling a bicycle.

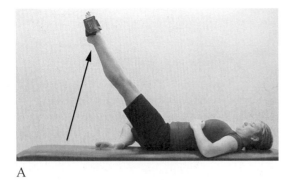

A

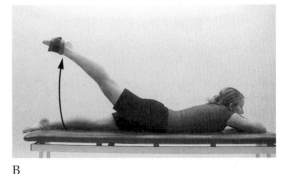

B

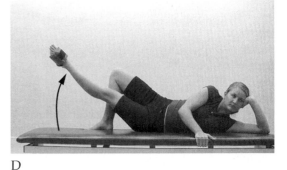

C   D

FIGURE 5-39. LEG LIFTS.

A, Front; B, Back; C, Side (leg up); D, Side (leg down).
Purpose: strengthen A, Hip flexors; B, Hip extensors; C, hip abductors; D, Hip adductors.
Muscles: A, Iliopsoas; B, Gluteus maximus; C, Gluteus medius; D, Adductor group.
Repetitions: beginner 10 each leg; intermediate 15 each leg; advanced 20 each leg.
Instructions: Raise the exercising leg up as far as possible in each position.

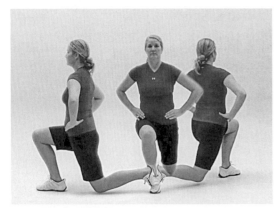

FIGURE 5-40. LUNGES.

Joints affected: hip and knee.
Movement: Forward lunge.
Position: standing, take giant step forward bending knee in multiple directions.
Primary muscles: gluteal, hamstrings, quadriceps.

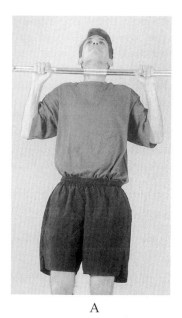
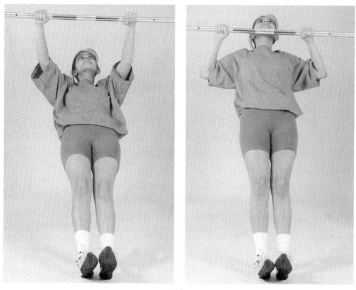

A   B

FIGURE 5-41. CHIN-UPS.
A, Chin-ups. B, Modified chin-ups.
Purpose: strengthening and stretch of shoulder joint.
Muscles: biceps, brachialis, and latissimus dorsi.
Repetitions: beginner 7; intermediate 10; advanced 15.
Instructions: Pull up until chin touches top of bar.

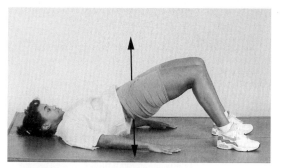

FIGURE 5-42. BUTTOCK TUCKS.
Purpose: strengthen muscles of buttocks.
Muscles: gluteus maximus, hamstrings.
Repetitions: beginner 10; intermediate 15; advanced 20.
Instructions: Lying flat on back with knees bent, arch back and thrust the pelvis upward.

purpose. If you do all the exercises, most of the major muscle groups in the body will be both stretched and contracted against resistance with the objective of improving strength, flexibility, and endurance. Each exercise can be done at your own pace, although the greater the pace, the greater the stress placed on the cardiorespiratory system. Thus it is recommended that you work quickly and move from one exercise to the next without delay. These exercises can be done to music if you so desire. Most people find it easier to exercise to fast-paced music with a hard, rhythmic beat. However, you should select the type of music most enjoyable to you.

ASSESSMENT OF MUSCULAR STRENGTH AND ENDURANCE

Lab Activities 5-1 through 5-3 will help you assess your levels of muscular strength, endurance, and power. On the worksheet on pages 140 and 141 you can monitor and record your progress on each of the exercises described in this chapter.

SUMMARY

- Muscular strength and endurance are important health-related components of fitness. Power is a skill-related component of fitness.
- The ability to generate force depends on the physical properties of the muscle as well as on the mechanical factors that dictate how much force can be generated through the lever system to an external object.
- Hypertrophy of a muscle is caused by increases in the size of the protein myofilaments, which result in an increased cross-sectional diameter of the muscle.
- The key to improving strength through resistance training is using the principle of overload.

- A number of different resistance-training techniques can improve muscular strength: progressive resistive exercise, isometric exercise, circuit training, functional strength training, plyometric training, calisthenic exercises, and core stabilization exercises.
- Muscular endurance tends to improve with muscular strength; thus, training techniques for these two components are similar.

SUGGESTED READINGS

Baechle, T. R. 2008. *Essentials of strength training and conditioning.* Champaign, IL: Human Kinetics.

Bompa, T. O., and L. J. Cornacchia. 2002. *Serious strength training.* Champaign, IL: Human Kinetics.

Bruce-Low, S., and D. Smith. 2007. Explosive exercises in sports training: A critical review. *Journal of Exercise Physiology* 10(1):21–33.

Chu, D. 1996. *Explosive strength and power.* Champaign, IL: Human Kinetics.

Clark, M. 2001. *Integrated training for the new millennium.* Calabasas, CA: National Academy of Sports Medicine.

Dunn-Lewis, C., and W. Kraemer. 2009. The basics of starting and progressing a strength-training program., *ACSM Fit Society Page* Winter issue:1.

Fahey, T. 2009. *Basic weight training for men and women,* New York: McGraw-Hill.

Flach, A., and E. O'Driscol. 2005. *The complete book of isometrics: The anywhere, anytime fitness book.* New York: Hatherleigh Press.

Fleck, S., and W. Kramer. 2004. *Designing resistance training programs.* Champaign, IL: Human Kinetics.

Folland, J., and A. Williams. 2007. The adaptations to strength training. *Sports Medicine* 37(2):145.

Gabriel, D., G. Kamen, and G. Frost. 2006. Neural adaptations to resistive exercise: Mechanisms and recommendations for training practices. *Sports Medicine* 36(2):133.

Garbutt, G., and N. T. Cable. 1998. Circuit weight-training. *Sports Exercise and Injury* 4(2/3):46–49.

Goldenberg, L., and P. Twist. 2006. *Strength ball training.* Champaign, IL: Human Kinetics.

Goldenberg, L., and P. Twist. 2006. Core stabilization. In *Strength ball training,* edited by L. Goldenberg. Champaign, IL: Human Kinetics.

Gravelle, B., and D. Blessing. 2000. Physiological adaptation in women concurrently training for strength and endurance. *Journal of Strength and Conditioning* 14(1):5.

Harrison, J. 2010. Bodyweight training: A return to basics., *Strength & Conditioning Journal* 32(2):52.

Hesson, J. 2010. *Weight training for life.* Belmont, CA: Brooks/Cole.

Heyward, V. H. 2010. Assessing strength and muscular endurance. In *Advanced fitness assessment and exercise prescription,* 6th ed., edited by V. H. Heyward. Champaign, IL: Human Kinetics.

Incledon, L. 2005. *Strength training for women.* Champaign, Il: Human Kinetics.

Knight, K. L., C. D. Ingersoll, and J. Bartholomew. 2001. Isotonic contractions might be more effective than isokinetic contractions in developing muscle strength. *Journal of Sport Rehabilitation* 10(2):124–31.

Komi, P. V. 2003. *Strength and power in sport,* 2nd ed. Oxford: Blackwell Science.

Kraemer, W., and S. Fleck. 2004. *Strength training for young athletes.* Champaign, IL: Human Kinetics.

Kraemer, W., K. Hakkinen, and W. Kraemer. 2001. *Strength training for sport.* Cambridge, MA: Blackwell Science.

Kraemer, W. J., and N. A. Ratamess, 2004. Fundamentals of resistance training: progression and exercise prescription. *Medicine and Science in Sports and Exercise* 36(4):574–688.

Leetun, D. T., M. L. Ireland, and J. D. Willson. 2004. Core stability measures as risk factors for lower extremity injury in athletes. *Medicine and Science in Sports and Exercise* 36(6):926–34.

Maguire, M., and J. Boult. 2010. Building a foundation of strength. *Rehab Management: The Interdisciplinary Journal of Rehabilitation* 23(6):20.

Mannie, K. 2004. Overloading without overtraining. *Coach and Athletic Director* 74(4):9–12.

McGill, S. 2001. Low back stability: From formal description to issues for performance and rehabilitation. *Exercise and Sport Science Reviews* 29(1):26–31.

Neporent, L. and S. Schlosberg. 2006. *Weight training for dummies.* Hoboken, NJ: Wiley and Sons.

Oliver, G., and H. Adams-Blair. 2010. Improving core strength to prevent injury. *JOPERD: The Journal of Physical Education, Recreation & Dance* 81(7):15.

Page, P., and T. Ellenbecker. 2010. *Strength band training.* Champaign, IL: Human Kinetics.

Pearl, B., and R. Goluke. 2006. *Getting stronger: Weight training for sports.* Bolinas, CA, Shelter Publications.

Plisk, S. S. 2001. Muscular strength and stamina. In *High-performance sports conditioning,* edited by B. Foran. Champaign, IL: Human Kinetics.

Radcliffe, J. C., and R. C. Farentinos. 2005. *High-powered plyometrics.* Champaign, IL: Human Kinetics.

Roetert, E. P. 1998. Facts and fallacies about strength training for women. *Strength and Conditioning* 20(6):172–78.

Sandler, D. 2005. Speed and strength through plyometrics. In Sandler, D. *Sports power,* Champaign, IL: Human Kinetics.

Schroeder, E. T., S. A. Hawkins, and S. V. Jaque. 2004. Musculoskeletal adaptations to 16 weeks of eccentric progressive resistance training in young women. *Journal of Strength and Conditioning Research* 18(2):227–35.

Stone, M., M. Stone and W. Sands. 2006. Maximum strength and strength training—A relationship to endurance? *Strength and Conditioning Journal* 28(3):44.

Verstegen, M., and P. Williams. 2008. *Core performance endurance: A new training and nutrition program that revolutionizes your workouts.* Emmaus, PA: Rodale Press Inc.

Young, W. 2006. Transfer of strength and power training to sports performance. *International Journal of Sports Physiology and Performance* 1(2):74.

Suggested Web Sites

Fitness-Mayo Clinic.com

This site contains good information about fitness in general and about strength training in specific. **http://www.mayoclinic.com/health/fitness/MY00396**

International Weightlifting Federation

The IWF is composed of the affiliated National Federations governing the sport of weightlifting on the basis of one federation per country and is the controlling body of all competitive lifting. The objectives of the IWF are to organize, control, and develop the sport of weightlifting on an international scale. **www.iwf.net**

National Council of Strength and Fitness

The NCSF Certification Agency strives to develop the most knowledgeable professional trainers by maintaining the highest standards in the industry. **www.ncsf.org**

National Strength and Conditioning Association Home Page

The NSCA sponsors this site. **www.nsca-lift.org**

USA Weightlifting

USA Weightlifting (USAW) is the national governing body (NGB) for Olympic weightlifting in the United States. USAW is a member of the United States Olympic Committee (USOC) and a member of the International Weightlifting Federation (IWF). As the NGB, USAW is responsible for conducting Olympic weightlifting programs throughout the country. **www.usaweightlifting.org**

Name   Section   Date

PURPOSE   To test muscular endurance.

PROCEDURE 1. *Men:* Begin in the standard push-up position with the weight supported on the hands and toes, with trunk and back straight (Figure 5-43). *Women:* Begin in the push-up position with the weight on the hands and knees (Figure 5-44).
2. Have a partner place his or her fist on the floor directly under your chest.
3. Lower yourself until your chest touches your partner's fist.
4. Count the number of consecutive correctly done push-ups.
5. Consult Table 5-3 to determine your score.

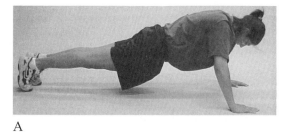

A

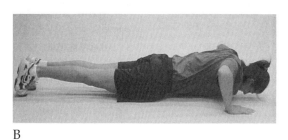

B

FIGURE 5-43. PUSH-UPS.

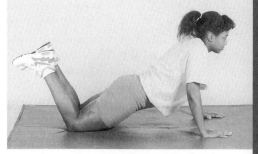

FIGURE 5-44. MODIFIED PUSH-UPS.

Push-Ups

TABLE 5-3
PUSH-UP MUSCULAR ENDURANCE TEST STANDARDS

	Age (Years)	Superior	Excellent	Very Good	Good	Average	Poor	Very Poor
				Fitness Level				
Males **Push-Up**	15–29	Above 55	51–54	45–50	35–44	25–34	20–24	15–19
	30–39	Above 45	41–44	35–40	25–34	20–24	15–19	8–14
	40–49	Above 40	35–39	30–34	20–29	14–19	12–13	5–11
	50–59	Above 35	31–34	25–30	15–24	12–14	8–11	3–7
	60–69	Above 30	26–29	20–25	10–19	8–9	5–7	0–4
Females **Modified** **Push-Ups**	15–29	Above 49	46–48	34–45	17–33	10–16	6–9	0–5
	30–39	Above 38	34–37	25–33	12–24	8–11	4–7	0–3
	40–49	Above 33	29–32	20–28	8–19	6–7	3–5	0–2
	50–59	Above 26	22–25	15–21	6–14	4–5	2–3	0–1
	60–69	Above 20	16–19	5–15	3–4	2–3	1–2	0

Pollock, M. L., J. H. Wilmore, and S. M. Fox. 1978. Health and fitness through physical activity. All rights reserved. Reprinted by permission of Allyn & Bacon.

Name   Section   Date

PURPOSE   To measure abdominal muscle endurance.

PROCEDURE
1. Lie flat on your back, and cross your arms across your chest, resting your hands on your shoulders. Knees should be bent to 90 degrees with the feet flat and 18 inches from the buttocks (Figure 5-45).
2. Count the number of sit-ups you are able to complete in 1 minute.
3. Consult Table 5-4 to determine your fitness level.

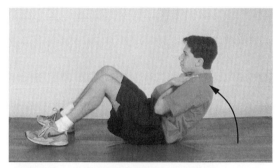

FIGURE 5-45. BENT-KNEE SIT-UPS.

Caution: It has been suggested by some experts on low back pain that sit-up exercises done with both bent and straight legs should be avoided due to the high compressive loads on the low back and spine. This is particularly true in individuals with existing low back pain. (McGill, 2001) While this view is not universally accepted, if sit-ups cause increased low back pain, they should be avoided.

TABLE 5-4
BENT-KNEE SIT-UPS SCORE

	Age (Years)	Superior	Excellent	Very Good	Good	Average	Poor	Very Poor
				Fitness Level				
Males	17–29	55+	51–55	48–50	42–47	36–41	17–35	0–17
	30–39	48+	44–48	39–43	33–38	27–32	13–26	0–13
	40–49	43+	39–43	34–38	28–33	23–27	11–22	0–11
	50–59	38+	34–38	29–33	22–28	17–21	8–16	0–8
	60–69	35+	31–35	25–30	18–24	13–17	6–12	0–6
Females	17–29	47+	43–47	36–42	33–35	29–32	14–28	0–14
	30–39	45+	41–45	35–40	29–34	23–28	11–22	0–11
	40–49	40+	35–40	31–34	24–30	19–23	9–18	0–9
	50–59	35+	31–35	25–30	18–24	13–17	6–12	0–6
	60–69	30+	26–30	21–25	15–20	11–14	5–10	0–5

*The values for ages over 30 are estimated.

_____   _____   _____
Name   Section   Date

PURPOSE   To test general levels of muscular endurance.

EQUIPMENT   Chinning bar and a 16-inch bench.
NEEDED

PROCEDURE   1. Perform the following exercises as indicated:
Men: Bent-leg sit-ups, push-ups, static push-ups, pull-ups, bench jumps.
Women: Bent-leg sit-ups, static push-ups, flexed arm hang, modified pull-ups, bench jumps.
Bent-leg sit-ups. Hands on shoulders, knees flexed to 90 degrees. One elbow must touch knee. Fingers must touch the floor between repetitions. Record total number in 1 minute (Figure 5-46).
Push-ups. Standard push-up position. Chest must touch floor during each repetition. Record total number performed consecutively. (Refer to Figure 5-33).
Static push-up. From a standard push-up position, lower the body until the elbow is flexed at 90 degrees or less. Record the number of seconds this position can be maintained without the body touching the floor or losing the proper form (Figure 5-47).

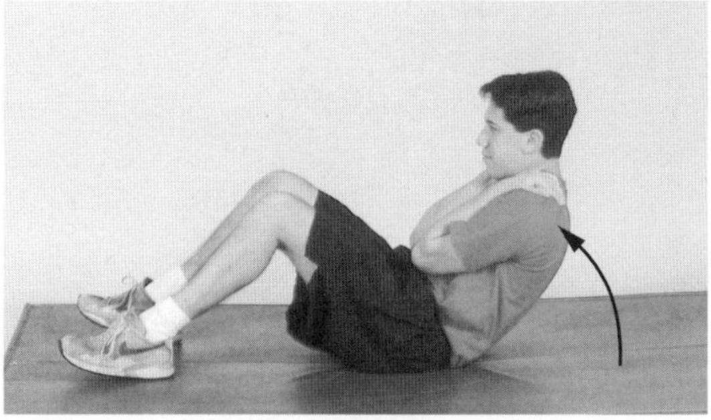

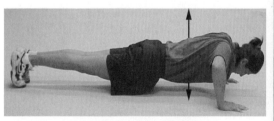

FIGURE 5-46. BENT-LEG SIT-UPS.

FIGURE 5-47. STATIC PUSH-UP.

Caution: It has been suggested by some experts on low back pain that sit-up exercises done with both bent and straight legs should be avoided due to the high compressive loads on the low back and spine. This is particularly true in individuals with existing low back pain. (McGill, 2001) While this view is not universally accepted, if sit-ups cause increased low back pain they should be avoided.

Pull-ups. Subject grasps bar. The body is raised until the chin is above the bar and lowered until the arms are fully extended. Record the number of repetitions to failure (Figure 5-48).

Flexed-arm hang. Using an overhand grip, raise the body until the chin is above the bar. Record the number of seconds the chin can be held above the level of the bar (Figure 5-49).

Modified pull-ups. Chinning bar is lowered to the height of the chest. Heels remain in contact with the floor underneath the bar. Arms are fully extended. Then pull up until chin touches bar. Record maximum number of repetitions (Figure 5-50).

Bench jumps. Using a 16-inch bench, record the number of times the subject can either jump or step up onto the bench in a 1-minute period (Figure 5-51).

2. Record the information as indicated on the worksheet.
3. Determine the percentile rank for each exercise by consulting Table 5-5.
4. Determine the overall percentile rank as indicated in the worksheet.

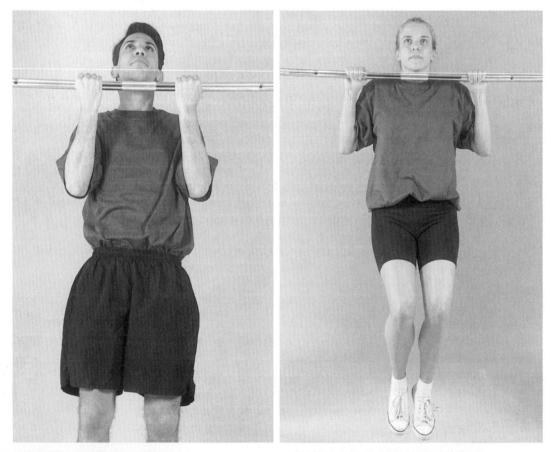

FIGURE 5-48. PULL-UPS.   **FIGURE 5-49. FLEXED-ARM HANG.**

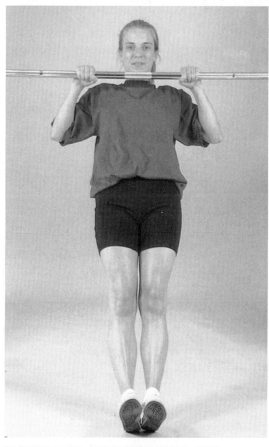

FIGURE 5-50. MODIFIED PULL-UPS.

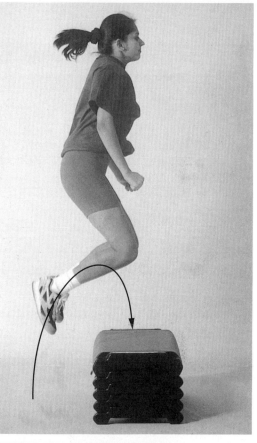

FIGURE 5-51. BENCH JUMPS.

Worksheet					
Women				**Men**	
Exercise	*Score*	*Percentile*	*Exercise*	*Score*	*Percentile*
Bent-leg sit-ups	____	____	Bent-leg sit-ups	____	____
Static push-ups	____	____	Push-ups	____	____
Flexed-arm hang	____	____	Static push-ups	____	____
Modified pull-ups	____	____	Pull-ups	____	____
Bench jumps	____	____	Bench jumps	____	____
Total of all five percentiles ____			Total of all five percentiles ____		
Overall percentile rank ____ (divide by 5)			Overall percentile rank (divide by 5)		

Muscular Endurance Test

TABLE 5-5
MUSCULAR ENDURANCE SCORING TABLE

	Percentile Rank	Bent-Leg Sit-Ups (1 Minute Maximum)	Static Push-Ups (Women); Push-Ups (Men)	Flexed Arm Hang (Women); Static Push-Ups (Men)	Modified Pull-Ups (Women); Pull-Ups (Men)	Bench Jumps
Men	95	50	53	77	14	38
	90	47	49	72	12	36
	80	44	44	67	10	34
	70	41	41	63	9	33
	60	39	38	60	8	31
	50	37	35	57	7	30
	40	35	32	54	6	29
	30	33	29	51	5	27
	20	30	26	47	4	26
	10	27	21	42	2	24
	5	24	17	37	0	22
Women	95	36	38	34	43	28
	90	33	35	28	40	26
	80	30	32	19	36	24
	70	28	30	14	33	22
	60	26	28	10	30	21
	50	24	26	8	28	20
	40	22	24	6	26	19
	30	20	22	4	23	18
	20	18	20	2	20	16
	10	15	17	1	16	14
	5	12	14	0	13	12

CHAPTER 6

Increasing Flexibility Through **Stretching**

Objectives

After completing this chapter, you should be able to do the following:

- Define flexibility and describe its importance as a health-related component of fitness.
- Identify factors that limit flexibility.
- Differentiate between active and passive range of motion.
- Explain the difference between dynamic, static, and PNF stretching.
- Describe stretching exercises that may be used to improve flexibility at specific joints throughout the body.
- Discuss Pilates and yoga as two alternative stretching techniques.

WHY IS IT IMPORTANT TO HAVE GOOD FLEXIBILITY?

Flexibility may best be defined as the range of motion possible about a given joint or series of joints. Flexibility can be discussed in relation to movement involving only one joint, such as the knee, or movement involving a whole series of joints, such as the spinal vertebral joints, which must all move together to allow smooth bending, or rotation, of the trunk. Flexibility is specific to a given joint or movement. A person may have good range of motion in the ankles, knees, hips,

back, and one shoulder joint. However, if the other shoulder joint lacks normal movement, then a problem exists that needs to be corrected before that person can function normally.

Flexibility was identified in Chapter 1 as a health-related as opposed to performance-related component of fitness, although for most

---

flexibility: the range of motion possible about a given joint or series of joints

---

KEY TERMS

flexibility	*static stretching*
active range of motion	*proprioceptive*
passive range of motion	*neuromuscular facilitation (PNF)*
agonist muscle	*dynamic stretching*
antagonist muscle	*Pilates exercise*
ballistic stretching	*yoga*

of us it may be considered important for both. The ability to move a joint or series of joints smoothly and easily throughout a full range of motion is certainly essential to healthy living. The arthritic person who suffers from degeneration in one or more joints loses the capacity of painless, nonrestricted motion and is hampered in the performance of daily acts of healthful living. Lack of flexibility may result in uncoordinated or awkward movements and may predispose a person to muscle strain. Low back pain is frequently associated with tightness of the musculature in the lower spine and also of the hamstring muscles.

If you are physically active, a lack of flexibility will likely impair your performance. For example, if you are a power walker with tight, inelastic hamstring muscles, you may have a problem walking at a fast pace, because tight hamstrings restrict your ability to flex the hip joint, thus shortening your stride length. Most activities you engage in require relatively "normal" amounts of flexibility. However, some activities, such as ballet, karate, tai chi, yoga, and gymnastics require increased flexibility for superior performance (Figure 6-1). Increased flexibility may increase one's performance through improved balance and reaction time. Experts in the field of training and the development of physical fitness generally agree that good flexibility is essential to successful physical performance, although their ideas are based primarily on observation rather than on scientific research.

While many studies over the years have suggested that stretching improves performance, several recent studies have found that stretching causes decreases in performance parameters such as strength, endurance, power, and reaction times. The same can be said when examining the relationship between flexibility and reducing the incidence of injury. While it is generally accepted that good flexibility reduces the likelihood of injury, a true cause–effect relationship has not been clearly established in the literature.

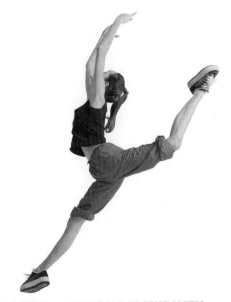

FIGURE 6-1. EXTREME FLEXIBILITY.
Certain dance and athletic activities require extreme flexibility for successful performance.

WHAT STRUCTURES IN THE BODY CAN LIMIT FLEXIBILITY?

A number of different anatomical structures may limit the ability of a joint to move through a full, unrestricted range of motion.

Normal bone structure, fat, and skin or scar tissue may limit the ability to move through a full range of motion. Muscles and their tendons are most often responsible for limiting range of motion. When performing stretching exercises for the purpose of improving a particular joint's flexibility, you are attempting to take advantage of the highly elastic properties of a muscle. Over time, it is possible to increase elasticity, or the length that a given muscle can be stretched. Individuals who have a good deal of movement at a particular joint tend to have highly elastic and flexible muscles.

Ligaments function to connect bone to bone and help provide stability around a joint. If a joint is immobilized (in a cast or splint) for a period of time, ligaments will lose some of their inherent elasticity and actually shorten. This condition is most commonly seen after surgical repair of an unstable joint, but it can also result from long periods of inactivity. Stretching will have a positive effect on muscles, tendons, and ligaments.

On the other hand, it's also possible for a person to have relatively slack ligaments. These people are generally referred to as being "loose-jointed." Examples of this would be an elbow or knee that hyperextends beyond 180 degrees (beyond straight). Frequently there is instability associated with loose-jointedness that may be as great a problem in movement as a joint that is too tight.

ACTIVE AND PASSIVE RANGE OF MOTION

When a muscle actively contracts, it produces a joint movement through a specific range of motion. However, if passive pressure is applied to an extremity, it is capable of moving farther in the range of motion. **Active range of motion** refers to that portion of the total range of motion through which a joint can be moved by an active muscle contraction. Your ability to move through the active range of motion is not necessarily a good indicator of the stiffness or looseness of a joint because it applies to the ability to move a joint efficiently, with little resistance to motion. **Passive range of motion** refers to the portion of the total range of motion (beyond the active range of motion) through which a joint may be moved passively. No muscle contraction is needed to move a joint through a passive range of motion. Passive range of motion begins at the end of and continues beyond active range of motion.

While it is important that an extremity be capable of actively moving through a non-restricted range of motion, passive range of

motion is important for injury prevention. There are many situations in which a muscle is forced to stretch beyond its normal active limits. If the muscle does not have enough elasticity to compensate for this additional stretch, it is likely that the muscle or its tendon will be injured.

AGONIST VERSUS ANTAGONIST MUSCLES

Before discussing the three different stretching techniques, it is essential to define the terms **agonist muscle** and **antagonist muscle**. Most joints in the body are capable of more than one movement. The knee joint, for example, is capable of flexion and extension. Contraction of the quadriceps group of muscles on the front of the thigh causes knee extension, whereas contraction of the hamstring muscles on the back of the thigh produces knee flexion. The muscle that contracts to produce a movement, in this case the quadriceps, is referred to as the agonist muscle. Conversely, the muscle

active range of motion: that portion of the total range of motion through which a joint can be moved by an active muscle contraction

passive range of motion: that portion of the total range of motion (beyond active range of motion) through which a joint may be moved passively without muscle contraction producing the movement

agonist muscle: the muscle that contracts to produce a movement

antagonist muscle: the muscle being stretched in response to contraction of the agonist muscle

being stretched in response to contraction of the agonist muscle is called the antagonist muscle. In this example of knee extension, the antagonist muscle would be the hamstring group.

Some degree of balance in strength must exist between agonist and antagonist muscle groups. This is necessary for normal, smooth, coordinated movement as well as for reducing the likelihood of muscle strain due to the muscular imbalance. Understanding the relationship between agonist and antagonist muscles is essential for a discussion of the three techniques of stretching.

WHAT ARE THE DIFFERENT STRETCHING TECHNIQUES?

Maintaining a full, nonrestricted range of motion has long been recognized as an essential component of physical fitness. Flexibility is important not only for successful physical performance but also in the prevention of injury. The goal of any effective flexibility program should be to improve the range of motion around a given joint by altering the extensibility of the muscles and tendons that produce movement at that joint. It is well documented that exercises that stretch these muscles and tendons over a period of time will increase the range of movement possible about a given joint.

Stretching techniques for improving flexibility have evolved over the years. The oldest technique for stretching is called **ballistic stretching,** which makes use of repeated bouncing movements. Ballistic stretching is seldom used because it is likely to cause delayed onset muscle soreness, particularly in sedentary, unfit individuals. A second technique, known as **static stretching,** involves stretching a muscle to the point of discomfort and then holding it at that point for an extended time. This technique has been used for many years. More recently, another group of stretching techniques known collectively as **proprioceptive**

neuromuscular facilitation (PNF), involving alternating contractions and stretches, has also been recommended. Currently, the most widely used and recommended technique of stretching is **dynamic stretching,** which was discussed earlier in Chapter 3 as part of the warm-up. Researchers have had considerable discussion about which of these techniques is most effective for improving range of motion.

BALLISTIC STRETCHING

With ballistic stretching, repetitive contractions of the agonist muscle are used to produce quick stretches of the antagonist muscle. Over the years, many fitness experts have questioned the safety of the ballistic stretching technique. Their concerns have been primarily based on the idea that ballistic stretching creates somewhat

ballistic stretching: technique involving repetitive contractions of the agonist muscle that are used to produce quick stretches of the antagonist muscle

static stretching: technique involving passively stretching a given antagonist muscle by placing it in a maximal position of stretch and holding it there for an extended time

proprioceptive neuromuscular facilitation (PNF): a group of stretching techniques including slow-reversal-hold-relax, contract-relax, and hold-relax techniques, all of which involve some combination of alternating contraction and relaxation of both agonist and antagonist muscles

dynamic stretching: uses hopping, skipping, and bounding activities and active muscular effort to stretch a muscle

uncontrolled forces within the muscle that can exceed the extensibility limits of the muscle fiber, thus producing small tears within the muscle. Certainly this might be true in sedentary individuals or perhaps in athletes who have sustained muscle injuries.

STATIC STRETCHING

The static stretching technique is an extremely effective and popular technique of stretching. This technique involves contracting the agonist muscle to passively stretch a given antagonist muscle by placing it in a maximal position of stretch and holding it there for an extended time. Recommendations for the optimal time for holding this stretched position vary, ranging from as short as 3 seconds to as long as 60 seconds. Data are inconclusive at present; however, it appears that 30 seconds may be a good time. The static stretch of each muscle should be repeated three or four times. Much research has been done comparing ballistic and static stretching techniques for the improvement of flexibility. Both static and ballistic stretching are effective in increasing flexibility, and there is no significant difference between the two. However, with static stretching there is less danger of exceeding the extensibility limits of the involved joints because the stretch is more controlled. Ballistic stretching may cause muscular soreness if performed too aggressively, whereas static stretching generally does not and is commonly used in injury rehabilitation of sore or strained muscles.

Static stretching is certainly a much safer stretching technique, especially for sedentary or untrained individuals. However, many physical activities involve dynamic movement. Thus in physically active individuals who routinely engage in dynamic activities, dynamic stretching is likely the technique of choice, particularly during a warm-up.

PROPRIOCEPTIVE NEUROMUSCULAR FACILITATION (PNF) TECHNIQUES

PNF techniques were first used by physical therapists for treating patients who had various types of neuromuscular paralysis. Only recently have PNF stretching exercises been used as a stretching technique for increasing flexibility. A number of different PNF techniques are currently being used for stretching, including slow-reversal-hold-relax, contract-relax, and hold-relax techniques. All involve some combination of alternating contraction and relaxation of both agonist and antagonist muscles (a 10-second pushing phase followed by a 10-second relaxing phase).

Using a hamstring stretching technique as an example (Figure 6-2), the slow-reversal-hold-relax technique would be done as follows. Lying on your back with the knee extended and the ankle flexed to 90 degrees, a partner passively flexes your leg at the hip joint to the point at which you feel slight discomfort in the muscle. At this point you begin pushing against your partner's resistance

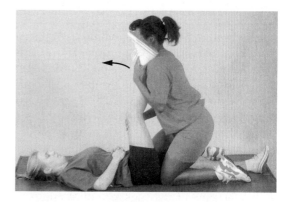

FIGURE 6-2. SLOW-REVERSAL-HOLD-RELAX TECHNIQUE.
This technique stretches hamstring muscles.

by contracting the hamstring muscle. After pushing for 10 seconds, the hamstring muscles are relaxed and the agonist quadriceps muscle is contracted while your partner applies passive pressure to further stretch the antagonist hamstrings. This should move the leg so that there is increased hip joint flexion. The relaxing phase lasts for 10 seconds, at which time you again push against your partner's resistance, beginning at this new joint angle. The push-relax sequence is repeated at least three times.

The contract-relax and hold-relax techniques are variations on the slow-reversal-hold-relax method. In the contract-relax method, the hamstrings are isotonically contracted so that the leg actually moves toward the floor during the push phase. The hold-relax method involves an isometric hamstring contraction against immovable resistance during the push phase. During the relax phase, both techniques involve relaxation of hamstrings and quadriceps while the hamstrings are passively stretched. This same basic PNF technique can be used to stretch any muscle in the body. PNF stretching techniques are perhaps best performed with a partner, although they may also be done using a wall as resistance.

DYNAMIC STRETCHING

Dynamic stretching uses movement, momentum, and active muscular effort to stretch a muscle, as compared with static stretching, which is performed with limited and controlled stretching of the muscle. It uses hopping, skipping, and bounding activities. Most physical activities require dynamic movements. For example, forcefully kicking a soccer ball 50 times involves a repeated dynamic contraction of the agonist quadriceps muscle. The antagonist hamstrings are contracting eccentrically to decelerate the lower leg. Dynamic stretching of the hamstring muscle before engaging in this type of activity should

allow the muscle to gradually adapt to the imposed demands and reduce the likelihood of injury. Because dynamic stretching is more functional, it should be integrated into a flexibility program and is in fact recommended for any physically active individual who is involved in dynamic activity. Figure 6-3 provides an example of a dynamic stretching technique.

PRACTICAL APPLICATION

Although all four stretching techniques have been demonstrated to effectively improve flexibility, there is still considerable debate as to which technique produces the greatest increases in range of movement. The ballistic technique is seldom recommended in sedentary individuals because of the potential for causing muscle soreness. It should be added that in highly trained individuals, it is unlikely that ballistic stretching will result in muscle soreness. Static stretching has perhaps been the most widely used technique for many years. It is a simple technique and does not require a partner. A full nonrestricted range of motion can be attained through static stretching over time. PNF stretching techniques are capable of producing dramatic increases in range of motion during one stretching session. Studies comparing static and PNF stretching suggest that PNF stretching is capable of producing greater improvement in flexibility over an extended training period. The major disadvantage of PNF stretching is that a partner is required to help you stretch, although stretching with a partner may have some motivational advantages. It appears that dynamic stretching has become the technique of choice primarily because it is more functional or more closely related to the dynamic movement associated with physical activity. Safe Tip 6-1 offers guidelines and precautions for stretching.

IS THERE A RELATIONSHIP BETWEEN STRENGTH AND FLEXIBILITY?

We often hear about the negative effects that strength training has on flexibility. For example, someone who develops bulk through strength training is often referred to as muscle-bound. The expression *muscle–bound* has negative connotations regarding that person's ability to move. We tend to think of people who have highly developed muscles as having lost much of their ability to move freely through a full range of motion.

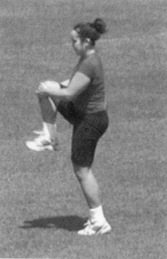

A

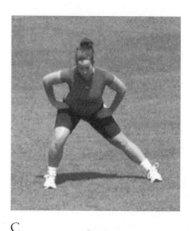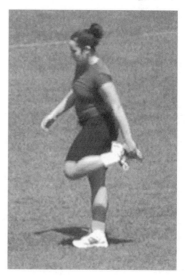

C

B

D

FIGURE 6-3. DYNAMIC STRETCHING TECHNIQUE.
A, *Walking lunge with rotation.* **B,** *Walking knees to chest.* **C,** *Walking lateral lunge.*
D, *Walking quadriceps stretch.*

SAFE TIP 6-1

Guidelines and Precautions for Stretching

The following guidelines and precautions should be incorporated into a sound stretching program:

- Warm up using a slow jog or fast walk before stretching vigorously.
- To increase flexibility, overload or stretch the muscle beyond its normal range but not to the point of pain.
- Stretch only to the point where you feel tightness or resistance to stretch or perhaps some discomfort. Stretching should not be painful.
- Increases in range of motion will be specific to whatever joint is being stretched.
- Exercise caution when stretching muscles that surround painful joints. Pain is an indication that something is wrong and should not be ignored.
- Avoid overstretching the ligaments that surround joints.
- Exercise caution when stretching the low back and neck. Exercises that compress the vertebrae and their discs may cause damage.
- Stretch those muscles that are tight and inflexible.
- Strengthen those muscles that are weak and loose.
- Always stretch with control regardless of the stretching technique.
- Be sure to continue normal breathing during a stretch. Do not hold your breath.
- Static and PNF techniques are most often recommended for individuals who want to improve their range of motion.
- Ballistic stretching should be done only by those who are already flexible and/or are accustomed to stretching and only after static stretching.
- Dynamic stretching appears to be the most effective technique to use as a warm-up prior to engaging in physical activity.
- Stretching should be done at least three times per week to see minimal improvement. It is recommended that you stretch between five and six times per week to see maximum results.

Occasionally a person develops so much bulk that the physical size of the muscle prevents a normal range of motion. When strength training is not properly done, movement can be impaired. However, there is no reason to believe that weight training, if done properly through a full range of motion, will impair flexibility. Proper strength training probably improves dynamic flexibility and, if combined with a rigorous stretching program, can greatly enhance powerful and coordinated movements that are essential for success in many activities. In all cases a heavy weight training program should be accompanied by a strong flexibility program (Figure 6-4).

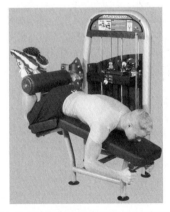

FIGURE 6-4. STRENGTH TRAINING AND FLEXIBILITY.

If strength training is combined with flexibility exercise, a full range of motion may be maintained.

STRETCHING EXERCISES

Figures 6-5 to 6-17 illustrate stretching exercises that may be used to improve flexibility at specific joints throughout the body. The exercises described may be done statically or with slight modification; they may also be done with a partner using a PNF technique.

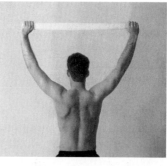

A

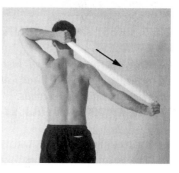

B

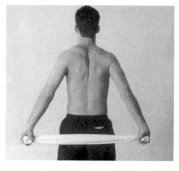

C

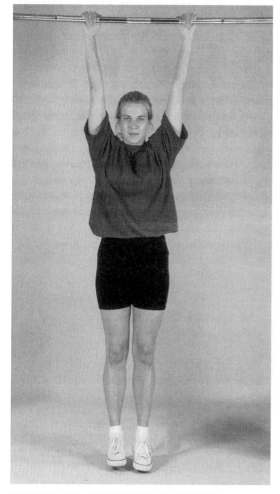

FIGURE 6-5. ARM HANG EXERCISE.
Muscles stretched: entire shoulder girdle complex.
Instructions: Using a chinning bar, simply hang with shoulders and arms fully extended for 30 seconds. Repeat five times.

FIGURE 6-6. SHOULDER TOWEL STRETCH EXERCISE.
Muscles stretched: internal and external rotators.
Instructions: A, Begin by holding towel above head shoulder-width apart. B, Try to pull towel down behind back, first with left hand then with right; you should end up in position C. Reverse order to get back to position A. Repeat five times on each side.

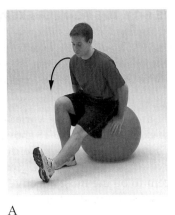

A

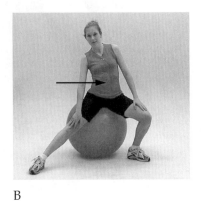

B

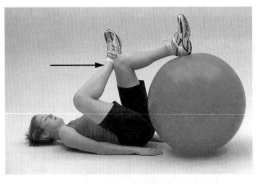

C

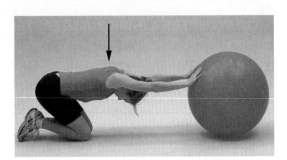

D

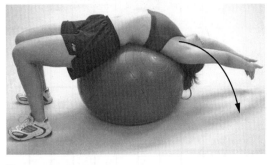

E

FIGURE 6-18. STATIC STRETCHING USING A STABILITY BALL.
A, Hamstrings. B, Hip adductors. C, piriformis muscle. D, latissimus dorsi. E, abdominal muscles.

checklist that can help you monitor your stretching program.

Regardless of the stretching exercise or technique you are using, the same principles of overload and progression that were discussed in Chapter 5 relative to strength training must be applied to stretching. To see improvement in range of motion, the muscle must be "overloaded" or stretched to a point where there is some discomfort, but stretching should stop short of causing pain. As the muscle gradually accommodates to the demands of a stretching

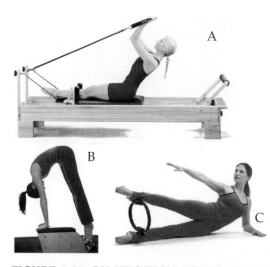

FIGURE 6-20. PILATES TECHNIQUES USING EQUIPMENT.
A, *Reformer.* *B*, *Wunda chair.* *C*, *Magic ring.*

illness is related to poor mental attitudes, posture, and diet. Practitioners of yoga maintain that stress can be reduced through combined mental and physical approaches. Yoga can help an individual cope with stress-induced behaviors like overeating, hypertension, and smoking. Yoga's meditative aspects are believed to help alleviate psychosomatic illnesses. Yoga aims to unite the body and mind to reduce stress. Various body postures and breathing exercises are used in this activity.

Hatha-yoga uses a number of positions through which the practitioner may progress, beginning with the simplest and moving to the more complex (Figure 6-21). The various positions are intended to increase mobility and flexibility. However, caution must be used when selecting yoga positions. Some positions

> **Yoga:** body postures and breathing exercises used to help reduce stress

exercise, the intensity of the stretch should be progressively increased. Over time, this gradual progression will lead to an increase in the range of motion.

ALTERNATIVE STRETCHING TECHNIQUES

Two exercise techniques, Pilates exercises and yoga, integrate some elements of stretching and flexibility into their philosophies of mind/body control.

THE PILATES METHOD

The Pilates method is a somewhat different approach to improving flexibility. This method has become extremely popular and widely used among personal fitness trainers and physical therapists. Pilates is an exercise technique devised by German-born Joseph Pilates, who established the first Pilates studio in the United States before World War II. The Pilates method is a conditioning program that improves muscle control, flexibility, coordination, strength, and tone. The basic principles of **Pilates exercise** are to make people more aware of their bodies as single integrated units, to improve alignment and breathing, and to increase efficiency of movement. Unlike other exercise programs, the Pilates method does not require the repetition of exercises but instead consists of a sequence of carefully performed movements (Figure 6-19) some of which are carried out on specially designed equipment (Figure 6-20). Each exercise is de-

> **Pilates exercise:** a sequence of carefully performed movements that stretch and strengthen muscles

signed to stretch and strengthen the muscles involved. There is a specific breathing pattern for each exercise to help direct energy to the areas being worked while relaxing the rest of the body.

The Pilates method works many of the deeper muscles together, improving coordination and balance, to achieve efficient and graceful movement. Instead of seeking an ideal or perfect body, the goal is for the practitioner to develop a healthy self-image, through the attainment of better posture, proper coordination, and improved flexibility. This method concentrates on alignment, lengthening all of the muscles of the body into a balanced whole, and building endurance and strength without putting undue stress on the lungs and heart. Pilates instructors believe that problems such as soft-tissue injuries can cause bad posture, which can lead to pain and discomfort. Pilates exercises aim to correct this.

Normally a beginner sees a Pilates instructor on a one-to-one basis for the first session. The instructor assesses the client's physical condition and asks the client about any problems and about the client's lifestyle. The client is then shown a series of exercises that take joints and muscles through a range of movement that is appropriate based on the client's needs. A class in a studio might involve working on specially designed equipment, primarily using resistance against tensioned springs, in order to isolate and develop specific muscle groups. Matwork classes utilize a repertoire of exercises on a floor mat only. This type of class has become very popular in health clubs and gyms and is often compared to other forms of body conditioning. In fact, the Pilates mat exercises are generally more subtle than mat exercises in most other conditioning classes.

YOGA

Yoga originated in India approximately 6,000 years ago. Its basic philosophy is that most

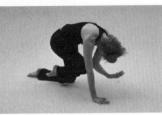

Start

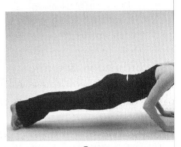

Start

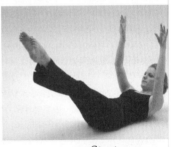

Start

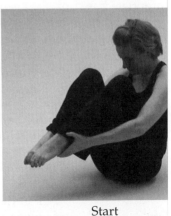

Start

FIGURE 6-19. PILATES FLOOR EXERCIS

A, Alternating arm, opposite leg extensions.
B, Push-up to a side plank. C, Alternating leg

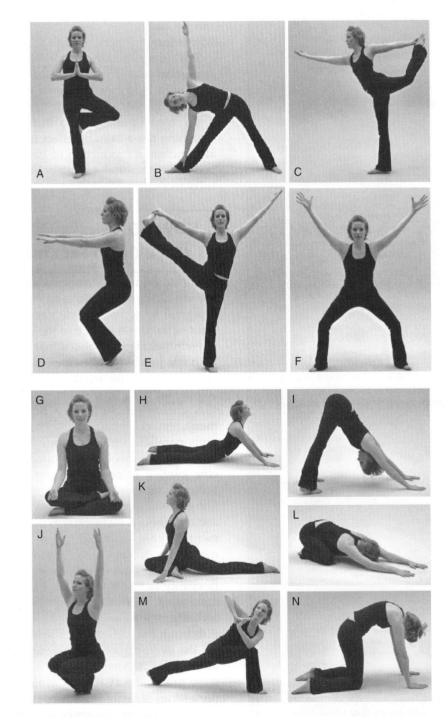

FIGURE 6-21. YOGA POSITIONS.
A, Tree. B, Triangle. C, Dancer. D, Chair. E, Extended hand to big toe. F, Big mountain. G, Lotus. H, Cobra.
I, Downward facing dog. J, Static squat. K, Pigeon. L, Child. M, Runner's lunge with twist. N, Cat.

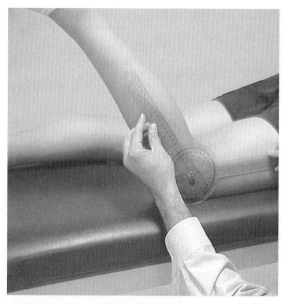

FIGURE 6-22. GONIOMETRIC MEASURE-MENT OF KNEE JOINT FLEXION.

good estimation of your overall flexibility. Lab Activities 6-1 through 6-3 will help you assess your existing flexibility.

SUMMARY

- Flexibility is the ability to move a joint or a series of joints smoothly through a full range of motion.
- Flexibility may be limited by fat or defects in bone structure, skin, connective tissue, ligaments, or muscles and tendons.
- Passive range of motion refers to the degree to which a joint may be passively moved to the end points in the range of motion, whereas active range of motion refers to movement through a portion of the range of motion resulting from active contraction.
- An agonist muscle is one that contracts to produce joint motion; the antagonist muscle is stretched with contraction of the agonist.
- Ballistic, static, proprioceptive neuromuscular facilitation (PNF) techniques, and

dynamic stretching have all been used as stretching techniques for improving flexibility.
- Pilates exercise and yoga offer two alternative approaches to stretching for improving flexibility.
- Strength training, if done correctly through a full range of motion, will probably improve flexibility.
- Measurement of joint flexibility is accomplished through the use of a goniometer.

SUGGESTED READINGS

Alter, M. J. 2004. *The science of flexibility,* 3rd ed. Champaign, IL: Human Kinetics.

Alpkaya, U., and D. Koceja. 2007. The effects of acute static stretching on reaction time and force. *Journal of Sports Medicine and Physical Fitness* 47(2):147–50.

Anderson, B. 2010. *Stretching.* Bolinas, CA: Shelter.

Bernardo, L. 2007. The effectiveness of Pilates training in healthy adults: An appraisal of the research literature. *Journal of Bodywork and Movement Therapies* 11(2): 106–10.

Blahnik, J. 2010. *Full body flexibility.* Champaign, IL: Human Kinetics.

Burke, D. G., C. J. Culligan, and L. E. Holt. 2000. The theoretical basis of proprioceptive neuromuscular facilitation. *Journal of Strength and Conditioning Research* 14(4):496–500.

Davis, R. 2010. Pilates and the science of human movement. *IDEA Fitness Journal.* 7(8):92.

De Deyne, P. G. 2001. Application of passive stretch and its implications for muscle fibers. *Physical Therapy* 81(2):819–27.

Dykema, R. 2011. *Yoga for fitness and wellness.* Florence, KY: Brooks Cole.

Ferreira, G., T. Nunes, and L. Teixeira. 2007. Gains in flexibility related to measures of muscular performance: Impact of flexibility on muscular performance. *Clinical Journal of Sport Medicine* 17(4):276–81.

Fitzgerald, M. 2001. Strength, endurance, flexibility: A Pilates home workout will leave you all three. *Men's Fitness* 17(10):74–79.

Hedrick, A. 2000. Dynamic flexibility training. *Strength and Conditioning Journal* 22(5):33–38.

Heyward, V. H. 2010. Assessing flexibility and designing stretching programs. In *Advanced fitness assessment and exercise prescription,* 6th ed. edited by V. H. Heyward. Champaign, IL: Human Kinetics.

Iyengar, B. 2008. *Yoga: The path to holistic health.* New York: Dorling Kindersley.

Kaplan, B., and M. Pierce. 2008.*Yoga for your life: A practice manual of breath and movement for everybody.* New York; Sterling Publishing.

Kirk, M., and B. Boon. 2005. *Hatha yoga illustrated.* Champaign, IL: Human Kinetics.

Kokkonen, J., A. Nelson, and C. Eldredge. 2007. Chronic static stretching improves exercise performance. *Medicine and Science in Sports and Exercise* 39(10): 1825-31.

Kovacs, M. 2009. *Dynamic stretching: The revolutionary new warm-up method to improve power, performance and range of motion.* Berkley, CA: Ulysses Press.

Kurz, T. 2003. *Stretching scientifically: A guide to flexibility training.* Island Port, VT: Stadion.

Lemay, M. 2003. *Essential stretch.* New York: Perigee Trade.

Mann, D., and C. Whedon. 2001. Functional stretching: Implementing a dynamic stretching program. *Athletic Therapy Today* 6(3):10–13.

Manoel, M., M. Harris-Love, J. Danoff 2008. Acute effects of static, dynamic, and proprioceptive neuromuscular facilitation stretching on muscle power. *Journal of Strength & Conditioning Research* 22(5):1528.

Markil, N., and C. Geithner. 2010. Hatha Yoga. *ACSM's Health & Fitness Journal* 14(5):19.

McAtee, R. E. 2007. *Facilitated stretching.* Champaign, IL: Human Kinetics.

Mueller, D. 2002. Yoga therapy. *ACSM's Health and Fitness Journal* 6(1):18–24.

Nelson, R. T., and W. D. Bandy. 2004. Eccentric training and static stretching improve hamstring flexibility of high school males. *Journal of Athletic Training* 39(3):254–58.

Newson, A. 2010. *Get fit for free with home workouts: Yoga and Pilates: workout routines to build strength, increase flexibility, enhance your vitality and save money,* Reader's Digest.

Parragon Publishing complete guide to pilates, yoga, meditation & stress relief. 2004. New York: Parragon Publishing.

Page, P. 2010. *Pilates illustrated.* Champaign, IL: Human Kinetics.

Pilates, J., and W. Miller. 2006 *A pilates' primer: The millennium edition: Return of life through contrology and your health.* New York: Bodymind Publishing.

Power, K., D. Behm, and F. Cahill. 2004. An acute bout of static stretching: Effects on force and jumping performance. *Medicine and Science in Sports and Exercise* 36(8):1389–96.

Riewald, S. 2004. Stretching the limits of our knowledge on stretching. *Strength and Conditioning Journal* 26(5):58–59.

Rubini, E., A. Costa, and P. Gomes. 2007. The effects of stretching on strength performance. *Sports Medicine* 37(3): 213.

Santana, J. C. 2004. Flexibility: More is not necessarily better. *Strength and Conditioning Journal* 26(1):14–15.

Siler, B. 2005. *Your ultimate pilates challenge: At the gym. on the mat and on the move.* New York, Broadway Books.

Small, K. 2008. A systematic review into the efficacy of static stretching as part of a warm-up for the prevention of exercise-related injury. *Research in Sports Medicine* 16(3):213.

Stewart, K. 2001. Pilates for beginners. New York: Harper Resource.

Tracker, S. B., D. F. Gilchrist, D. F. Stroup, and C. D. Kimsey Jr. 2004. The impact of *stretching* on sports injury risk: A systematic review of the literature. *Medicine and Science in Sports and Exercise* 36(3):371–78.

Tubecki, E. 2002. The world of Pilates. *Women's Fitness and Sport* 8(2):31–32.

Ungaro, A. 2010. *Pilates practice companion.* New York: Dorling Kindersley.

Yoga and pilates more popular on their own. 2007. *IDEA Finess Journal* 4(5): 18.

Young, W. 2007. The use of static stretching in warm-up for training and competition. *International Journal of Sports Physiology & Performance* 2 (2): 212.

SUGGESTED WEB SITES

Brad Appleton's Stretching and Flexibility FAQ

This site presents frequently asked questions with answers on flexibility and stretching. It tells you everything you ever wanted to know.
www.stretching.bradapp.net

STOTT PILATES the contemporary approach to . . . Pilates exercise

This site provides information on Pilates equipment, educational programs, registered instructors, and a forum for posing questions about Pilates.
www.stottpilates.com

The Yoga Site—Web site directory

This online yoga resource center features a free teacher directory, posture info, Yoga Therapy Report, style guide, Q and A, retreats, books, links, and more.
www.yogasite.com

Welcome to Pilates

The Pilates Method is a conditioning program that improves muscle control, flexibility, coordination, strength and tone.
www.pilates.com

Name   Section   Date

PURPOSE   This test measures the flexibility of the lower back muscles and the hip extensors (that is, the hamstrings and gluteals).

PROCEDURE   Sit with the legs together, knees flat on the floor, and feet flat against some vertical surface. Bend forward at the waist and reach as far forward as possible with fingers (Figure 6-23).

Your score is determined by measuring the number of inches you can reach either in front of or beyond the vertical surface.

To determine your classification, see Table 6-2.

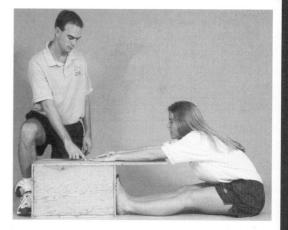

FIGURE 6-23. TRUNK AND HIP FLEXION TEST.
Feet are placed flat against a box with head up.

TABLE 6-2 FLEXIBILITY IN TRUNK AND HIP FLEXION (SIT AND REACH)		
Classification	**Men**	**Women**
Poor	0 in	0 in
Average	1–3 in	2–4 in
Good	4–6 in	5–7 in
Excellent	7 in	8 in

Name   Section   Date

PURPOSE   This test measures the flexibility of the abdominal and hip flexor muscles.

PROCEDURE   Lie in a prone position on the floor. Have a partner hold the legs and hips to the ground. Grasp your hands behind the neck, inhale, lift the upper trunk as high off the floor as possible, and hold (Figure 6-24).

Your score is determined by measuring the distance from the chin to the floor. To determine your classification, see Table 6-3.

Caution: This test should be avoided for a student who has back pain.

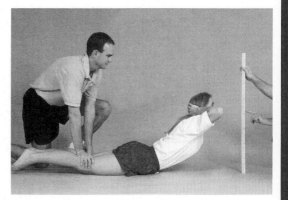

FIGURE 6-24. TRUNK EXTENSION TEST.

TABLE 6-3 FLEXIBILITY IN TRUNK AND HIP FLEXION (SIT AND REACH)		
Classification	**Men**	**Women**
Poor	16 in	17 in
Average	17–18 in	18–19 in
Good	19–21 in	20–23 in
Excellent	22 in	24 in

Name   Section   Date

PURPOSE   This test measures the flexibility of the shoulder flexors.

PROCEDURE Lie prone on the floor with arms extended over the head while holding the hands together. Raise hands as high as possible, with the face and chest kept flat on the floor; hold (Figure 6-25).

Your score is determined by measuring the distance from the hands to the ground. To determine your classification, see Table 6-4.

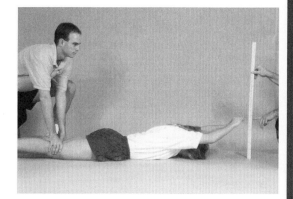

FIGURE 6-25. SHOULDER LIFT TEST.

TABLE 6-4		
FLEXIBILITY OF THE SHOULDER JOINT		
Classification	**Men**	**Women**
Poor	0–19 in	0–20 in
Average	20–22 in	21–23 in
Good	23–25 in	24–26 in
Excellent	26 in	27 in

CHAPTER 7

Eating Right

Objectives

After completing this chapter, you should be able to do the following:

- Identify the six classes of nutrients.
- Describe the major function of the nutrients.
- Analyze your diet for nutritional quality using U.S. Dietary Guidelines and MyPlate.
- Explain the relationship of nutrition to physical performance.

WHY DO YOU NEED TO KNOW ABOUT NUTRITION?

"**S**ports drinks," "anabolic amino acids," "antioxidants," "fat burners" —it seems that every day you read or hear about the health benefits of some nutrition-related product or service. **Nutrition** "experts" promote their latest books on radio talk shows, salespeople in health food stores praise the virtues of nutrient supplements, and friends give advice about diets that guarantee to melt pounds fast. Nutrition appears to be the key that unlocks the door to a healthy, more attractive body. How true are all of the nutrition claims about foods, nutrients, or diet plans? What role does nutrition play in maximizing fitness? Lab Activity 7-1 will help you determine how much you know about nutrition. By understanding the basics of nutrition, you will be more likely to recognize the many forms of nutritional misinformation. And, armed with some

basic nutrition information, you will be able to identify "weak" areas of your diet and work to strengthen them. Are you eating a nutritious diet now? Lab Activity 7-2 will help you assess your eating patterns and find out whether or not you are currently eating a nutritious diet.

> **nutrition:** the science of certain food substances

KEY TERMS

nutrition	*overnutrition*
diet	*diuretics*
nutrients	*nutrient dense*
macronutrients	*requirement*
micronutrients	*recommendation*
deficiencies	*foodborne illness*

BASIC PRINCIPLES OF NUTRITION

What do you think of when you hear the word *diet?* Although many people think of losing weight, **diet** actually refers to your usual food selections. Everyone is on a diet! When a person eats less food in an effort to lose weight, he or she is on a weight reduction diet. Nutrition is the science of certain food substances, **nutrients,** and what they do in your body. Nutrients perform three major roles:

1. Growth, repair, and maintenance of all body cells
2. Regulation of body processes
3. Supply of energy for cells

Fit List 7-1 summarizes the various nutrients, which are categorized into six major classes: carbohydrates, fats (often called lipids), proteins, vitamins, minerals, and water. Carbohydrates, fats and proteins are most often referred to as **macronutrients,** from which energy is derived. Vitamins, minerals, and water are classified as **micronutrients,** which are necessary for regulating bodily functions. Most foods are actually mixtures of these nutrients. Although we think of bread as being a carbohydrate food, it supplies fats, proteins, and other nutrients too. Some nutrients can be made by the body; an *essential* nutrient must be supplied by the diet. Not all substances in foods are considered nutrients. For example, caffeine is found in some foods and beverages. Caffeine has definite effects on the body, but we can live without it. Furthermore, there is no such thing as a perfect food; that is, no single natural food contains all of the nutrients needed for health.

Without an adequate supply of nutrients, cells soon lose their ability to perform their jobs. Eventually the rest of the body is affected, and various health disorders called nutritional **deficiencies** develop. Thanks to our varied food supply, cases of people suf-

FIT LIST 7-1

Essential Nutrients

Macronutrients

- Carbohydrates
- Fat
- Protein

Micronutrients

- Vitamins
- Minerals
- Water

fering from nutritional deficiencies are uncommon in the United States. Nevertheless, some Americans consume diets that are borderline deficient in certain nutrients. Occasionally, days with hectic schedules often result in careless eating or skipped meals. If your usual diet is good, it is unlikely that a few "off days" will lead to the development of a nutritional deficiency disease. However, if your diet is consistently of low quality, you run the risk of not being able to function at your peak level. Also, you could develop a deficiency disorder.

diet: refers to the types of food substances consumed

nutrients: perform three major roles including growth, repair, and maintenance of all body cells; regulation of body processes; and supplying energy for cells

macronutrients: carbohydrates, fats, proteins which provide energy

micronutrients: vitamins, minerals, and water which regulate bodily functions

deficiencies: consuming an inadequate supply of nutrients eventually affects the cells' ability to function and disease results

Just as low levels of nutrients can lead to health problems, nutrient excesses create trouble for your body. **Overnutrition,** eating too much food or specific nutrients, is common in the United States. Eating more food than needed can lead to obesity, which will be discussed in Chapter 8. Many nutrients are toxic (poisonous) when taken in large doses. However, it is difficult to obtain toxic levels of nutrients by consuming a varied diet. Most cases of nutrient overdoses are the result of overzealous self-treatment with vitamin/mineral supplements. People think that nutrient supplements are foods and therefore perfectly safe to consume in large quantities. However, the body is designed to obtain its nutrients from foods, not supplement pills or powders.

Running your body requires energy. This energy is supplied by the carbohydrates, fats, and proteins found in foods. Alcohol also provides energy, but it is not a nutrient. The energy value of food is measured by calories. Fats are the most concentrated source of calories in our diet. A gram of fat (there are about 28 grams in an ounce) supplies 9 calories. Carbohydrates and proteins each contribute 4 calories per gram. Alcohol, the nonnutrient, supplies 7 calories per gram. Water, vitamins, and minerals do not supply any calories and therefore no energy. Most Americans eat too much fat and too little carbohydrate. Scientists recommend that we alter the proportions of fat and carbohydrate in diets (Figure 7-1). Later in this chapter, we'll focus on energy use during physical activity.

overnutrition: eating too much food or taking too many supplements can have negative effects on your body

It is recommended that the diet consist of:
55% Carbohydrate
30% Fat
15% Protein

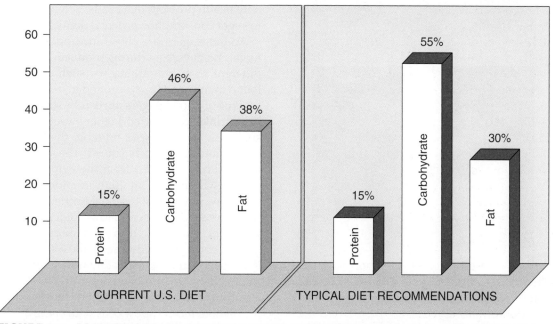

FIGURE 7-1. COMPARISON OF CALORIES FROM CARBOHYDRATES, FATS, AND PROTEINS.

THE MACRONUTRIENTS

▶Carbohydrates (CHO)

The major role of carbohydrates is to provide energy for the body. Although muscles run on fats and carbohydrates, nerve tissue, especially brain cells, prefer to burn carbohydrates for energy. People should consume at least 55 percent of their total caloric needs from carbohydrates. Both children and adults should consume at least 130 grams of carbohydrate each day. Carbohydrates are classified as simple (sugars) or complex (starch, glycogen, and most forms of fiber). Figure 7-2 shows the different sources of carbohydrates. Let's take a

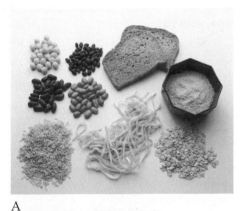

A

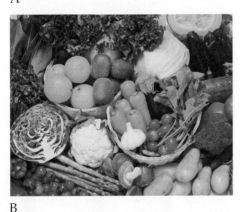

B

FIGURE 7-2. SOURCES OF CARBOHYDRATE.
A, Beans, bread, whole cereal, rice, pasta.
B, Raw fruits and vegetables.

closer look at some of the more important carbohydrates.

Sugars. Sugars are simple carbohydrates that occur as single-sugar or double-sugar chemical units. Glucose (blood sugar) is needed for fueling all cells. It is crucial for the body to maintain normal blood sugar levels. Food sources of glucose include fruits, syrups, and honey. Fructose (fruit sugar) occurs naturally in honey and is added to processed foods. Honey is often promoted as a substitute for sugar. However, honey supplies the same simple carbohydrates as table sugar, so there is no nutritional advantage in using honey as a sweetener. Milk sugar (lactose) and table sugar (sucrose) are double sugars. Table sugar is made from sugarcane and sugar beets, and it is nearly 100 percent pure carbohydrate. Because it contributes no other nutrients besides carbohydrate, you should limit the amount of table sugar eaten to no more than 10 percent of your total calories. If too much sugar is eaten, it displaces more nutritious foods from your diet. That's why sugary foods are referred to as "empty calories." Although table sugar has been blamed for causing hyperactivity in children, criminal behavior, and allergies, the only health problem that can be actually linked to sugar consumption is dental decay.

Added sugars are those incorporated into foods and beverages during production and are different from natural sugars, such as lactose found in milk and fructose found in fruits. Major sources of added sugars are candy, soft drinks, fruit drinks, pastries, and other sweets. Added sugars should comprise no more than 10 percent of total calories consumed. The suggested maximum level stems from the evidence that people whose diets are high in added sugars have lower intakes of essential nutrients.

Sugars are often referred to as "quick" energy. However, you really don't obtain energy the instant you eat a candy bar. While it's true that it takes more time to break down starches, table sugar still has to be broken down and its single-sugar units have to be absorbed by the digestive tract before it can supply cells with energy.

Starches. Starches are called complex carbohydrates because they consist of long chains of glucose units. Plants make starches, such as those found in whole cereal grains, potatoes, and beans. During digestion, the long starch chains are broken down, releasing individual glucose units that are absorbed. Individual glucose units combine to form glycogen, which is stored in muscle and the liver. When cells need energy, glycogen is broken down to release glucose.

Fiber. Your grandparents knew the importance of eating plenty of roughage to stay "regular" (avoid constipation). We now call roughage "fiber." There are many different types of fiber, but they share the common characteristic of being from plant foods. Although most forms are complex carbohydrates, fiber cannot be digested in the small intestine, so it moves through the digestive tract relatively unchanged. Rich sources of fiber include raw fruits, raw vegetables, whole grain breads and cereals, nuts, beans, and peas.

Researchers believe that our diet does not supply enough fiber. They think that low-fiber diets may be responsible for intestinal problems, such as hemorrhoids, colon cancer, and diverticulosis. A common health problem, hemorrhoids are swollen rectal veins that can cause pain and bleeding. Colon cancer (cancer of the large intestine) is a major cause of cancer deaths in the United States. Diverticulosis is a common condition in which small "blowouts" (pouches) form in the wall of the large intestine. These pouches can become infected (diverticulitis) and cause serious health problems.

Fiber may help prevent these conditions because certain forms attract water. This helps to form large, bulky stools that are easier to eliminate during bowel movements. People consuming diets rich in fiber are not as likely to experience constipation. Therefore, instead of relying on laxatives for simple cases of constipation, just eat more fiber-rich foods!

Besides helping to prevent constipation, certain forms of fiber may help lower blood cholesterol levels. High blood cholesterol levels are a major risk factor for cardiovascular diseases. The fiber from whole oats, and raw fruits and vegetables is recommended for its cholesterol-lowering ability. These forms of fiber seem to interfere with cholesterol absorption from the intestinal tract. When less cholesterol is absorbed, less enters the bloodstream and causes trouble in your arteries. The recommended daily intake for total fiber for adults 50 years and younger is set at 38 grams for men and 25 grams for women. The fiber recommendations are based on studies that show an increased risk for heart disease among people whose diets are low in fiber are consumed.

"Total fiber" is defined as the combination of "dietary" and "functional" fiber. Dietary fiber is the edible, nondigestible component of carbohydrates and lignin naturally found in plant food. Foods with dietary fiber include whole cereal bran, flaked corn cereal, sweet potatoes, legumes, and onions. Functional fibers are fiber sources that have been shown to have health benefits similar to those of dietary fiber, but these fibers are isolated or extracted from natural sources or are synthetic. An example would be pectin extracted from citrus peel and used as a gel as the basis for jams and jellies. The definition of functional fiber aims to exclude fiberlike products, whether extracted or synthesized, that cannot be shown to have proven health benefits.

▶ Fats

Recently, fat has received a lot of negative publicity for a nutrient that is extremely important in the diet. Extra calories supplied by dietary carbohydrates, proteins, and fats may all be converted to triglyceride and stored in adipose cells as body fat for future energy needs. These body fat deposits cushion organs and give the body rounded contours (especially in women). Fat supplies a major portion of the energy used by muscles. Furthermore, certain types of fat cannot be formed by the body and are essential for health. We like to include fat in our meals because it makes eating more enjoyable by contributing flavor and texture. However, most Americans eat too much fat, a major factor in the development of obesity and cardiovascular diseases.

Saturated versus Unsaturated Fats. Depending on their chemical nature, fats may be either saturated or unsaturated. In general, unsaturated fat is from plants and is liquid at room temperature. Canola, peanut, olive, and vegetable oils from corn, cottonseed, sunflower, and soybean sources are rich in unsaturated fat.

Monounsaturated and polyunsaturated fatty acids reduce blood cholesterol levels and thus lower the risk of heart disease when they replace saturated fats in the diet. However, polyunsaturates lower the "good" type of cholesterol or high-density lipoprotein (HDL) rather than the "bad" type called low-density lipoprotein (LDL) and thus monounsaturated fatty acids are a better choice. People must get two types of polyunsaturated fatty acids, known as omega-3 fatty acid and omega-6 fatty acid, from the foods they consume because neither is synthesized in the body. A lack of either one will result in symptoms of deficiency, including scaly skin and dermatitis. Recommended intakes for omega-3 fatty acid, which is present in high levels in vegetable oils such as safflower oil or corn oil, in fish oil, in salmon, black cod, and in walnuts and pumpkin seeds are 17 grams per day for men 12 grams per day for women (about 1 tablespoon) based on average intakes in the United States. For omega-6 fatty acid, which is found in milk, nuts and seeds, and some vegetable oils such as soybean and flaxseed oils, the recommendations are 1.6 and 1.1 grams per day (less than ½ teaspoon) for men and women, respectively.

Saturated fats are derived mainly from animal sources. These include the fat in meats, such as beef, pork, and lamb, as well as much of the fat in eggs and dairy products—cream, butter, milk, and cheese. Coconut and palm

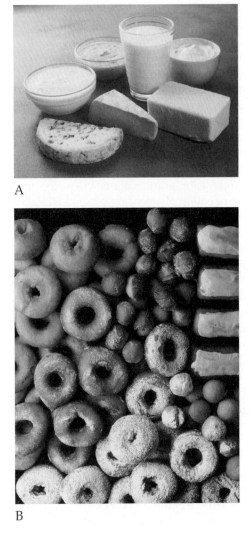

A

B

FIGURE 7-3. FOOD SOURCES OF FAT.
A, Oils, creams, buttermilk, and cheese. B, Cookies and doughnuts are high in transfat.

oils, unlike most plant oils, are highly saturated (Figure 7-3).

Cholesterol. Saturated fat and cholesterol are believed to be responsible for creating blocked arteries that lead to cardiovascular diseases. Cholesterol is a fat-related substance that is only found in animal foods. People think that cholesterol is "bad," but actually it is very important. Even if you avoid all foods that contain cholesterol, your body would make what it needs. The body makes vitamin D and its own steroid hormones from cholesterol. However, when low-density cholesterol (LDL) becomes too high, the risk of developing cardiovascular diseases also increases. Saturated fat can raise the amount of low-density lipoprotein (LDL) and the level of "bad" cholesterol, thus increasing their risk for heart disease.

Trans fatty acids have physical properties generally resembling saturated fatty acids, and their presence tends to harden oils. Often found in cookies, doughnuts, crackers, dairy products, meats, and fast foods, trans fatty acids increase the risk of heart disease by boosting levels of LDL (Figure 7-3B). Because they are not essential and provide no known health benefit, there is no safe level of trans fatty acids and people should eat as little of them as possible while consuming a nutritionally adequate diet.

Many studies show that eating trans fat, saturated fat, and cholesterol seems to increase blood cholesterol levels. Beef, milk, butter, and cheese are rich sources of saturated fat. Also, foods from animal sources, including dairy products, egg yolks, liver, and meats, contribute lots of cholesterol. Margarine made from plant fats (oils) is a good substitute for butter because all plant oils are cholesterol-free. Unsaturated fats do not raise blood cholesterol levels like saturated fats. Because certain kinds of saturated fats contribute to the development of high blood cholesterol levels, it is wise to reduce your consumption of foods made with tropical oils.

Fat Intake. Most experts believe it is more important to cut back on your total fat intake than worry about eating specific types of fats. The typical American gets about 40 percent of total calories from fat. Experts think that this is too much and recommend levels of about 25 to 30 percent. These experts also suggest that cholesterol intake be limited to around 300 milligrams a day. Considering that one egg yolk

has about 250 milligrams of cholesterol, this recommendation may be tough to meet if you like to eat eggs or products made from eggs every day. The American Heart Association recommends that you eat no more than four eggs a week. The good news is that food consumption surveys show that we have cut back on our saturated fat and cholesterol consumption. This appears to be helping to reduce the number of cardiovascular deaths, especially in younger people. Although not all of this decline is due to eating fewer eggs and drinking more skim milk, reducing overall fat consumption is believed to be partially responsible.

▶ Protein

Protein is needed for growth, repair, and maintenance of all cells. Major body structures, such as bone, muscles, and organs, are made of protein. Your skin, hair, and nails are made up of protein. Proteins are needed to make the enzymes that speed up chemical reactions, certain hormones, and components of the immune system. A small amount of protein can be used for energy, too. However, the body prefers to use carbohydrate and fat for energy, conserving protein for its other important functions.

Your body's need for protein increases during periods of growth. For example, protein needs are very high in infancy, during childhood and adolescent growth spurts, and during pregnancy. Breast-feeding women need more protein to supply their nursing infant's needs. During active body-building, athletes have a greater need. However, the typical American diet contains plenty of protein to meet an athlete's needs.

The recommended amount of protein is based on body weight; the typical adult recommendation is 0.8 gram of protein per kilogram of body weight. To determine how many grams of protein are recommended for your weight, take your weight in pounds and divide by 2.2 to obtain your weight in kilograms. Multiply that number times 0.8 to obtain the grams of protein that meet recommended levels of intake. Dietary surveys show that Americans eat more protein than needed, well over 100 grams per day. Much of that protein is from fatty animal sources. Your diet should contain about 12 to 15 percent of its calories from protein.

Proteins are made up of smaller units called amino acids. There are about 20 amino acids in the body. Nine essential amino acids must be supplied by the diet; the remainder can be made by the body. In order to grow, you need to have all of the essential amino acids available. If the diet is protein-deficient, growth slows or stops. During digestion, food proteins are broken down and amino acids are released and absorbed. Most animal proteins, such as those found in meat, fish, poultry, and eggs, contain ample amounts of the essential amino acids and are called complete or high-quality proteins (Figure 7-4).

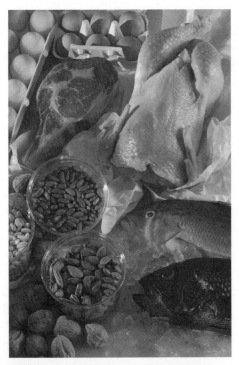

FIGURE 7-4. SOURCES OF PROTEIN.
Meat, chicken, fish, eggs, and nuts.

Plant proteins, such as those found in beans, peas, nuts, seeds, and cereals, also contribute protein to the diet. For example, a slice of bread supplies 2 grams of protein. Plant food proteins are incomplete; that is, they are not good sources of the essential amino acids. However, in combination with each other, plant proteins can be good sources of the essential amino acids. The quality improves further when they are mixed with proteins from animal sources of food. Many of our favorite food combinations, such as cereal and milk, macaroni and cheese, chili con carne, and tuna or chicken noodle casserole, combine small amounts of high-quality animal proteins with larger amounts of plant proteins. You do not have to eat large portions of animal foods to obtain enough protein.

Vegetarianism is an alternative to the usual American diet that is rich in animal sources of food. All vegetarians use plant foods to form the foundation of their diets; animal foods are either excluded or included to varying degrees. People who choose to follow vegetarian diets can certainly get all the nutrients they need, but to do so they must eat a wide variety of foods to meet their nutritional needs. Generally vegetarian diets tend to be a healthier choice than the typical American diet. Vegetarian diets are usually lower in fat and higher in fiber and antioxidant nutrients than typical American food selections.

THE MICRONUTRIENTS

▶Water

Water is the most essential nutrient (Figure 7-5). You can live for weeks, months, even years without the other nutrients, but you will perish after a few days without water. About 60 percent of the adult's body weight is water. Many materials used in the body are water soluble, that is, dissolved in water. Although water does not supply any calories, an adequate supply of water is needed for energy

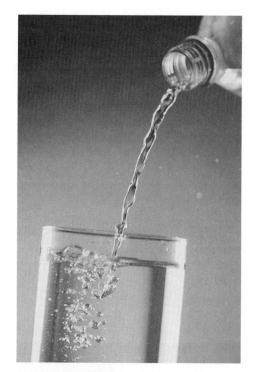

FIGURE 7-5. WATER.
Water is the single most essential nutrient.

production. Water also takes part in digestion and maintaining the proper environment inside and outside of cells. When your body burns fuels for energy, it produces a great deal of heat energy. Sweating is how your body uses water to keep itself from overheating.

A gross estimate is that an average adult requires a minimum of 2.5 liters, or about 10 glasses, of water a day. Because it is so vital, the healthy body carefully manages its internal water levels. When body water weight drops by 1 to 2 percent, you begin to feel thirsty. By drinking water, you help your internal water levels return to normal. If you ignore thirst signals and body water continues to decrease, dehydration results. People who are dehydrated cannot generate energy and feel weak. Other symptoms include nausea, vomiting, and

fainting. If water losses become too great, the individual dies.

Dehydration is more likely to occur when you are outdoors and heavily sweating while engaging in some strenuous activity. To prevent dehydration, make sure you replace the lost water by drinking plenty of fluids. Don't rely on thirst as a signal that it's time to have a drink. Many people ignore their thirst, or, if they do heed it, they don't drink enough. Avoid replacing water with caffeinated beverages and alcohol; these fluids act as **diuretics,** pulling more vital water out of your body.

Most adults can benefit from drinking more water. You don't need to buy canned or bottled waters. Drinking tap water may not impress people but it will quench your thirst for a lot less money.

Sport Drinks. Do you need to drink special sport beverages? These sport drinks are very popular and are widely marketed to the American public.

During physical activity it is essential to replace fluids lost through sweating. Replacing lost fluids with a sport drink is more effective than using water alone. Research has shown that because of the flavor you are likely to drink more sport drinks than water. Sport drinks quickly replace both fluids and electrolytes lost in sweat that provide energy to the working muscles. Water is a good "thirst quencher," but it is not a good "rehydrator" because water "turns off" your thirst before you're completely rehydrated. Water also "turns on" the kidneys prematurely so you lose fluid in the form of urine much more quickly than when drinking a sport drink. A small amount of sodium and an even smaller amount of potassium allows your body to hold onto the fluid you consume rather than losing it through urine.

diuretics: foods or chemicals that eliminate natural fluids from your body

Not all sport drinks are the same. How a sport drink is formulated dictates how well it works in providing rapid rehydration and energy. The optimal level of carbohydrate is 14 grams per 8 ounces of water for quickest absorption and energy. It has been shown that a sport drink can be effective in improving performance during both endurance activities and short-term high-intensity activities such as soccer, basketball, and tennis that last from 30 minutes to an hour. Table 7-1 compares the amount of calories, carbohydrates, sodium, and potassium in a variety of fluid replacement drinks.

Oxygenated Bottled Water. Bottled waters with added oxygen are a recent trend in the beverage market. Athletes have touted the benefits of different brands, and such advertising attempts to persuade us that this extra oxygen will lead to improved performance.

What's the reason for adding oxygen to water, and does the extra oxygen do anything for sport performance? According to manufacturers, oxygenated water delivers extra oxygen to the body to enhance metabolism and improve endurance. The bottom line is that manufacturers' claims have lots of theory and very little substance. Human physiology and science show us that oxygenated water won't elevate oxygen levels in the blood or muscle. Such claims are enticing, but they don't hold up when it comes to improving muscle metabolism and performance.

▶ Vitamins

Like carbohydrates, proteins, and fats, vitamins are organic compounds that are essential for health. Although required in very small amounts, vitamins perform many roles, prima-

TABLE 7-1
FLUID REPLACEMENT BEVERAGES

Beverage (per 8 oz. serving)	Calories	Carbohydrates (CHO gms)	CHO %	Sodium (mg)	Potassium (mg)	Carbohydrate Ingredient
Gatorade®	50	14	6	110	30	Sucrose, glucose, fructose
Powerade®	70	19	8	55	30	High fructose corn syrup, glucose polymers
AllSport®	70	19	8	55	55	High fructose corn syrup
Exceed®	70	17	7	50	45	Glucose polymers, fructose
Coca-Cola®	103	27	11	6	0	High fructose corn syrup, sucrose
Orange Juice	104	25	10	6	436	Fructose, sucrose, glucose

Modified from http://www.nutritionexpert.com/sportsdrinks.html

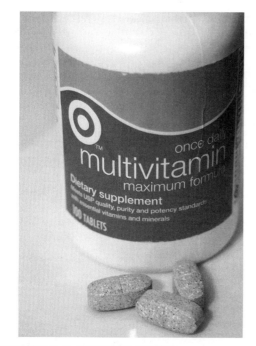

FIGURE 7-6. MULTIVITAMINS.
Vitamins in very small amounts are essential for regulating the bodily processes.

rily as regulators of body processes. Humans need 13 vitamins for health (Figure 7-6). You are probably familiar with their letter names, such as vitamins A, B_1, and C. Today, many are referred to by their chemical names. For example, *thiamin* is the chemical name for vitamin B_1. During the past 50 years, no new vitamins have been discovered, but scientists are still learning about their many roles.

People mistakenly think that vitamins provide energy. In fact, the body cannot break them down to release energy. However, many of the B-vitamins participate in the various chemical steps that release energy from carbohydrate, fat, and protein. Table 7-2 provides information about vitamins, including rich food sources, deficiency symptoms, and toxicity potential from high doses.

Vitamin deficiencies are uncommon in the United States. A few groups of people, such as the elderly, alcoholics, and those who severely restrict their food intake, are at risk of developing vitamin deficiency diseases. However, nutrition experts are concerned that many people are nutritionally on the "borderline," that is, close to being deficient. We may be too busy to plan nutritious meals, and we rely too much on vending machines or fast food restaurants. Furthermore, many young people are smoking cigarettes and drinking alcoholic beverages, behaviors that increase vitamin and other nutrient needs.

Fat-Soluble Vitamins. Vitamins are grouped according to the ability to dissolve in water or fat. Vitamins A, E, D, and K dissolve in fat rather than water. Extra amounts of the fat-soluble vitamins are not easy to eliminate from the body in urine, which is mostly water. Instead they are stored in the liver or body fat until needed. This feature makes them potentially toxic, so be careful if you choose to take supplements of these vitamins. See Table 7-2 for information about the fat-soluble vitamins, including their toxicity potential.

Water-Soluble Vitamins. The water-soluble vitamins, B-complex and C, dissolve in water. This feature makes it easier for the body to eliminate excesses in urine. Many of the B-vitamins help produce energy from carbohydrates, proteins, and fats. When these vitamins are unavailable, every cell cannot generate energy to perform its numerous jobs. The result is feeling tired. Don't think that by taking extra amounts of the B-vitamins that you'll have more energy. Once your cells have enough of the B-vitamins, any additional doses will not make cells generate extra amounts of energy. Although excesses of most water-soluble vitamins are excreted in urine, high doses of certain water-soluble vitamins have been linked to toxic effects. See Table 7-2 for information about the water-soluble vitamins, including their toxicity potential.

Antioxidant Nutrients. Nutrition experts have generated excitement and controversy over reports that certain nutrients, called

TABLE 7-2
VITAMINS

Vitamin	Major Function	Most Reliable Sources	Deficiency	Excess (Toxicity)
A	Maintains skin and other cells that line the inside of the body; bone and tooth development; growth; vision in dim light	Liver, milk, egg yolk, deep green and yellow fruits and vegetables	Night blindness, dry skin, growth failure	Headaches, nausea, loss of hair, dry skin, diarrhea
D	Normal bone growth and development; helps with absorption of calcium	Exposure to sunlight; fortified dairy products; eggs and fish liver oils	"Rickets" in children—defective bone formation leading to deformed bones	Appetite loss, weight loss, failure to grow
E	Prevents destruction of polyunsaturated fats caused by exposure to oxidizing agents; protects cell membranes from destruction	Vegetable oils, some in fruits and vegetables, whole grains	Breakage of red blood cells leading to anemia	Nausea and diarrhea; interferes with vitamin K if vitamin D is also deficient. Not as toxic as other fat-soluble vitamins
K	Production of blood-clotting substances	Green leafy vegetables; normal bacteria that live in intestines produce K that is absorbed	Increased bleeding time	
Thiamin	Needed for release of energy from carbohydrates, fats, and proteins	Cereal products, pork, peas, and dried beans	Lack of energy, nerve problem	
Riboflavin	Energy from carbohydrates, fats, and proteins	Milk, liver, fruits and vegetables, enriched breads and cereals	Dry skin, cracked lips	

Continued

TABLE 7-2
VITAMINS—CONT.

Vitamin	Major Function	Most Reliable Sources	Deficiency	Excess (Toxicity)
Niacin	Energy from carbohydrates, fats, and proteins	Liver, meat, poultry, peanut butter, legumes, enriched breads and cereals	Skin problems, diarrhea, mental depression, and eventually death (rarely occurs in U.S.)	Skin flushing, intestinal upset, nervousness, intestinal ulcers
B_6	Metabolism of protein; production of hemoglobin	White meats, whole grains, liver, egg yolk, bananas	Poor growth, anemia	Severe loss of coordination from nerve damage
B_{12}	Production of genetic material; maintains central nervous system	Foods of animal origin	Neurological problems, anemia	
Folate (Folic acid)	Production of genetic material	Wheat germ, liver, yeast, mushrooms, green leafy vegetables, fruits	Anemia	
C (Ascorbic acid)	Formation and maintenance of connective tissue; tooth and bone formation; immune function; helps with absorption of iron	Fruits and vegetables	"Scurvy" (rare); swollen joints, bleeding gums, fatigue, bruising	Kidney stones, diarrhea
Pantothenic acid	Energy from carbohydrates, fats, proteins	Widely found in foods	Not observed in humans under normal conditions	
Biotin	Use of fats	Widely found in foods	Rare under normal conditions	

antioxidants, may prevent premature aging, certain cancers, heart disease, and other health problems. An antioxidant protects vital cell components from the destructive effects of certain agents, including oxygen. Vitamin C, vitamin E, and beta carotene are antioxidants. Beta carotene is a plant pigment that is found in dark green, deep yellow, or orange fruits and vegetables. The body can convert beta carotene to vitamin A. Since the early 1980s, evidence has accumulated about the benefits of a diet rich in the antioxidant nutrients. Fit List 7-2 lists foods rich in the antioxidant nutrients.

Some experts believe people should increase their intake of antioxidants, even if it means taking supplements. Others are more cautious. Excess beta carotene pigments circulate throughout the body and may turn your skin yellow. However the pigment is not believed to be toxic like its nutrient cousin, vitamin A. On the other hand, increasing your intake of vitamins C and E is not without some risk. Excesses of vitamin C are not well absorbed; the excess is irritating to the intestines and causes diarrhea. Although less toxic than vitamins A or D, too much vitamin E causes health problems, as indicated in Table 7-2.

▶ Minerals

More than 20 mineral elements must be supplied by the diet. These include the minerals listed in Table 7-3. Other mineral elements are found in the body. The role of minerals is unclear. Minerals are needed for a variety of jobs, such as forming strong bones and teeth, helping to generate energy, activating enzymes, and maintaining water balance. Most minerals are stored in the body, especially in the bones and liver. Vitamins are stored in the liver, too. That explains why liver usually leads the list of most nutritious foods. Vitamins and minerals interact with one another—if you don't get enough of one, the other may not work the way it is supposed to.

Calcium. You are probably aware that calcium is needed for building strong bones and teeth, but it is also needed for nerve and muscle function. Milk products are rich in calcium, but many people do not like to drink milk. For young women, poor food choices and efforts to lose weight are believed to be responsible for low intakes of calcium. Over a lifetime, this may lead to osteoporosis, a condition in which the bones become less dense and break easily.

FIT LIST 7-2

Foods Rich in Antioxidants

Beta Carotene Foods

- Sweet potatoes
- Pumpkin
- Squash
- Carrots
- Red bell peppers
- Dark green vegetables
- Apricots
- Mango
- Cantaloupe

Vitamin C Foods

- Kiwi fruit
- Citrus fruits
- Berries
- Cantaloupe
- Honeydew
- Bell peppers
- Tomatoes
- Cabbage
- Broccoli

Vitamin E Foods

- Vegetable oils
- Nuts
- Seeds
- Margarine
- Wheat germ
- Olives
- Leafy greens
- Asparagus

Osteoporosis leads to loss of height, a humped-shaped upper back, and hip fractures that can result in disabling injuries and even death. The most-affected bones are those in the wrist, hip, and spine. Factors contributing to osteoporosis include heredity, cigarette smoking, menopause, lack of physical activity, and a lifetime of poor calcium intake.

The calcium in milk products is well absorbed by the body. To increase your dietary

TABLE 7-3
MINERALS OF MAJOR CONCERN

Vitamin	Major Function	Most Reliable Sources	Deficiency	Excess (Toxicity)
Calcium	Bone and tooth formation; blood clotting; muscle contraction; nerve function	Dairy products	May lead to osteoporosis	Calcium deposits in soft tissues
Phosphorus	Skeletal development; tooth formation	Meats, dairy products, and other protein-rich foods	Rarely seen	May contribute to the development of hypertension
Sodium	Maintenance of fluid balance	Salt (sodium chloride) added to foods and sodium-containing preservatives	Muscle cramps; fluid imbalance	Can cause death in children from supplement overdose
Potassium	Maintains functioning of muscle and nerve tissues; maintains heart beat	Whole cereals, coffee, fresh fruits, meat, vegetables, whole-grain flour	General muscle paralysis; metabolic disturbances	May lead to: arrhythmia, metabolic disturbances
Iron	Formation of hemoglobin; energy from carbohydrates, fats, and proteins	Liver and red meats, enriched breads and cereals	Anemia	Nausea and vomiting
Magnesium	Strengthens bones; improves enzyme function and nerve and heart function	Wheat germ, vegetables, nuts, chocolate	Weakness, muscle pain, poor heart function, osteoporosis	Kidney failure
Copper	Formation of hemoglobin	Liver, nuts, shellfish, cherries, mushrooms, whole grain breads and cereals	Skin problems, delayed development, growth problems	Interferes with copper use; may decrease HDL levels
Zinc	Normal growth and development	Seafood and meats	Mental and growth retardation; lack of energy	
Iodine	Production of the hormone thyroxin	Iodized salt, seafood		
Fluorine	Strengthens bones and teeth	Fluoridated water	Teeth are less resistant to decay	Damage to tooth enamel

calcium intake without eating too much fat, choose low-fat cheeses, milks (skim or 1 percent), or yogurt products. Although cottage cheese is made from milk, it is not a good source of calcium because the mineral is lost from the milk during processing. Calcium can also be found in broccoli, spinach, kale, cabbage, and mustard greens. Vitamin D helps with the absorption of calcium; thus it is important that vitamin D intake meet the minimum recommended levels.

Iron. Iron is needed to form the oxygen-carrying pigment in red blood cells called hemoglobin. When hemoglobin picks up oxygen in the lungs, it turns the blood bright red. In cases of iron-deficiency anemia, red blood cells are smaller and do not contain enough hemoglobin. The cells cannot get the oxygen needed to make energy. As a result, one feels tired and looks pale. Iron-deficiency anemia is a fairly common disorder, especially for young women who experience menstrual blood losses and who avoid eating meat. This deficiency can be due to a lack of iron in the diet, a deficiency of vitamin C (which aids in the absorption of iron), or excessive blood losses. Donating blood is a worthwhile activity, but it increases the need for iron as the body replaces red blood cells. Among the best food sources of iron are red meats, which contain a type of iron that is well absorbed. However, some people need to take iron pills to treat the anemia. Furthermore, some people absorb too much iron, which causes health problems. Keep in mind that there are many possible causes of anemia; iron-deficiency anemia is just one type of the disorder. Also, if you feel fatigued, you should not automatically assume that your iron levels are low. A blood test will indicate whether you have low iron.

Others. The other minerals are just as important, but the body needs so many minerals that it is beyond the scope of this text to delve further. Review Table 7-3 to learn more about calcium, iron, and several other minerals known to play important roles in the body.

PRODUCTION OF ENERGY

Energy is produced when cells break down the chemical units of glucose, fats, or amino acids to release energy stored in these compounds. Glycogen is not used directly for energy; it must first be broken down to release its supply of glucose units. This process is often referred to as "burning" the energy-supplying nutrients for energy. It is similar to burning a log, except your cells are the "fireplaces." Cellular combustion releases heat energy that maintains your body temperature and generates a form of energy that allows your cells to do work. For example, muscle cells need energy to keep moving, brain cells for thinking, and bone cells for building bone.

Logs cannot burn without oxygen; cells cannot produce much energy without oxygen, too. In Chapter 4, we discussed how anaerobic and aerobic conditions influence the amount of energy that can be generated. Recall that under aerobic conditions, muscle can generate more energy, especially from fat. Figure 7-7 shows the relative proportions of carbohydrate, fat, and protein fuels used for different kinds of physical activity. As shown in the graph, the proportions of nutrient fuels that are burned at any time depend on the type, duration, and intensity of the activity. These factors influence the amount of oxygen that cells need to generate energy.

When sitting around watching TV or reading, oxygen needs are low, and the body runs mostly on fat. As you can see in Figure 7-7, carbohydrates provide the major proportion of energy for short-term, high-intensity muscular contractions. As the duration and the intensity of the activity increase, breathing also increases, supplying more oxygen for the cells and maximizing energy production. When the activity is prolonged, such as in an endurance type of sport, the percentage of fat and carbohydrate used for fuel is similar. Under usual conditions, proteins supply less than about 5 percent of

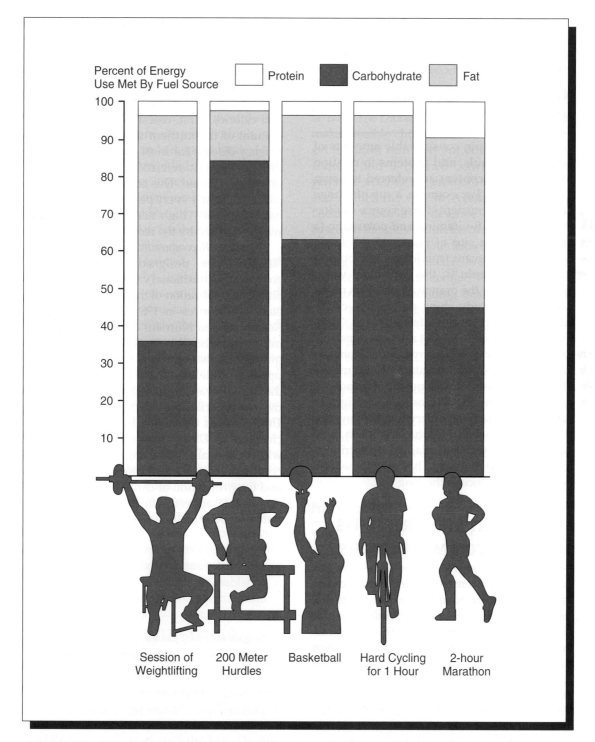

FIGURE 7-7. THE RELATIVE PROPORTIONS OF CARBOHYDRATES, FAT, AND PROTEIN FUELS USED FOR PHYSICAL ACTIVITY.

HEALTH LINK 7-1

2010 Dietary Guidelines

Balancing calories to Manage weight

- Prevent and/or reduce overweight and obesity through improved eating and physical activity behaviors.
- Control total calorie intake to manage body weight. For people who are overweight or obese, this will mean consuming fewer calories from foods and beverages.
- Increase physical activity and reduce time spent in sedentary behaviors.
- Maintain appropriate calorie balance during each stage of life—childhood, adolescence, adulthood, pregnancy and breastfeeding, and older age.

Foods and Food Components to Reduce

- Reduce daily sodium intake to less than 2,300 milligrams (mg) and further reduce intake to 1,500 mg among persons who are 51 and older and those of any age who are African American or have hypertension, diabetes, or chronic kidney disease. The 1,500 mg recommendation applies to about half of the U.S. population, including children, and the majority of adults.
- Consume less than 10 percent of calories from saturated fatty acids by replacing them with monounsaturated and polyunsaturated fatty acids.
- Consume less than 300 mg per day of dietary cholesterol.
- Keep trans fatty acid consumption as low as possible by limiting foods that contain synthetic sources of trans fats, such as partially hydrogenated oils, and by limiting other solid fats.
- Reduce the intake of calories from solid fats and added sugars.
- Limit the consumption of foods that contain refined grains, especially refined

grain foods that contain solid fats, added sugars, and sodium.
- If alcohol is consumed, it should be consumed in moderation—up to one drink per day for women and two drinks per day for men—and only by adults of legal drinking age.

Foods and Nutrients to Increase

- Individuals should meet the following recommendations as part of a healthy eating pattern while staying within their calorie needs.
- Increase vegetable and fruit intake.
- Eat a variety of vegetables, especially dark-green and red and orange vegetables and beans and peas.
- Consume at least half of all grains as whole grains. Increase whole-grain intake by replacing refined grains with whole grains.
- Increase intake of fat-free or low-fat milk and milk products, such as milk, yogurt, cheese, or fortified soy beverages.[6]
- Choose a variety of protein foods, which include seafood, lean meat and poultry, eggs, beans and peas, soy products, and unsalted nuts and seeds.
- Increase the amount and variety of seafood consumed by choosing seafood in place of some meat and poultry.
- Replace protein foods that are higher in solid fats with choices that are lower in solid fats and calories and/or are sources of oils.
- Use oils to replace solid fats where possible
- Choose foods that provide more potassium, dietary fiber, calcium, and vitamin D, which are nutrients of concern in American diets. These foods include vegetables, fruits, whole grains, and milk and milk products.

Continued

HEALTH LINK 7-1

2010 Dietary Guidelines-CONT

Building healthy eating Patterns

- Select an eating pattern that meets nutrient needs over time at an appropriate calorie level.
- Account for all foods and beverages consumed and assess how they fit within a total healthy eating pattern.
- Follow food safety recommendations when preparing and eating foods to reduce the risk of foodborne illnesses.

Recommendations for specific population groups
Women capable of becoming pregnant

- Choose foods that supply heme iron, which is more readily absorbed by the body, additional iron sources, and enhancers of iron absorption such as vitamin C-rich foods.
- Consume 400 micrograms (mcg) per day of synthetic folic acid (from fortified foods and/or supplements) in addition to food forms of folate from a varied diet.[8]

Women who are pregnant or breastfeeding[7]

- Consume 8 to 12 ounces of seafood per week from a variety of seafood types.
- Due to their high methyl mercury content, limit white (albacore) tuna to 6 ounces per week and do not eat the following four types of fish: tilefish, shark, swordfish, and king mackerel.
- If pregnant, take an iron supplement, as recommended by an obstetrician or other health care provider.

Individuals ages 50 years and older

- Consume foods fortified with vitamin B12, such as fortified cereals, or dietary supplements.

http://www.cnpp.usda.gov/Publications/DietaryGuidelines/2010/PolicyDoc/ExecSumm.pdf

HEALTH LINK 7-2

Healthy Cooking—Improve Your Health and Diet with These Tips

There's much you can do about healthy cooking, starting with the ingredients you use.

- Select low-fat or reduced-fat items.
- Buy polyunsaturated margarine instead of butter.
- Include as little meat as possible in your menu.
- White meat such as fish and poultry is always healthier than red meat.
- Always buy lean meat, and trim off any fat.
- When using cooking oil, try to use olive oil and canola oil.
- When you take your food out of the oven or fryer, place it on several napkins to drain the oil.

- Try cooking fewer high-fat, high-calorie foods such as burgers and pizzas, and cook healthier foods such as salads, soups, and stir-fries.
- Cooking methods such as basting, grilling, and deep-frying are less healthy than steaming, poaching, and stir-frying.
- When basting or grilling, don't use the fat from the grilled item, use vegetable oil instead.
- Eat out less, and eat less fast food.

www.healthycookingrecipes.com/cookinghealthyarticles/healthycooking.htm

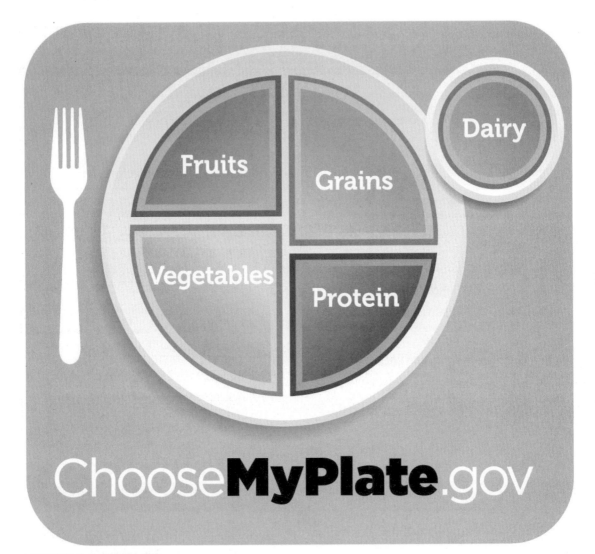

FIGURE 7-8. MYPLATE.

A new website, ChooseMyPlate.gov has been developed to provide practical information to several groups including individual Americans, health professionals, nutrition educators, and the food industry to help these consumers build healthier diets. Resources and tools for dietary assessment, nutrition education, and other user-friendly nutrition information can also be found on this web site. Because the American population is experiencing epidemic rates of overweight and obesity, the hope is that the online resources and tools can empower people to make healthier food choices for themselves, their families, and their children. Hopefully this approach will help to eliminate frustration among consumers over what they report as hearing contradictory nutrition information.

The 2010 Dietary Guidelines for Americans form the basis of the federal government's

individual
tion. Even
quate leve
as calcium
planning. .
rich in an
agreement
ing antioxi
taking sup
is warrant
the followi
some peop

Calcium
strengthen
women, to
their norm
mature ost
but the hor
normal to p
check with
supplemen
that magne
cium for pr

Iron. The
anemia, sp
occurs in th
distance ru
not this is
mildly aner
performanc
of iron-rich
serious, a p
advice rega

▶**Creatin**

Creatine is
pound mad
creas. Crea
meat and f
mentation w
performanc
exercise. Cr
metabolism

There ar
creatine an

nutrition education programs, federal nutrition assistance programs, and dietary advice provided by health and nutrition professionals. Action oriented messages will help professionals and the media to understand and deliver relevant nutrition information to help people in their daily lives.

The Guidelines messages include several actionable messages including:

Balance Calories
- Enjoy your food, but eat less.
- Avoid oversized portions.

Foods to Increase
- Make half your plate fruits and vegetables.
- Switch to fat-free or low-fat (1%) milk.
- Make at least half your grains whole grains

Foods to Reduce
- Compare sodium (salt) in foods like soup, bread, and frozen meals, and choose foods with lower numbers.
- Drink water instead of sugary drinks.

READING LABELS

Over the past 20 years, food labels have provided helpful nutritional information for consumers. In 1994, a new nutritional labeling format changed the look and importance of food product packaging. People were becoming concerned over the amount of fat, cholesterol, sodium, and fiber in the typical American diet, thus producing the drive for a more health-conscious label. Health educators believe that the new format has made it easier for consumers to make more informed, healthful food selections. In 2004, the FDA mandated that trans fat be added to the label.

Examine the sample label shown in Figure 7-9. The manufacturer must list the total number of calories per serving, and include information about the number of total calories contributed by fat. Unfortunately, you have to do some

Nutrition Facts

Serving Size 1 cup (228g)
Servings Per Container 2

	% Daily Value*
Total Fat 12g	**18%**
Saturated Fat 3g	**15%**
Trans Fat 3g	
Cholesterol 30mg	**10%**
Sodium 470mg	**20%**
Total Carbohydrate 31g	**10%**
Dietary Fiber 0g	**0%**
Sugars 5g	
Protein 5g	
Vitamin A	**4%**
Vitamin C	**2%**
Calcium	**20%**
Iron	**4%**

*Percent Daily Values are based on a 2,000 calorie diet. Your Daily Values may be higher or lower depending on your calorie needs.

	Calories:	2,000	2,500
Total Fat	Less than	65g	80g
Sat Fat	Less than	20g	25g
Cholesterol	Less than	300mg	300mg
Sodium	Less than	2,400mg	2,400mg
Total Carbohydrate		300g	375g
Dietary Fiber		25g	30g

Ingredients: Corn, Vegetable Oil,
Contains one or more of the following: Canola, Corn, Cheeses (Cheddar from cow's milk) Salt, Buttermilk, Garlic Powder, Dextrose, Sugar

FIGURE 7-9. LABEL INDICATING NUTRITION INFORMATION PER SERVING.

math to
calories
trying t
diet to
Further
formati
based o
2,000 ca
Figure
ing con
value o
of the v
your da
80 perc
dients l
exactly
ents are
nance.
ones th
tom of
trace an
tions, n
include
isfied v
ultimat

WHA

Interes
very hi
that ce
their fi
pendin
athletes
explore
examin
about t
cal perf

NUTF

You ma
eral, a

SUGAR

In the past it was believed that eating large quantities of simple carbohydrates, such as those supplied by candy bars, honey, or pure sugar, immediately before physical activity had a negative impact on performance. However, recent evidence indicates that for most healthy, active people, the effects of eating carbohydrates before activity are more beneficial than negative. Some people find that large quantities of fructose lead to intestinal upset and diarrhea. (Sources of fructose include honey, fruit, and table sugar.) Therefore, it is wise to avoid fructose or, for that matter, any food that upsets your stomach, before engaging in physical activity.

CAFFEINE

Caffeine is a stimulant found in coffee, tea, chocolate, and carbonated beverages. Although small amounts of caffeine may benefit physical performance, too much can cause headaches, nervousness, irritability, and increased heart rate. Olympic officials have ruled that athletes' blood caffeine levels should not exceed the amount that results from drinking six cups of coffee.

ALCOHOL

Alcohol is a depressant drug that supplies 7 calories per gram. However, alcoholic beverages offer little nutritional value other than energy. In fact, alcohol actually raises triglyceride levels which contributes to increased body fat. The depressant effects of alcohol include reductions in physical coordination, slowed reaction times, and decreased mental alertness. Alcohol also has a diuretic effect, resulting in body water losses. Therefore, it is not wise to replace water losses from physical activity by using alcoholic beverages, such as beer. Too much alcohol is harmful, destroying the liver and brain cells and potentially causing negative effects in your personal life.

HERBS

The use of herbs as natural alternatives to drugs and medicines has clearly become a trend among American consumers. Most herbs, as edible plants, are safe to take as foods, and they are claimed to have few side effects. One herb that has potentially dangerous side effects is ephedrine. Ephedrine is a central nervous system stimulant that has been linked to a variety of potentially life-threatening conditions. In 2003, ephedrine was banned by the Food and Drug Administration.

Hundreds of herbs are widely available today at all quality levels. They are readily available at health food stores. However, unlike both food and medicine, no federal or governmental controls regulate the sale and ensure the quality of the products being sold. The research-based information regarding the use of herbal supplements is limited and thus claims relative to the efficacy of using a specific herb to achieve a medicinal effect should be viewed by the consumer with skepticism and caution.

Relative to nutrition, herbs can offer the body nutrients that are reported to nourish the brain, glands, and hormones. Unlike vitamins that work best when taken with food, it is not necessary to take herbs with other foods.

Herbs in their whole form are not drugs. As medicine, herbs are essentially body balancers that work with the body functions, so that the body can heal and regulate itself. Herbal formulas can be general for overall strength and nutrient support, or specific to a particular ailment or condition.

Table 7-4 lists the most popular and widely used herbal products sold in health food stores. Some additional potent and complex herbs, such as capsicum, lobelia, sassafras, mandrake tansy, canada snake root, wormwood, woodruff, poke root, and rue, may be useful in small amounts and as catalysts but should not be used alone.

TABLE 7-4
MOST WIDELY USED HERBS AND PURPOSES FOR USE
Cayenne—for weight loss
Cascara—as a laxative, can cause dehydration
Dong quai—to treat menstrual symptoms
Echinacea—to promote wound healing and strengthen the immune system
Fever few—to prevent and relieve migraine headaches, arthritis, and PMS
Garlic—as an antibiotic, antibacterial, antifungal agent to prevent and relieve coronary artery disease by reducing total blood cholesterol and triglyceride levels and raising HDL levels
Garcina cambagia—to promote loss of fat
Ginkgo biloba—to improve blood circulation especially in the brain
Ginseng—to reduce impotence, weakness, lethargy, and fatigue
Guarana—as a stimulant, contains large amounts of caffeine, often in weight loss products
Kava—to reduce anxiety, relax muscle tension, produce analgesic effects, act as a local anesthetic, provide antibacterial benefit
Ma huang (ephedrine)—derived from the ephedra plant, it has been used in China for medicinal purposes including increased energy, appetite suppression, increased fat burning, and preservation of muscle tissue from breaking down. It is a central nervous system stimulant drug used in many diet pills. In 1995, the FDA revealed adverse reactions to ephedrine such as heart attacks, strokes, paranoid psychosis, vomiting, fever, palpitations, convulsions, and comas, and in 2003 banned its use.
Mate—CNS stimulant
Saw palmetto—to treat inflamed prostate; also used as a diuretic and as a sexual enhancement agent
Senna—as a laxative, can cause water and electrolyte loss
St. John's wort—used as an antidepressant; also used to treat nervous disorders, depression, neuralgia, kidney problems, wounds, and burns
Valerian—to treat insomnia, anxiety, stress
Yohimbe—to increase libido and blood flow to sexual organs in the male

THE PROBLEM WITH EATING FAST FOODS

Eating fast food is a way of life in American society. Most Americans have grown up as fast-food "junkies." Aside from occasional problems with food flavor, the biggest concern in consuming fast foods, as can be seen in Table 7-5, is that 40 to 50 percent of the calories consumed are from fats. To compound this problem, these already sizable meals are now being "supersized" at a more affordable price for those who want maximum fat, salt, and calories in a single sitting (Figure 7-10).

Fast-food restaurants have supposedly broadened their menus to include whole-wheat breads and rolls, salad bars, and low-fat milk

TABLE 7-5
FAST-FOOD CHOICES AND NUTRITIONAL VALUE

Food	Calories	Protein (g)	CHO (g)	Fat (g)	Calories from Fat (%)	Cholesterol (mg)	Sodium (mg)
Hamburgers							
McDonald's hamburger	263	12.4	28.3	11	38.6	29.1	506
Dairy Queen single hamburger w/cheese	410	24	33	20	43.9	50	790
Hardee's 1/4 pound cheeseburger	506	28	41	26	46.2	61	1,950
Wendy's double hamburger, white bun	560	4.1	24	34	54.6	125	575
McDonald's Big Mac	570	24.6	39.2	35	55.2	83	1045
Burger King Whopper sandwich	640	27	42	41	57.6	94	842
Chicken							
Arby's chicken breast sandwich	592	28	56	27	41.0	57	1,340
Burger King chicken sandwich	688	26	56	40	52.3	82	1,423
Dairy Queen chicken sandwich	670	29	46	41	55.0	75	870
Church's Crispy Nuggets (one; regular)	55	3	4	3	49.0	—	125
Kentucky Fried Chicken Nuggets (one)	46	2.82	2.2	2.9	56.7	11.9	140
Fish							
Church's Southern Fried Catfish	67	4	4	4	53.7	—	151
Long John Silver's Fish & More	978	34	82	58	53.3	88	2,124
McDonald's Filet-O-Fish	135	14.7	35.9	25.7	53.1	45.2	799
Others							
Hardee's hot dog	346	11	26	22	57.2	42	744
Taco Bell Beef Burrito Supreme	440	17	52	18	36	35	1,220

Continued

TABLE 7-5
FAST-FOOD CHOICES AND NUTRITIONAL VALUE—CONT.

Food	Calories	Protein (g)	CHO (g)	Fat (g)	Calories from Fat (%)	Cholesterol (mg)	Sodium (mg)
Taco Bell chicken soft taco	240	14	21	11	42	45	490
Taco Bell taco salad	830	29	66	51	55	60	1,760
Arby's roast beef sandwich (regular)	350	22	32	15	38.5	39	590
Hardee's roast beef sandwich	377	21	36	17	40.5	57	1,030
French Fries							
Arby's french fries	211	2	33	8	34.1	6	30
McDonald's french fries (regular)	220	3	26.1	11.5	47.0	8.6	109
Wendy's french fries (regular)	280	4	35	14	45.0	15	95
Shakes							
Dairy Queen	710	14	120	19	24.0	50	260
McDonald's							
Vanilla	352	9.3	59.6	8.4	21.4	30.6	201
Chocolate	383	9.9	65.5	9	21.1	29.7	300
Strawberry	362	9	62.1	8.7	22.3	32.2	207
Soft Drinks							
Coca Cola	154	—	40	—	—	—	6
Diet Coke	0.9	—	0.3	—	—	—	16
Sprite	142	—	36	—	—	—	45
Tab	1	—	1	—	—	—	30
Diet Sprite	3	—	0	—	—	—	9

products. The nutritional value of these "improvements" to the menu, though, is still questionable. Many of the larger fast-food restaurants provide nutritional information for consumers upon request or from well-stocked racks. Safe Tip 7-1 provides suggestions for eating more healthfully at fast-food restaurants.

PRE-EVENT MEAL

People engaging in competitive sports are often very concerned with the kinds of foods selected for pre-event meals. However, they should be more concerned with their eating patterns well before the day of the event. The purpose of the

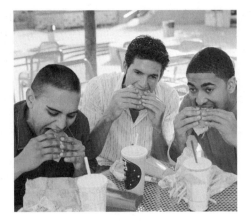

FIGURE 7-10. FAST FOODS.
*Fast foods generally contain a lot of fat, especially
if they are "supersized."*

pre-event meal is to supply the competitor with enough energy and fluids for competition. The meal should be easily digestible as well. Most experts recommend a light meal (around 300 calories) that is rich in carbohydrate about 2 to 4 hours before the event. A full stomach is uncomfortable, so avoid fatty or greasy meals that take longer to digest. Preloading on extra water is a good idea to keep well hydrated. Individuals vary in their ability to tolerate various foods, but it is advisable to avoid known gas-forming foods or any food the athlete believes contributes to intestinal upset.

VEGETARIANISM

Vegetarians use plant foods to form the foundation of their diet; animal foods are either totally excluded or included in a variety of

SAFE TIP 7-1

Tips for Selecting Fast Foods

- Limit deep fried foods such as fish and chicken sandwiches and chicken nuggets, which are often higher in fat than plain burgers are. If you are having fried chicken, remove some of the breading before eating.
- Order roast beef, turkey, or grilled chicken, where available, for a lower fat alternative to most burgers.
- Choose a small order of fries with your meal rather than a large one, and request no salt. Add a small amount of salt yourself if desired. If you are ordering a deep-fat-fried sandwich or one that is made with cheese and sauce, skip the fries altogether and try a plain baked potato (add butter and salt sparingly) or a dinner roll instead of a biscuit; or try a side salad to accompany your meal instead.
- Choose regular sandwiches instead of "double," "jumbo," "deluxe," or "ultimate." And order plain types rather than those with the works, such as cheese, bacon, mayonnaise, and special sauce. Pickles, mustard, ketchup, and other condiments are high in sodium. Choose lettuce, tomatoes, and onions.
- At the salad bar, load up on fresh greens, fruits, and vegetables. Be careful of salad dressings, added toppings, and creamy salads (potato salad, macaroni salad, coleslaw). These can quickly push calories and fat to the level of other menu items or higher.
- Many fast-food items contain large amounts of sodium from salt and other ingredients. Try to balance the rest of your day's sodium choices after a fast-food meal.
- Alternate water, low-fat milk, or skim milk with a soda or a shake.
- For dessert, or a sweet-on-the-run, choose low-fat frozen yogurt where available.
- Remember to balance your fast-food choices with your food selections for the whole day.

eating patterns. People who choose to become vegetarians do so for economic, philosophical, religious, cultural, or health reasons. The U.S. Dietary Goals that recommend eating less fat, cholesterol, salt, and sugar while increasing fiber intake easily support a vegetarian eating pattern.

Types of vegetarians include the following:

- *Total vegetarians or vegans:* People who consume plant but no animal foods; meat, fish, poultry, eggs, and dairy products are excluded. This diet has been found to be adequate for most adults if they give careful consideration to obtaining enough calories; sources of vitamin B_{12}; and the minerals calcium, zinc, and iron. It is not recommended for pregnant women, infants, or children because of the difficulty in consuming the quantity of plant foods necessary to meet the caloric and nutritional needs during these life stages.
- *Lactovegetarians:* Individuals who consume milk products along with plant foods. Meat, fish, poultry, and eggs are excluded. Iron and zinc levels can be low in people who practice this form of vegetarianism.
- *Lacto-ovo-vegetarians:* People who consume dairy products and eggs in their diet, along with plant foods. Meat, fish, and poultry are excluded. Again, iron could be a problem.
- *Semivegetarians:* People who consume animal products but exclude red meats. Plant products still form an important part of the diet. This diet is usually adequate.

FOOD SAFETY

Safety in preparing and consuming food is important not only when eating out in restaurants but also when preparing and eating food at home. While the food supply in the United States is one of the safest in the world, it is estimated that every year approximately 76 million people get sick, more than 300,000 are hospitalized, and 5,000 die from eating contaminated food. Bacteria are the most common cause of **foodborne illness.** Foods may have some bacteria on them when you buy them. Raw foods are the most common source of foodborne illnesses because they are not sterile; examples include raw meat and poultry that may have become contaminated during slaughter. Fruits and vegetables may become contaminated when they are growing or when they are processed. Seafood may become contaminated during harvest or through processing. But contamination can also happen in your kitchen if you leave food out for more than 2 hours at room temperature. Parasites and bacteria are less likely to cause a foodborne illness. Safe Tip 7-2 lists fundamental practices to maintain sanitary hygiene with food handling and preparation.

Foodborne illness can cause the following mild to serious symptoms:

- Upset stomach
- Abdominal cramps
- Nausea and vomiting
- Diarrhea
- Fever
- Dehydration

The treatment in most cases is increasing your fluid intake. For more serious illness, you may need treatment at a hospital.

Food scientists and food technolgists are engaged in an ongoing effort to develop ways to process, preserve, package, distribute, or store food, according to industry and government specifications and regulations that can help minimize the risks of foodborne illnesses.

SUMMARY

- The classes of nutrients are carbohydrates, fats, proteins, vitamins, minerals, and water.

- Carbohydrates, fats, and proteins are macronutrients that provide the energy required for muscular work. Vitamins, minerals, and water are micronutrients that play a role in the function and maintenance of body tissues.
- Vitamins are substances found in foods that have no caloric value but are necessary to regulate body processes.
- Antioxidants are nutrients that protect the body against various destructive agents.
- Minerals are also involved in regulation of bodily functions and are used to form important body structures.
- Water is the most essential nutrient and should be the drink of choice.
- The 2010 U.S. Dietary Guidelines are designed to help you plan meals that are healthy.
- The pre-event meal should be (1) higher in carbohydrates, (2) easily digested, (3) eaten 2 to 4 hours before an event, and (4) acceptable to the athlete.
- Vegetarians use plant foods as the basis of their diet.

SUGGESTED READINGS

Antonio, J. 2008. *Essentials of sports nutrition and supplements,* Clifton, NJ: Humana Press.

Brodney, S., R. S. McPherson, R. A. Carpenter, D. Welten, and S. N. Blair. 2001. Nutrient intake of physically fit and unfit men and women. *Medicine and Science in Sports and Exercise* 33(3):459–67.

Brouns, F. 2002. *Essentials of sports nutrition,* 2nd ed. New York: John Wiley and Sons.

Brukner, P., K. Khan, K. Inge, and S. Crawford. 2002. Maximizing performance: nutrition. In *Clinical sports medicine,* 2nd rev. ed., edited by P. Brukner. New York: McGraw-Hill.

Burke, L. 2009. *Clinical sports nutrition.* 4th ed. New York: McGraw-Hill.

Burke, L. M., B. Kiens, and J. L. Ivy. 2004. Carbohydrates and fat for training and recovery. *Journal of Sports Sciences* 22(1):15–30.

Byrd-Bredbenner, C., and J. Berning. 2009. *Wardlaw's perspectives in nutrition.* New York: McGraw-Hill.

Clark, N. 2008. *Nancy Clark's sports nutrition guide book.* Champaign, IL: Human Kinetics.

Coleman, E. 2001. Carbohydrate during stop-and-go sports. *Sports Medicine Digest* 23(12):142–43.

Coleman, E. 2001. Nutrition update: Position stand on nutrition and athletic performance. *Sports Medicine Digest* 23(5):54–55.

Cooper, K. 2004. *Antioxidant revolution.* Nashville: Thomas Nelson.

Daniels, D. 2008. *Exercises for osteoporosis: A safe and effective way to build bone density and muscle strength and improve posture and flexibility.* 3rd ed. New York: Hatherleigh Press.

Eberle, S. 2007. *Endurance sports nutrition.* Champaign, IL: Human Kinetics.

Eberle, S. G. 2004. Vegetarian diets for endurance athletes. *Strength and Conditioning Journal* 26(4):60–61.

Froiland, K., W. Koszewski, and J. Hingst. 2004. Nutritional supplement use among college athletes and their sources of information. *International Journal of Sport Nutrition and Exercise Metabolism* 14(1):104–20.

Gleeson, M., D. C. Nieman, and B. K. Pedersen. 2004. Exercise, nutrition and immune function. *Journal of Sports Sciences* 22(1):115–25.

Haas, R. 2005. *Eat to win for the 21st century: The sports nutrition bible for a new generation.* East Rutherford, NJ: Penguin Group.

Hedrick, H., A. Mikesly, and L. Burgoon. 2006. *Practical applications in sports nutrition.* Boston: Jones and Bartlett.

Hunt, B. P., and A. Gillentine. 2001. Dietary supplement knowledge and information sources among college students. *Journal of the International Council for Health, Physical Education, Recreation, Sport, and Dance* 37(3):53–56.

Insel, P., E. Turner, and D. Ross. 2010. *Nutrition.* Sudbury, MA: Jones and Bartlett Publishers.

Izquierdo, M., J. Ibanez, J. J. Gonzalez-Badillo, and E. M. Gorostiaga. 2002. Effects of creatine supplementation on muscle power, endurance, and sprint performance. *Medicine and Science in Sports and Exercise* 34(2):332–43.

Kleiner, S. 2001. The scoop on protein supplements. *Athletic Therapy Today* 6(1): 52–53.

Kleiner, S. M., and M. Greenwood-Robinson. 2006. Performance herbs. In *Power eating,* 3rd ed., edited by S. M. Kleiner. Champaign, IL: Human Kinetics.

Kleiner, S. M., and M. Greenwood-Robinson. 2006. Vitamins and minerals for strength trainers. In *Power eating,* 3rd ed., edited by S. M. Kleiner. Champaign, IL: Human Kinetics.

Larson-Duyff, R. 2002. *The American Dietetic Association's complete food and nutrition guide.* New York: John Wiley.

Litt, A. (ed.) 2004. *Fuel for young athletes.* Champaign, IL: Human Kinetics.

Manore, M. M. 2004. Nutrition and physical activity: Fueling the active individual. *President's Council on Physical Fitness and Sports Research Digest* 5(1):1–8.

Maughan, R. J. 2002. *Sports nutrition.* Malden, MA: Blackwell Science.

Maughan, R., and R. Murray. 2001. *Sports drinks: Basic science and practical aspects.* Boca Raton, FL: CRC Press.

Maughan, R. J., D. S. King, and T. Lea. 2004. Dietary supplements. *Journal of Sports Sciences* 22(1):95–113.

McArdle, W. D. 2009. *Exercise physiology: Energy, nutrition, and human performance.* 7th ed. Philadelphia: Lippincott Williams & Wilkins.

McArdle, W., F. Katch, and V. Katch. 2008. *Sports and exercise nutrition.* Philadelphia: Lippincott, Williams and Wilkins.

McVicar, J. 2008. *The complete herb book.* Westport, CT: Firefly Books.

Platen, P. 2001. The importance of sport and physical exercise in the prevention and therapy of osteoporosis. *European Journal of Sport Science* 1(3):237–44

Powers, S. K., K. C. DeRuisseau, and J. Quindry. 2004. Dietary antioxidants and exercise. *Journal of Sports Sciences* 22(1):81–94.

Ryan, M. 2007. *Sports nutrition for endurance athletes.* Boulder, CO: VeloPress.

Schlosser, E. 2005. *Fast food nation: The dark side of the all-American meal.* New York: Harper Perennial.

Sen, C. K. 2001. Antioxidants in exercise nutrition. *Sports Medicine* 31(13):891–908.

Sforzo, G. A. 2002. Sports supplements [Review]. *Medicine and Science in Sports and Exercise* 34(1):183.

Sharkey, B. J. 2006. Nutrition and health. In *Fitness and health,* 5th ed., edited by B. J. Sharkey. Champaign, IL: Human Kinetics.

Spriet, L. L., and M. J. Gibala. 2004. Nutritional strategies to influence adaptations to training. *Journal of Sports Sciences* 22(1):127–41.

Stevenson, S. W., and G. A. Dudley. 2001. Creatine loading, resistance exercise performance and muscle mechanics. *Journal of Strength and Conditioning Research* 15(4):413–19.

Stout, J., and J. Antonia. 2010. *Essentials of creatine in sports and health.* Clifton, NJ: Humana Press.

Tribole, E. (ed.) 2004. *Eating on the run,* 3rd ed. Champaign, IL: Human Kinetics.

U.S. Department of Agriculture. 2010. *Dietary guidelines for Americans.* Washington, DC: U.S. Government Printing Office.

U.S. Department of Agriculture and U.S. Department of Health and Human Services. 2010. *Nutrition and your health: Dietary guidelines for Americans.* 6th edition. Washington, DC.

Welsh, R. S., J. M. Davis, J. R. Burke, and H. G. Williams. 2002. Carbohydrates and physical/mental performance during intermittent exercise to fatigue. *Medicine and Science in Sports and Exercise* 34(4):723–31.

Weil, A. 2008. *Eating well for optimal health: The essential guide to food, diet and nutrition.* London: Sphere.

Williams, M. 2009. *Nutrition for health, fitness, and sport.* St. Louis: McGraw-Hill.

Suggested Web Sites

American Dietetic Association

This site educates individuals about how making informed food choices can help them decrease the risk of heart disease, breast cancer, osteoporosis, diabetes, and obesity; it advocates nutrition research.
www.eatright.org

American Heart Association

Complete with comprehensive nutrition guidelines, the American Heart Association is a great resource for health practitioners and laypersons.
www.heart.org

American Institute for Cancer Research

Visit this site for the latest cancer prevention research in diet and nutrition. Read the "Diet and Cancer link" and their dietary guidelines on "Reducing Your Cancer Risk" position pages.
www.aicr.org

American School Food Service Association

The ASFSA is dedicated to healthy meals for school food service, with a membership of 60,000 professionals committed to child nutrition integrity. It is good for parents, students, and school officials.
www.asfsa.org

Center for Food Safety and Applied Nutrition—FDA

Timely fact sheets and press releases are available from Food and Drug Administration.
http://cfsan.fda.com

CNN's Health News: Diet & Fitness

This site presents NEWS and helpful tips on topics related to diet and nutrition.
http://cnn.com/HEALTH/diet.fitness

International Food Information Council Foundation (IFIC)

The IFIC Foundation site is an industry-sponsored foundation that steers a middle road in the debates about nutrition. This useful and cautious perspective includes some very good information on diet.
www.ific.org

Mayo Clinic Diet and Nutrition Resource Center

Mayo Clinic nutrition experts offer practical advice, creative encouragement, and healthy recipes to cut fat, cholesterol, sodium, and calories and improve your diet. This site includes a Q&A section with Mayo dietitians.
www.mayoclinic.com/health/food-and-nutrition/ NU99999

MyPlate

Government web site designed to help consumers adopt healthy eating habits consistent with the 2010 Dietary Guidelines
http://www.choosemyplate.gov/

The Diet Channel

Cutting-edge diet information on weight loss, sports nutrition, heart disease, cancer, and preventative nutrition is

presented. You can request a professional diet analysis or browse through 600 links to reliable nutrition information on the Web.
www.thedietchannel.com

U.S. Dietary Guidelines

This site details the revised 2010 U.S. Dietary Guidelines for Americans.
www.healthierus.gov/dietaryguidelines

USDA's FNIC

The USDA's Food and Nutrition Information Center is a valuable resource for any nutrition topic.
http://fnic.nal.usda.gov

Vegetarian Diet: MedlinePlus

Provides a wealth of information and links to other Web sites that deal with vegetarian diets.
www.nlm.nih.gov/medlineplus/vegetariandiet.html

Nutritional Knowledge Survey

_____ _____ _____
Name   Section   Date

PURPOSE   To test your knowledge about nutrition.

PROCEDURE   Consider the following statements and answer true or false in the space to the left of the statement. Answers and an explanation are on the next page, as well as information on how to interpret your score.

_____ 1. Butter has more calories than the same amount of margarine.
_____ 2. Carbohydrates are fattening.
_____ 3. Vitamins provide energy for the body.
_____ 4. Excessive amounts of certain vitamins can cause health problems.
_____ 5. Cholesterol is dangerous and should be avoided.
_____ 6. If your serum cholesterol levels are low, you don't have to worry about heart disease.
_____ 7. Millions of Americans suffer from hypoglycemia.
_____ 8. Sugar offers no nutritional value.
_____ 9. Sugar causes hyperactive behavior and attention span disorders in children.
_____ 10. Protein supplements are unnecessary for body builders.
_____ 11. Zinc supplements will improve your sex drive.
_____ 12. Honey is more nutritious than sugar.
_____ 13. Meat is essential for a nutritious diet.
_____ 14. Fasting removes toxic wastes that build up in your body from dietary sources.
_____ 15. Organically grown foods are nutritionally superior to conventionally grown ones.

ANSWERS

1. False   Each has 100 calories per tablespoon. The nature of the fat is different; butter contains more saturated fat than margarine. Butter also contains cholesterol; margarine does not. However, these differences do not affect the number of calories per serving.

2. False   Carbohydrates contribute 4 calories per gram, the same as a gram of protein. What is added to the carbohydrate-rich food to make it tasty often piles on the calories. These include fatty spreads, sauces, and gravies.

3. False   Vitamins cannot be broken apart and used for energy. However, many do participate in chemical reactions that extract energy from carbohydrate, protein, and fat.

4. True   Excesses of the fat-soluble vitamins are toxic, and vitamin B_6, niacin, and ascorbic acid can cause health problems if taken in large amounts.

5. False   Cholesterol has many important uses in the body. It is used to make steroid hormones and bile, which is needed for proper fat digestion.

6. False   Although a high serum cholesterol level is associated with the development of heart disease, low serum cholesterol levels are no guarantee of protection. If too much is in the LDL form, the risk of heart disease is higher than it is for someone who has a higher total cholesterol level but more in the HDL form.

7. False   When you haven't eaten, blood sugar drops and you feel hungry. Eating raises blood sugar levels. Hypoglycemia (low blood sugar) associated with metabolic abnormalities is rare. Medical experts consider hypoglycemia a fad disease in most cases.

8. False   Refined white sugar is almost 100 percent carbohydrate. It is digested into very simple sugars that are used for energy by the body.

9. False   Despite many personal reports, sugar does not cause behavioral problems in children or adults. As the answer to #8 explains, it is a simple chemical that is broken down and used for energy. Often, sugar-laden foods also contain caffeine and related stimulants, which may explain the association of sugar with hyperactive behavior.

10. True   Protein supplements are unnecessary because most Americans obtain plenty of protein in their normal diet. Exercise builds muscles, not extra protein. More protein than needed is processed by the body and used for energy or converted to fat.

11. False   Severe zinc deficiency leads to poor growth and failure to develop sexually. However, this is extremely rare in the U.S.

12. False   Honey contains large amounts of the simple sugar, fructose. Fructose is one of the components of table sugar. The body converts fructose to glucose irrespective of the source. Considering how much honey is used and the tiny amounts of nutrients it contains, honey is just a more expensive choice as a sweetener.

13. False   The iron in red meat is more easily absorbed than the iron in plant foods. However, fish and chicken contribute iron, too. Thus, red meat is not essential as a food.

14. False   Fasting actually creates metabolic wastes that must be eliminated, since more body fat is burned for energy than under fed conditions. There are no health benefits derived from fasting.

15. False   Studies have demonstrated no nutritional superiority of foods grown with natural fertilizers and without pesticides.

Scoring: Give yourself one point for each correct response and total your points.
Total: _____

Score	Rating	Comments
13–15	Superior	You have sound knowledge of the subject.
9–12	Good	Good start; you may want to read reliable nutrition books to enhance your knowledge.
6–8	Fair	Read Chapter 7 again for more information.
<5	Poor	You have accumulated some misinformation about nutrition; try locating some reliable reading material and study Chapter 7.

Assessing Your Nutritional Habits

_____ _____ _____
Name   Section   Date

PURPOSE   To identify the number that best describes the frequency of your food-related behaviors.

PROCEDURE   Indicate the number that best describes the frequency of your food-related behaviors.

Point Values
0 = never   1 = rarely   2 = occasionally   3 = often   4 = always

_____ 1. Every day I eat a nutritious breakfast.
_____ 2. I try to include recommended servings from each of the food groups in my daily diet.
_____ 3. I eat food without salting it.
_____ 4. When I snack, I choose fruits, vegetables, low-fat yogurt, or cheese.
_____ 5. I try to include mostly fresh and less processed foods in my daily diet.
_____ 6. I avoid fatty foods and trim off the visible fat from meats.
_____ 7. I include foods containing fiber, such as fruits, vegetables, whole-grain products, and beans, in my diet.
_____ 8. I drink skim milk instead of whole or 2% milk.
_____ 9. I consume fish at least once a week.
_____ 10. I avoid foods that contain large amounts of honey and sugar.
_____ 11. For reliable nutrition information, I ask a qualified nutritionist instead of relying on the popular press.
_____ 12. I do not drink alcoholic beverages.
_____ 13. I keep my weight within acceptable limits.
_____ 14. I obtain my nutrients through foods rather than rely on nutritional supplements.

_____ Total Points

Modified from Allen R, Hyde R: Investigation in stress control, Minneapolis, 1981, Macmillan.

INTERPRETATION

Score

50–60	Excellent	Your food-related behaviors should contribute to your ability to maintain good health. Keep it up!
45–49	Good	If you make some minor improvements to your food-related behaviors, it should be easy to move into the excellent rating category.
39–44	Fair	Analyze the statements to determine which had the lowest scores. Then think about actions you can take to improve your nutritional behaviors.
<39	Poor	You need to make major changes in your food related behaviors to improve your nutritional status and your overall health. Analyze your responses to the statements and read Chapter 7 carefully.

| Name | | Section | | Date |

PURPOSE   To determine your eating habits during a 7-day period.

PROCEDURE   For a 7-day period, Monday through Sunday, assign yourself the points indicated when each dietary requirement is met. Record your points in the appropriate column for each day. Total your daily and weekly points. Negative points for junk food consumption should be subtracted from your daily and weekly totals.

Food	Points	Maximum Score	Daily Score M	T	W	T	F	S	S
Milk and Milk Products		15							
One cup of milk or equivalent	5								
Second cup of milk or equivalent	5								
Third serving	5								
Vegetables		25							
Three to five servings deep green or yellow	5 each								
Fruits		20							
Two to four servings whole or juices	5 each								
Bread and Cereals		30							
Six or more servings of whole-grain or enriched cereals or breads	5 each								
Protein-Rich Foods		10							
One serving of egg, meat, fish, poultry, cheese, dried beans, or peas	5								
One or two additional servings of egg, meat, fish, poultry, or cheese	5								

Continued

7-Day Diet Analysis

Food	Points	Maximum Score	Daily Score						
			M	T	W	T	F	S	S
Junk Foods (or Negative Point Value Foods)									
Sweet rolls	−5								
Fruit pies	−5								
Potato chips, corn chips, or cheese twists	−5								
Candy	−5								
Nondiet sodas	−5								
Total		100							

Point Record
Weekly point total_____
Negative point total _____
Adjusted weekly _____
   point total

Interpretation
600–700   Excellent dietary practices
450–599   Adequate dietary practices
300–449   Poor dietary practices
Below 300 Very poor dietary practices

ASSESSING YOUR DIETARY PRACTICES

1. On which day of the week was it most difficult for you to eat a balanced diet? Why?

    _____

    _____

    _____

2. Approximately what percentage of your total points was from foods purchased in a restaurant? _____

    _____

3. Approximately how much money did you spend on food during this 7-day period?

    _____

4. Was this a typical 7-day period in terms of the types of food eaten? If not, describe how a more typical 7-day period would appear. _____

    _____

5. Your instructor may prepare a dietary profile of the class against which you can evaluate your personal 7-day diet assessment.

CHAPTER 8

Limiting Your Body Fat Through
Diet & Exercise

Objectives

After completing this chapter, you should be able to do the following:

■ Explain the distinction between body weight and body composition.
■ Analyze the principle of caloric balance and how imbalances lead to gain or loss of body fat.
■ Identify various methods for losing body fat.
■ Assess the importance of lifestyle modification for long-term weight control.
■ Develop a program of weight loss or maintenance consistent with your needs.

WHY SHOULD YOU BE CONCERNED ABOUT BODY FAT?

It seems that virtually all Americans at one time or another have been concerned about their body fat. Most look in the mirror and study the "roll" of fat that spreads around their midsection or the dimpled fat on their thighs and wonder how to eliminate it. Wearing a bathing suit becomes an act of courage. Our desire to achieve a more ideal appearance makes us easy targets for those interested in profiting from our concern.

The battle against excess body fat has turned into a multibillion-dollar industry that presents various diet plans, exercise studios, and countless gimmicks and gadgets guaranteed to help you lose that extra body fat and inches. One thing they don't guarantee is that you will be able to maintain the loss of body fat. Most people who do lose body fat eventually regain it and even some extra fat. So, why bother to try and lose body fat?

Many people decide to try and lose fat because they are dissatisfied with their appearance. However, there is little question that being overweight can lead to a number of health-related problems. If you are overly fat, you run an increased risk of developing heart

KEY TERMS

overweight	*caloric balance*
obesity	*calories*
body mass index (BMI)	*kilocalorie*
adipose cell	*basal metabolic rate*
subcutaneous fat	*set point theory*
body composition	*spot reducing*
lean body weight	*bulimia nervosa*
	anorexia nervosa

disease, hypertension, atherosclerosis, stroke, diabetes, infections of the respiratory tract, cancer, and disorders of the kidneys. If you are moderately overweight, you have a 40 percent higher risk of premature death. Individuals who are obese have a death rate 70 percent higher than normal. Obviously, you must be concerned about the amount of body fat you have.

THE AMERICAN LIFESTYLE

There are many reasons why our American lifestyle makes controlling the development of body fat difficult. It is virtually impossible to do anything socially without having something to eat or drink. We associate food with dating, weddings, birthdays, and funerals.

Technology has allowed the American lifestyle to become increasingly sedentary as more "labor-saving" devices are invented. The purpose of devices such as escalators and elevators, garage door openers and remotes for video and audio equipment is to make life and work easier, but there are few associated training effects from pressing a button or moving a joystick (Figure 8-1).

We do little in our lifestyle that increases physical activity levels. We try to park as close to the entrance as possible so we don't waste time and energy walking back and forth. It is easier to hop on an elevator or escalator than to walk up flights of stairs. Most are not aware of how their behaviors conserve energy rather than burn it.

In this country the problem with people having excess body fat has reached epidemic proportions. However, it must be emphasized that you should not assume that an individual who has either normal weight or normal body fat is also fit and healthy. A person who has some excess body fat relative to bone structure and height is said to be **overweight.** An individual who has a lot of excess body fat is said to be **obese.** Whether an individual with excess body fat is considered to be overweight or is considered to be obese is generally determined by their **body mass index (BMI).** BMI is determined by using a ratio of a person's body weight to height (Figure 8-2). A BMI between 18.5 and 25 is considered a range for healthy body weight. An individual with a BMI between 25 and 30 is considered overweight. If the BMI is greater than 30, that individual is considered to be obese. Lab Activity 8-1 will help you precisely calculate your BMI.

According to the latest information from the Centers for Disease Control and Prevention (CDC), about two of three U.S. adults over age 20 (64 percent) have a BMI greater than 25 and thus are either overweight or obese. Thirty percent have a BMI greater than 30 and are considered to be obese. The total economic cost of obesity in the United States is about $117 billion per year, including more than $50 billion in avoidable medical costs. Clearly the problem of having excess body fat is a major health problem in the United States.

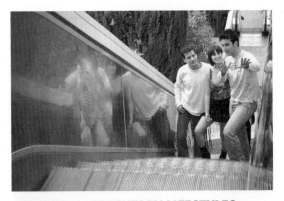

FIGURE 8-1. SEDENTARY LIFESTYLES.
Technology has allowed our lifestyle to become more sedentary.

overweight: having excess body weight relative to bone structure and height

obesity: an excessive amount of body fat

body mass index (BMI): Body mass index: ratio of body weight to height

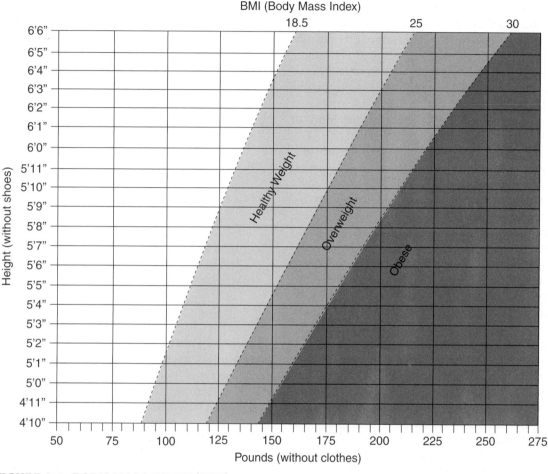

FIGURE 8-2. BODY MASS INDEX (BMI).

Source: Report of the Dietary Guidelines Advisory Committee on the Dietary Guidelines for Americans 2000.

What is the best way to minimize the development of body fat? Most people tend to panic when they realize that they have put on a little extra fat. They either go on starvation diets or become exercise fanatics, neither of which is particularly enjoyable or provides a long-term solution to the problem. The key to being able to limit your body fat is to have the motivation to alter your lifestyle in ways that you can live with. You need to make a commitment to changing your lifestyle so that you burn off extra energy and consume less food. The cumulative effect of these mod-ifications will make it easier for you to minimize the development of body fat. This approach should become an integral part of your lifestyle rather than a behavior you adopt from time to time.

HOW IS FAT STORED AND WHERE DO YOU FIND IT?

Fat is found in all of the body's cells. Some essential fat is necessary for cushioning organs, regulating temperature, and storing energy for future needs. Nonessential fat gradually accumulates when your food intake exceeds your energy demands. A special type of cell, the adipose cell, stores fat. The **adipose cell** stores triglyceride (a liquid form of fat), which moves in and out of the cell according to energy needs. The greater the amount of triglyceride contained in the adipose cells, the greater the amount of total body weight that is composed of fat.

There are two types of body fat: **subcutaneous fat** lies just below the skin, and visceral fat is generally found around the organs deep in the abdomen. Women have a genetic predisposition for depositing subcutaneous fat in the abdomen. Extra fat around the abdominal and pelvic areas provides a cushion that prevents trauma on a developing baby. Men tend to store visceral fat deep in their abdomen. After age 30, testosterone production tends to go down, causing reduced lean muscle mass and a higher rate of accumulation of abdominal fat. It becomes considerably more difficult to lose weight. The fat distribution in adults tends to follow particular patterns that are largely inherited. In general, people tend to have large stores of fat in the abdominal area; women tend to store more fat in their hips and thighs than men. A useful estimate of overweight, obesity, and body fat distribution involves measurement of waist circumference (Figure 8-3). It appears that the location of fat on the body is significant. If the majority of fat is found around the waist, you are more likely to develop health problems than if most of your fat is in your hips and thighs. This is true even if your BMI falls within the normal range. Males with a waist measurement of more than 40 inches or females with a waist measurement

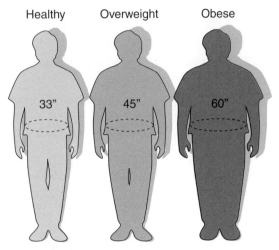

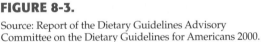

FIGURE 8-3.

Source: Report of the Dietary Guidelines Advisory Committee on the Dietary Guidelines for Americans 2000.

of greater than 35 inches may have a higher disease risk than people with smaller waist measurements because of where the majority of their fat is found (Figure 8-4).

The term *cellulite* is often used in magazines and advertisements to identify a type of fat that appears to be dimpled and usually is deposited in the buttocks, upper thighs, and upper arms. Cellulite is a nonmedical term for the ordinary adipose tissue that is found in these sites. Losing weight and exercising will reduce all body fat, including cellulite.

WHAT DETERMINES HOW MUCH FAT YOU HAVE?

►Fat Cell Theory

Two factors determine the amount of fat found in the body: (1) the number of adipose cells and (2) the size of the adipose cell. The number of adipose cells increases before birth and continues to rise until puberty. Children who become obese at an early age are believed to have too many fat cells (hyperplasia). Adolescents who

---

adipose cell: a type of cell that stores triglyceride, a liquid form of fat

subcutaneous fat: the fat that is found directly under the skin

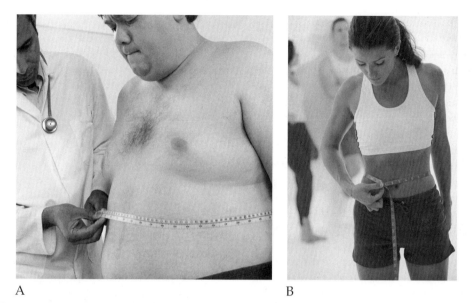

A   B

FIGURE 8-4. WAIST CIRCUMFERENCE.
Waist measurement is directly related to obesity and overweight.

become overweight seem to develop a greater number of fat cells than those of normal weight. It has been thought that by early adulthood the number of fat cells becomes fixed. However, most recent evidence suggests that fat cell number may increase under certain conditions during adulthood.

In addition to cell number, cell size is a factor in obesity. The size of the adipose cell depends on the amount of fat stored within it. Fat cell size increases (hypertrophies) until early adulthood. In the mature adult, fat cell size fluctuates as a function of caloric balance. If more calories are consumed than are needed, the excess is converted to fat and stored in the adipose cells. Under this condition, adipose cells swell with fat. When the energy from fat is needed to fuel activities, the fat cells lose stored fat and shrink in size.

The aging process generally leads to increased percentage of body fat and reduced quantities of lean muscle mass. With aging, metabolism changes, and there is a tendency to easily store fat around the midsection. A research study has shown that as age progresses, muscle thickness decreases while subcutaneous fat increases around the abdomen in both males and females, with the rate of change in both measures being higher in women than in men. Also, subcutaneous fat is a more significant factor affecting waist circumference than muscle thickness, irrespective of age or gender.

Contrary to popular belief, a fat baby does not necessarily become a fat child or fat young adult. However, after the age of two, a child begins to adopt the eating behaviors and activity patterns of his or her family members. If this child is still too fat by the time he or she starts school, then it is more likely that he or she will become a fat adolescent and adult. In fact the chances of this happening are three times greater in the obese child than in children of normal body weight.

In children who become obese at an early age, weight increases are primarily due to increases in the number of fat cells. In adults, weight loss or gain is primarily a function of the changes in fat cell size, not cell numbers. Thus obese adults tend to exhibit a great deal of adipose cell hypertrophy.

WHAT IS BODY COMPOSITION?

Body composition refers to both the fat and the nonfat components of the body. The portion of total body weight that is composed of fat tissue is referred to as the percentage body fat. **Lean body weight** is made up by every type of body tissue that is not fat (i.e., bone, muscle, tendon, ligament, connective tissue, nerves, skin, hair, etc.). Generally, the goal is to maximize the percentage of total body weight that is composed of lean tissue, and minimize the percentage of total body weight composed of fat. Assessment of body composition is perhaps a bit more difficult than simply stepping on a scale and measuring actual body weight in pounds. **However, body weight as determined by a scale does not take into account how much of the weight is lean tissue and how much of the weight is fat.** Body composition measurements are more accurate in attempting to determine precisely how much weight a person may gain or lose.

In the traditional college student age range, between 20 and 25 percent of the average female's total body weight is made up of fat. The average male has between 15 and 20 percent body fat. However, persons who engage in strenuous physical activities on a regular basis tend to have a lower percentage body fat. Male endurance athletes may get their fat percentage as low as 8 to 12 percent, and female endurance athletes may reach 12 to 18 percent body fat. It is recommended that body fat percentage not go below 5 percent in

body composition: the fat and nonfat components of the body

lean body weight: the portion of the total body weight that is composed of nonfat or lean tissue

men and 12 percent in women because a certain amount of body fat is necessary for good health. As age increases, average percent body fat for both males and females will also increase. Individuals whose body fat percentage is above these normal ranges are said to be overfat while those below the normal ranges are referred to as underfat.

HOW DO YOU MEASURE BODY COMPOSITION?

There are several methods of assessing body composition:

1. Hydrostatic (underwater) weighing involves placing a subject in a specially designed underwater tank to determine body density. Accuracy +/−1.5 percent.
2. Measurement of electrical impedance predicts the percentage body fat by assessing resistance to the flow of electrical current through the body between selected points. Accuracy +/−3 percent.
3. DXA (dual energy X-ray absorptiometry) technology is the most recent and the most accurate technique of assessing body composition, but it is fairly expensive, costing around $300 per test. The instrument uses total body X-ray technique to look at the density of the body and can then estimate the amount of lean and fat tissue. Accuracy +/−1.5 percent.
4. The BOD POD Body Composition System uses the relationship between pressure and volume to derive the body volume of a subject seated in a fiberglass chamber. The principle is similar to hydrostatic weighing except instead of using water to measure body volume, the BOD POD uses air displacement to measure body volume. Accuracy +/−3 percent.
5. Measurement of skinfold thickness is the simplest and most commonly used method. Accuracy +/−3 percent.

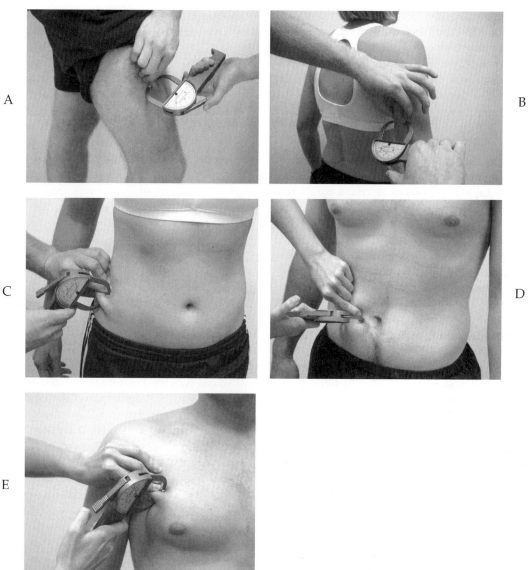

FIGURE 8-5. SKINFOLD MEASUREMENT SITES.
A, Thigh (males & females); B, Tricep (females only); C, Suprailiac (females only); D, Abdominal (males only); E, Chest (males only).

▶Measuring Skinfold Thickness

The last technique is based on the idea that about 50 percent of the fat in the body is subcutaneous (under the skin). By measuring the thickness of this layer of fat, the total percentage of body fat can be estimated. Skinfolds are measured at various body sites using skinfold calipers (see Figure 8-5). Men and women tend to develop fat deposits in different body areas; skinfold measurements must be taken at these specified places. A number of different methods for calculating percent body fat using skinfold measurements have been developed. The technique proposed by Jackson and Pollack will be used in Lab Activity 8-2 to determine body fat composition. Although skinfold measurement is a less accurate method than underwater weighing and a DXA scan, and about the same as electrical impedence, almost everyone can learn to perform this technique. Furthermore, the calipers are less costly and time-consuming to use than the other equipment.

When taking a series of skinfold measurements over time to determine changes, it is important that the same person take the measurements all the time. Due to the potential error that is always possible with caliper measures, having the same person take repeated measurements will minimize errors and give a more accurate indication of absolute changes in body composition.

Once you have calculated the percentage of your total body weight that is made up of fat tissue, you may determine that you have too much fat. It would be helpful to determine how much weight you have to lose to achieve a normal percent body fat. Lab Activity 8-2 provides a worksheet to help you calculate your desired body weight.

HOW DO YOU ACHIEVE CALORIC BALANCE?

It is important to reemphasize that fat in the form of triglyceride moves in and out of the adipose cell according to energy demands. If you have been able to maintain your weight, you are in a state of **caloric balance.** That is, the number of **calories*** that you consume in food equals the number that you use or expend. If you are trying to gain weight, then you need to consume more calories than you expend. The extra calories will be stored, and you will gain weight (*positive caloric balance*). Conversely, if you want to lose weight, you need to expend more energy than you are consuming so that the body has to use its fat stores for energy (*negative caloric balance*). **Any excess of calories, whether from foods or supplements that contain the basic energy nutrients (protein, carbohydrates, or fat), can be converted to body fat and stored.** See Chapter 7 for a more detailed discussion of the various foodstuffs.

There are differences in the caloric content of these three foodstuffs.

> Carbohydrate = 4 calories per gram
> Protein = 4 calories per gram
> Fat = 9 calories per gram

It becomes extremely important to consider the implications of caloric values when considering programs for weight loss or gain. The percentage of total body weight that is composed of fat is highly related to the level of physical activity. Persons who have an excess of fat tend to be sedentary and therefore are in a positive calorie situation. In behavioral terms, the number of calories in food ingested and the number of calories expended can be modified. You can eat less and exercise more. However, for many who do not overeat, gradual weight gain often occurs as a result of decreased activity and muscle mass reduction that occurs with aging. The caloric expenditure of physical activities and resting metabolism declines with aging. It will become necessary to decrease caloric intake by about 2.5 percent for every 10 years over the age of 25. Thus, as you age, it

---

*A calorie is simply a measure of the energy value of a foodstuff. A calorie by defintion is the amount of energy necessary to raise the temperature of 1 gram of water 1°C. However, this unit is too small to be easy to use, so the term kilocalorie is more appropriate. A **kilocalorie** is equal to 1,000 calories. Thus subsequent mention to a specific number of calories in this text refers to kilocalories, which will be denoted as kcal or calories.

---

caloric balance: the number of calories consumed equals the number of calories expended

calories: a measure of the energy value of a foodstuff

kilocalorie: 1,000 calories

becomes increasingly important to either increase exercise levels or decrease caloric intake to avoid gaining body fat.

HOW MANY CALORIES DO YOU EXPEND EACH DAY?

Before you can plan your weight modification program, you need to know (1) how much energy you typically use each day (caloric expenditure) and (2) how much energy you consume in your diet each day. Physical activity, whether competitive or recreational, results in an increased need for energy. The goal is to consume enough nutritious foods to meet basic tissue needs plus an additional amount to meet increased energy needs for the activity. Generally, people who participate in physical activity need more energy supplied by the three foodstuffs but not additional vitamins or minerals. As they increase their activity, people usually increase their food intake, which meets nutritional needs (Figure 8-6).

If a physically active person's daily energy intake does not match the energy expenditure, body weight loss will occur. For individuals who want to maintain or alter their weight, some estimation of caloric expenditure and intake is necessary.

To estimate your total daily energy expenditure (TDEE) you must calculate both your **basal metabolic rate** (BMR) and the total energy required for all activities you are involved in throughout the course of a day. It is first necessary to determine the number of calories (energy) needed to support your basal metabolism. This is the minimal level of energy required to sustain the body's vital functions such as respiration, circulation, and maintenance of body temperature. The BMR is the rate at which calories are spent for these maintenance activities. Fit List 8-1 describes various factors that influence BMR. Lab Activity 8-3 will help you determine your BMR.

Once BMR has been determined, Lab Activity 8-4 will help you calculate energy

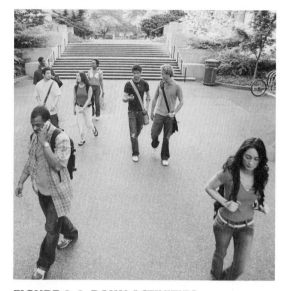

FIGURE 8-6. DAILY ACTIVITIES.
How many calories do you expend walking to class, exercising, studying, watching TV, or sleeping each day?

requirements of all activities done in a 24-hour period. There is a wide variation in energy output for different types of activity and thus there is some difficulty in achieving accuracy in this exercise. It is determined by the type, intensity, and duration of a physical activity. Body size is also a factor; heavier people expend more energy in an activity than lighter ones. Specific energy expenditures may be determined by consulting charts that predict energy used in an activity based on (1) the time spent in each activity in minutes and (2) the metabolic costs of each activity in kilocalories per minute per pound (kcal/min/lb) of body weight. If you were to carefully calculate energy costs of all daily activities such as sitting, walking, and studying, you can

basal metabolic rate: the rate at which calories are spent for carrying on the body's vital functions and maintenance activities

FIT LIST 8-1

Factors Influencing BMR

Age: In general, the younger the person, the higher the BMR.

Body surface area: The greater the amount of body surface area, the higher the BMR.

Gender: Men generally have a higher metabolic rate than women.

Diet: There is a dramatic and sustained reduction in BMR that occurs with very-low-calorie dieting.

Exercise: Consistent exercise tends to increase the BMR during the activity and for a period of time after the activity ceases.

estimate the amount of energy used in a day. By determining your caloric needs for BMR and daily activities, you can calculate your total daily energy expenditure.

HOW MANY CALORIES DO YOU EAT EACH DAY?

Once you have some idea of how many calories you expend each day, you need to determine how many calories you are consuming. A physically active person needs a sufficient number of calories from food to maintain body weight and composition. Determining caloric intake requires consulting food composition tables such as the ones in the USDA Nutrient Database (http://www.nal.usda.gov/fnic/foodcomp/search/). The USDA Nutrient Database indicates the nutritive value of commonly used foods. This chart identifies specific foods and indicates the number of calories per specified serving size. For example, you will see that 1 ounce of cheddar cheese provides 114 calories. Maintaining a daily food intake log like that in Lab Activity 8-5 can determine not only your caloric intake but also your eating patterns

and habits. Factors unrelated to nutrition often influence what kinds of foods are selected and how much is eaten. These factors include your mood and social environment at mealtimes. From this table you may calculate your daily caloric intake.

ASSESSING YOUR CALORIC BALANCE

If the daily logs for estimating caloric intake and caloric expenditure have been accurately kept, it will be relatively easy to compare the total caloric values to determine whether you are in caloric balance. It is not easy to maintain caloric balance on a daily basis. One reason is that schedules never seem to be the same from one day to the next. Eating meals may be inconsistent, as are times spent engaged in physical activity. Estimations of caloric intake range from between 1,000 to 5,000 calories per day. Estimations of caloric expenditure range from between 2,200 and 4,400 calories per day. Energy demands will be higher for those who are physically active and considerably higher for endurance-type athletes, who may require 7,000 calories or more per day. If you desire to lose weight, you must modify your behaviors so that you are burning more calories for energy than you are taking in. If you want to gain weight, you must consume more calories than you expend (Figure 8-7). The Worksheet for Estimating

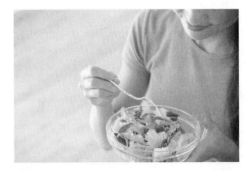

FIGURE 8-7. EATING.
How many calories do you consume each day?

Caloric Balance (page 211) will indicate whether you are in a state of positive or negative caloric balance based on your estimation of caloric intake and expenditure.

SET POINT THEORY OF WEIGHT CONTROL

If you completed the Lab Activities and kept track of your weight, you may have noticed that although your caloric balance fluctuated from day to day, your weight did not go up or down. **Set point theory** is intended to explain why it is so difficult to lose or gain weight. It is hypothesized that the body tends to maintain a certain level of body fat. This theory maintains that the body has a "set point" or some mechanism for maintaining a specific body weight. It operates like a thermostat that is set to control a house's temperature. When the temperature in the house drops below the set point, the furnace turns on. When the temperature warms to the setting, the furnace shuts off. For people, it may be that the body's fat level is set at a particular point, and the body resists attempts to reduce this level.

It is unclear how this set point is controlled. It may be that the fat cells tend to maintain a certain degree of fat stored within them and resist efforts to reduce their size. Exercise in combination with caloric restriction appears to be the only way to reduce the set point. In any case, the set point theory is just that, a theory that may explain why so many people are unsuccessful at keeping off the fat lost through dieting.

> **set point theory:** a mechanism for maintaining body weight at a specific level

WHAT CAN YOU DO TO LOSE BODY FAT?

There are many fat reduction techniques available; some are based on sound scientific and nutritional principles, and others are dangerous or a waste of money. Losing body fat boils down to creating a situation of negative caloric balance. First, food intake may be decreased by dieting. Second, caloric expenditure may be increased by increasing the amount of physical activity. Finally, a combination of approaches can be attempted.

LOSING BODY FAT BY DIETING

Fat loss through dieting alone is difficult (Figure 8-8). Much of what we choose to eat is influenced not by hunger but by other factors such as customs, advertising, our moods, and the attractiveness and availability of the food supply. Pizza can be delivered to your door with a phone call. Food has meaning to us; we associate sweet, "rich" desserts with rewards for good performances or just to make us feel

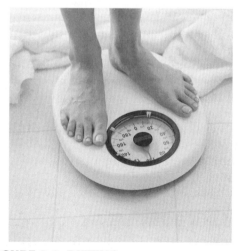

FIGURE 8-8. DIETING.
Losing fat and weight through dieting alone is difficult.

better. Furthermore, dieting is viewed as the deprivation and punishment one must endure for overindulgence. Every so often, we literally starve ourselves, lose a few pounds, and then promptly return to our old eating habits and regain the body fat that was lost. The behavior is repeated without achieving lasting weight control. Thus periodic dieting is ineffective. At best, long-term weight control by dieting alone is successful only 20 percent of the time.

Obviously, in any weight-loss program the goal is to lose fat, not lean tissue. Unfortunately, many popular diets, the so-called starvation diets, recommend reduction of caloric intake to dangerous levels. It is recommended that the minimum caloric intake for a female not go below 1,000 to 1,200 calories per day and for a male not below 1,200 to 1,500 calories per day. A minimum level of 1,200 calories may be needed to avoid entering a starvation metabolism. It should also be added that it is difficult to maintain adequate nutrition when caloric intake is at this level for long periods of time. Low-calorie eating plans require careful planning to avoid nutritional deficits.

Starvation diets that restrict caloric intake below these recommended levels may actually reduce metabolic rate, thus making losing fat more difficult. The body's metabolic rate goes into "low gear" and conserves calories. The ideal situation is to keep the metabolic rate at normal or raise it to burn more calories. The initial weight loss that occurs with severe caloric restriction for the first few days of the diet may be encouraging. However, the majority of this weight loss is not due to the loss of much fat but results from loss of water weight (dehydration). More moderate reductions of total calories are recommended to lose body fat.

LOSING BODY FAT BY EXERCISING

Clearly, dieting alone is not the answer to long-term weight control. However, the weight lost through exercise involves primarily loss of fat tissue (estimates are as high as 90 percent) and almost no loss of lean tissue. Establishing new behaviors that include daily physical activity takes a great deal of motivation. For most of us, exercise habits were established early in life. Physical activity in adolescence can prevent the formation of excess adipose tissue and results in an increase in lean body weight. At any age, physical activity, when combined with caloric reduction, can lead to substantial losses of body fat while preserving lean tissue (Figure 8-9). Keep in mind that physical activity in the sedentary college student may result in increases in muscle tissue, which is more dense and has greater weight than fat tissue. Thus, for anyone, initial attempts at weight loss through increased activity levels may be frustrating. You weigh yourself and see no change or even an increase in weight. Instead of relying on scales, which provide no information about changes in body composition, every few weeks you should measure skinfold thickness to determine fat loss.

It must be emphasized that the increase in muscle mass will eventually produce an increase in metabolism, which in the long term helps to burn fat stores.

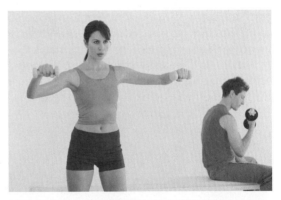

FIGURE 8-9. EXERCISE AND WEIGHT LOSS.
Weight loss through exercise involves primarily a loss of fat tissue and almost no loss of lean tissue.

▶ Moderate Intensity Aerobic Activity

To maximize weight loss during exercise you can turn to the FIT principle discussed in Chapter 4. For weight loss you should exercise using an aerobic activity at intensity of 60 percent to 70 percent of your maximum aerobic capacity or maximum heart rate. Certainly you want to expend calories during the activity. While exercising at an intensity above 70 percent of your maximum heart rate over an extended period of time may allow you to burn more calories, less of those calories will be from fat. If the body can't use your fat stores it begins to utilize lean muscle stores. For the most effective weight loss we want the calories to come from fat stores, not from lean muscle stores. Increasing the time of the exercise will help to expend additional calories. Therefore, slowing down and exercising longer is a quicker and more effective route to losing weight. It should be pointed out that once exercise ends, some additional calories are expended during that time the metabolic rate is returning to resting levels. This has been referred to as the recovery period. Clearly this would affect any estimate of the total number of calories expended in response to the energy demands of exercise and increased metabolism.

▶ Spot Reducing

Many try techniques for **spot reducing.** Trying to reduce the level of body fat at specific sites such as the waist or thighs is useless. During exercise, the energy is supplied from fat stores throughout the body, not just the muscles being moved. However, actively exercising a specific area may increase muscle tone and possibly muscle strength, although the fat in that area will not be reduced. You lose inches

> **spot reducing:** a useless attempt to reduce fat stored in a specific area

off your body, which makes clothing fit more comfortably. Nevertheless, the benefits of aerobic exercise on the entire body are important to overall health.

Losing fat through exercise alone is almost as difficult as losing weight through dieting. People trying to exercise solely for the purpose of losing fat are not likely to stick with an exercise program for a long time. However, it is essential to realize that physical exercise not only will result in weight reduction from losing body fat but also may enhance cardiorespiratory endurance, improve strength, and increase flexibility. For this reason, exercise has some distinct advantages over dieting in any weight-loss program.

LOSING BODY FAT BY DIETING AND EXERCISING

Undoubtedly the most efficient method of decreasing the percentage of body fat is through some combination of diet and exercise. A moderate caloric restriction combined with a moderate increase in caloric expenditure will result in a negative caloric balance. This method is relatively fast and easy compared with either of the others, especially if it focuses on changing eating habits and activity levels. You don't have to starve and run 6 miles a day. If you reduce caloric intake by 200 to 300 calories per day and increase caloric expenditure by 200 to 300 calories per day, over a 7-day period this will result in a loss of approximately 3,500 calories, or 1 pound of body fat.

> One Pound of Body Fat = 3,500 calories

In any weight-loss program, the maximum weight loss should be 1 to 2 pounds per week. The rate of weight loss depends on how much body fat the person has at the start of the period of caloric restriction. In general, the greater the amount of body fat, the more rapidly one loses while on a calorie-reduced diet. This explains why some people lose 4 pounds or more the

FIT LIST 8-2

Weight-Loss Strategies

A number of strategies may be involved in a behavior modification approach to weight loss. Some of these approaches include the following:

- Keeping a log of the times, settings, reasons, and feelings associated with your eating.
- Controlling negative emotions such as boredom, loneliness, anger, and frustration while eating.
- Setting realistic, long-term goals (for example, loss of a pound per week instead of 5 pounds per week).
- Avoiding the total deprivation of enjoyable foods (occasionally reward yourself with a small treat).
- Eating slowly and realizing that the sacrifices you are making are what *you* feel are important for *your* health and happiness.
- Putting more physical activity into your daily routine (taking stairs instead of elevators, or parking in the distant part of a parking lot, for example).
- Rewarding yourself when you reach your goals (with new clothes, sporting equipment, a vacation trip).
- Sharing your commitment to weight loss with your family and friends (then they can support your efforts).
- Keeping careful records of daily food consumption and weight change.
- Being prepared to deal with occasional plateaus and setbacks in your quest for weight loss.
- Cutting back consumption of "junk foods" and trying to adjust cooking habits (see the Health Links in Chapter 7).

From Payne, W., and D. Hahn. 2000. *Understanding your health.* St Louis: McGraw-Hill.

first week on a low-calorie diet. They had maintained their excess weight on relatively high-calorie levels, and the reduction creates a major need for energy from fat stores.

A slower rate of weight loss indicates that the person is making minor lifestyle changes, particularly in regard to eating and physical activity behaviors, that they can maintain over time. The adoption of new behaviors and attitudes takes time. Fit List 8-2 lists suggestions for weight-loss strategies to help keep one motivated in weight control efforts.

EMPHASIZING THE LONG-HAUL APPROACH TO MINIMIZING BODY FAT

In any program for losing body fat, the "long haul" must be emphasized. It generally took a long time to accumulate that extra body fat, and it will take time to lose it safely. This fact is frustrating to the impatient individual who wants results fast. Many of these people starve themselves to lose body fat, shed some pounds, then return to their former eating habits and experience weight gain, the so-called "yo-yo" effect. This behavior makes subsequent efforts to lose body fat even more difficult, since the body tends to protect its existing fat stores.

WEIGHT-LOSS GIMMICKS AND FADS

Even educated people will resort to almost anything in a desperate effort to lose weight. Each year (especially before the summer months), Americans spend billions of dollars trying to find any method that promises they will lose weight quickly and without much effort. People are willing to spend money and time on diet programs, creams, gadgets, books, and equipment that claim to "melt pounds fast." Claims are made for rubberized suits that are supposed to "sweat" off pounds, mechanical devices to shake, vibrate, or roll off the fat; and creams and powders to remove "cellulite." Many people resort to the use of diet pills. Advertisements display physically attractive people who are reported to have lost dozens of pounds while using a device or diet plan. Most weight-loss gimmicks are based on unsound nutritional information and have no basis in scientific fact. Although people may lose weight at first, they become bored with the technique and lose interest. Any weight that was lost is regained.

What about the numerous diet plans? It seems that a new diet plan appears in a book that makes the best-seller list monthly. It is not easy to determine whether or not a diet plan is reliable and safe to follow. Table 8-1 reviews some of the more popular weight-loss plans. You will continue to see or hear about unreliable methods as long as people are unable to make the lifestyle changes needed to maintain control over their body weight.

SETTING REALISTIC GOALS FOR WEIGHT LOSS

Once you have decided to change your lifestyle to decrease your percent body fat, you must set some weight-loss goals. First, determine a desirable weight that is realistic in terms of your age, height, and bone structure. Goals must be reasonable and attainable. If you set too high a goal, you may become dissatisfied with any degree of weight loss that does not meet the goal. Ultimately, your goal should be to reach the standards for at least achieving the "good" body fat percentages for your age group as

shown in Table 8-2. The second important goal is to determine a reasonable and safe rate of weight loss; it may be as low as ½ pound per week or as high as 2 pounds, depending on how much weight you have to lose. You may lose weight faster at first, but the rate slows and eventually averages out to become close to the goal rate within a few weeks.

HEALTH AT ANY SIZE

Health at Any Size (HAAS) is an approach to health and well-being that accepts natural diversity in body size, encouraging people to stop focusing on weight, dieting, or other weight loss efforts in favor of listening to and respecting their natural appetites for food, drink, sleep, rest, and recreation. This philosophy helps people live well without encouraging or reinforcing size/weight prejudices or phobias, poor body image, or eating disorders—or the negative health consequences of dieting-related weight loss and regain. HAAS and the similar group, Health at Every Size, base their ideas on research data suggesting that explicitly trying to achieve a weight in the standard recommended weight or body mass index range through dieting is not a desirable goal for individuals wishing to improve their health.

The basic principles of HAAS are:

- Accepting and respecting the diversity of body shapes and sizes.

- Recognizing that health and well-being are multidimensional and that they include physical, social, spiritual, occupational, emotional, and intellectual aspects.

- Promoting all aspects of health and well-being for people of all sizes.

- Promoting eating in a manner that balances individual nutritional needs, hunger, satiety, appetite, and pleasure.

TABLE 8-1
OVERVIEW OF DIET PLANS

Type of Diet	Advantages	Disadvantages	Examples
Low fat; Low cholesterol	High in fruit, vegetables; and whole grains; low-fat non-fat dairy Lowers cholesterol Lowers risk of stroke Lowers risk of heart disease Lowers risk of diabetes Lowers Blood pressure	Constipation	DASH Diet Mediterranean Diet Therapeutic Lifestyle Changes (TLC)
High-Protein, Low-Carbohydrate Diets Usually include all the meat, fish, poultry, and eggs you can eat Occasionally permit milk and cheese in limited amounts Prohibits fruits, vegetables, and any bread or cereal products	Rapid initial weight loss because of diuretic effect Very little hunger	Too low in carbohydrates Deficient in many nutrients—vitamin C, vitamin A (unless eggs are included), calcium, and several trace elements High in saturated fat, cholesterol, and total fat Will result in ketosis because the major energy sources are protein and fat—both dietary and body. Extreme diets of this type could cause death Impossible to adhere to these diets long enough to lose any appreciable amount of weight Dangerous for people with kidney disease Weight loss, which is largely water, is rapidly regained Diet does not develop a new and useful set of eating habits Expensive Unpalatable after first few days Difficult for dieter to eat out	Dr. Stillman's Quick Weight Loss Diet Calories Don't Count by Dr. Taller Dr. Atkin's Diet Revolution Scarsdale Diet Air Force Diet Mastering the Zone Diet Carbohydrate Addict's Lifespan Program South Beach Diet Protein Power Schwarzbein Principle Sugar Busters

From Guthrie, H.A. 1989. *Introductory nutrition,* St. Louis: Mosby.

Continued

TABLE 8-1 OVERVIEW OF DIET PLANS—CONT.			
Type of Diet	Advantages	Disadvantages	Examples
Low-Calorie, High-Protein Supplement Diets			
Usually a premeasured powder to be reconstituted with water or a prepared liquid formula	Rapid initial weight loss Easy to prepare—already measured Palatable for first few days Usually fortified to provide recommended amounts of micronutrients Must be labeled if >50% protein	Usually prescribed at dangerously low kilocalorie intake of 300 to 500 kcal Will result in ketosis Do not retrain dieters in acceptable eating habits Overpriced; initially, users are often urged to buy several large cans of different flavors of the diet food (which is usually non-fat dried milk) Low in fiber and bulk—constipating in short amount of time Frequently cause loss of potassium with resultant weakness and heart arrhythmias Often contain poor quality protein	Metracal Diet Cambridge Diet Liquid Protein Diet Last Chance Diet Diet Divas Oxford Diet
Restricted-Calorie, Balanced Food Plans			
	Sufficiently low in kilocalories to permit steady weight loss Nutritionally balanced Palatable Include readily available foods Reasonable in cost Can be adapted from family meals Permit eating out and social eating	Do not appeal to people who want a "unique" diet Do not produce immediate and large weight losses	Weight Watchers Diet Prudent Diet (American Heart Association) The I Love New York Diet UCLA Diet Time-calorie Displacement (TCD) Overeaters Anonymous The Beyond Diet

Continued

TABLE 8-1 OVERVIEW OF DIET PLANS—CONT.			
Type of Diet	**Advantages**	**Disadvantages**	**Examples**
	Promote a new set of eating habits		Take Off Pounds Sensibly (TOPS) Fit or Fat Target Diet Ediet
Fasting/Starvation Diet	Rapid inital loss	Nutrient deficient Danger of ketosis >60% loss is muscle <40% loss is fat Low long-term success rates	ZIP Diet 5-day Miracle Diet 3-day Diet
High-Carbohydrate Diet	Emphasizes grains, fruits, vegetables High in bulk Low in cholesterol	Limits milk, meat Nutritionally very inadequate for calcium, iron, and protein	Low Fat Diet New Beverly Hills Diet Quick Weight Loss Diet Pritikin Diet Carbohydrate Cravers Hilton Head Metabolism Diet
High-Fiber, Low-Calorie Diets	High satiety value Provide bulk	Irritating to the lower colon Decrease absorption of trace elements, especially iron Nutritionally deficient Low in protein	High Fiber Diet Volumetrics Pritikin Diet F Diet Zen Macrobiotic Diet Rice Diet Eat More, Weigh Less Heart Smart Diet

Continued

TABLE 8-1
OVERVIEW OF DIET PLANS—CONT.

Type of Diet	Advantages	Disadvantages	Examples
Protein-Sparing Modified Fats <50% protein: 400 kcal	Safe under supervision High-quality protein Minimize loss of lean body mass	Decreases BMR Monotonous Expensive	Optifast Medifast Cambridge Diet Last Chance Diet Slimfast Ultrafast
Premeasured Food Plans	Provides the pre-scribed portion sizes—little chance of too small or too large a portion Total food programs Some provide ade-quate calories (1,200) Nutritionally balanced or supplemented	Expensive Do not retrain dieters in accept-able eating habits Precludes eating out or social eating Often low in bulk Monotonous Low long-term success rates	NutriSystem Carnation Plan Jenny Craig Herbalife Genesis
Limited Food Choice Diets	Reduce the number of food choices made by the users Limited opportunity to make mistakes Almost certainly low in calories after the first few days	Deficient in many nutrients, de-pending on the foods allowed Monotonous—difficult to ad-here to Eating out and eating socially are difficult Do not retrain dieters in accept-able eating habits Low long-term success rates No scientific basis for these diets	Mayo Clinic Diet Cabbage Soup Diet Banana and Milk Diet Grapefruit and Cottage Cheese Diet Kempner Rice Diet Lecithin, Vinegar, Kelp, Vitamin B_6 Diet Beverly Hills Diet Fit for Life Low Sodium Diet Healthy Soy Diet

TABLE 8-2
PERCENT FAT BASED ON SKINFOLDS

Rating	9%–17% Men				Rating	17%–25% Women			
	Ages 20–29	Ages 30–39	Ages 40–49	Ages 50+		Ages 20–29	Ages 30–39	Ages 40–49	Ages 50+
Dangerously Low	<5	<5	<5	<5	Dangerously Low				
Excellent	5–8.9	5–10.9	5–11.9	5–12.9	Excellent	<12	<12	<12	<12
GOOD	9–12.9	11–13.9	12–15.9	13–16.9	GOOD	12–16.9	12–17.9	12–19.9	12–20.9
Fair	13–16.9	14–17.9	16–20.9	17–21.9	Fair	17–20.9	18–21.9	20–23.9	21–24.9
Poor	17–19.9	18–22.9	21–25.9	22–27.9	Poor	21–23.9	22–24.9	24–27.9	25–30.9
Very Poor	>19.9	>22.9	>25.9	>27.9	Very Poor	24–27.9	25–29.9	28–31.9	31–35.9
						>27.9	>29.9	>31.9	>35.9

- Promoting individually appropriate, enjoyable, life-enhancing physical activity, rather than exercise that is focused on a goal of weight loss.

WHAT IF YOU WANT TO INCREASE LEAN BODY MASS?

As a society we seem to be preoccupied with losing weight. However, there are people who would like to gain weight. The aim of a weight-gaining program should be to increase lean body mass—that is, muscle, as opposed to body fat. Muscle mass should be increased only by muscle work combined with an increase in food consumption. It cannot be increased by the intake of any special food or vitamin. Unfortunately, as was indicated in Chapter 7, muscle mass and weight may also be increased in an unsafe manner through the use of steroids or growth hormones.

The recommended rate of weight gain is a maximum of 1 to 2 pounds per week. This can be achieved through positive caloric balance. One pound of fat represents the equivalent of 3,500 calories. Lean body tissue, which contains less fat, more protein, and more water than fat tissue, represents approximately 2,500 calories. Therefore to gain 1 pound of muscle, a weekly excess of approximately 2,500 calories is needed. Adding 500 to 1,000 calories daily to the usual diet will provide the energy needs of gaining 1 to 2 pounds per week and fuel the increased energy expenditure of the muscle training program. Weight training must be part of the program; otherwise, the excess energy intake will be converted to fat. Safe Tip 8-1 offers suggestions for an individual concerned about a safe weight-gaining program. For recommendations regarding weight training, refer to Chapter 5.

Athletes in training for competition require very high-calorie diets. They often believe that more protein is needed to build bigger muscles. Actually, a relatively small amount

SAFE TIP 8-1

Guidelines for Gaining Weight

- Set a reasonable goal. An exercise program should begin in advance of the competing season. Rapid weight gain indicates increase in fat, not muscle.
- Follow an exercise program prescribed by a fitness professional and designed to develop the desired muscles (see Chapter 3).
- Determine the usual caloric intake, then estimate the additional calories needed daily to gain lean weight.
- For a young individual, an additional 500 to 1,000 calories per day may be needed to gain lean weight. Therefore it is important to plan both the composition and the timing of meals and snacks. The diet should be based on the food groups (see Chapter 7), with additional calories obtained from larger portions of foods rich in complex carbohydrates. It is recommended that the diet contain less than 25 percent of calories from fat. The fat component of the diet should be low in saturated fats and cholesterol.

of additional protein is needed for the muscles developed in a training program. Most Americans consume about twice the amount of protein needed; therefore, protein is obtained by eating natural food sources rather than by consuming protein supplements. Furthermore, protein supplements may have undesirable effects on the body including stomach trouble, dehydration, gout, and calcium loss, as well as damage to the liver and kidneys.

One should monitor body weight weekly to ensure a gradual weight gain. Having the same person measuring skinfold thickness regularly will detect any increases in body fat. An increase in the skinfold thickness indicates a need for a reduction in caloric intake or an increase in training, or both, until it is demonstrated that the percentage of body fat is not increasing.

WHAT IS DISORDERED EATING?

To this point we have been discussing the problems with and the consequences of being overweight and of obesity. Clearly diet and eating patterns that result in overweight and obesity are the most common forms of disordered eating. Obesity represents an extreme in the eating continuum. Unfortunately for many people in our society, both males and females, weight loss has become an obsession that poses a threat to health and well-being. The media bombard the public with an ideal body image that is super-model thin. This creates social and internal pressures, especially for young women, and some men to become overly concerned with the relationship of body image to self-image (Figure 8-10). At one time, concerns about body image were much more prevelent in females. However in today's society, one study has shown that 45 percent of men were dissatisfied with their physique while women were only slightly less satisfied at 55 percent. Pursuing an ideal body image, even one that is unrealistic and unhealthy, becomes an attainable goal. A person who believes that a thinner body is the key to becoming more satisfied with oneself is susceptible to adopting bizarre behaviors in an attempt to find happiness. Some people adopt such extreme dieting behavior that they literally starve themselves to death. The next sections describe some of the more common eating disorders associated with self-image problems. Also, Fit List 8-3 provides some clues to identifying those with dangerous weight-control behaviors.

BULIMIA NERVOSA

Bulimia nervosa, believed to be one of the more common eating disorders, involves recurrent episodes of binge-type eating ("pigging out") followed by purging (vomiting and laxative abuse). Usually the binge consists of foods high in calories from fat or sugar, such as bags of

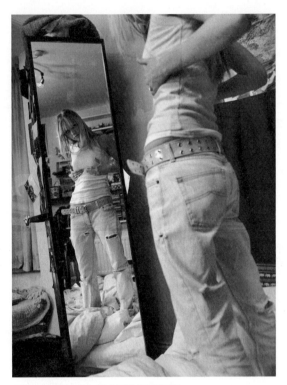

FIGURE 8-10. BODY IMAGE.
Many individuals with disordered eating tend to see an unrealistic distorted body image when they look at themselves in the mirror.

cookies, doughnuts, and chips. A typical binge involves the consumption of 1,000 calories or more during a 1- to 2-hour time period. These binges may occur once a month or, in severe cases, several times a day. To avoid gaining weight from the positive caloric situation, the person follows the binge with purging through vomiting, laxatives, or fasting. People who engage in such behavior tend to binge and purge in secret; in particular, the purging behavior is hidden from friends and family members.

bulimia nervosa: an eating disorder involving recurrent episodes of binge-type eating followed by purging

FIT LIST 8-3

Identifying Behaviors Associated with Disordered Eating

Reports or observation of the following signs or behaviors should arouse concern:

- Repeated expression of concerns about being or feeling fat even when weight is below average.
- Expressions of fear about being or becoming obese that do not diminish as weight loss continues.
- Refusal to maintain even a minimal normal weight consistent with the individual's sport, age, and height.
- Consumption of huge amounts of food not consistent with the person's weight.
- A pattern of eating substantial amounts of food, followed promptly by trips to the bathroom and resumption of eating shortly thereafter.
- Periods of severe calorie restriction or repeated days of fasting.
- Evidence of purposeless, excessive physical activity.
- Depressed mood and expression of self-deprecating thoughts after eating.
- Apparent preoccupation with the eating behavior of other people, such as friends, relatives, or teammates.
- Known or reported family history of eating disorders or family dysfunction.

Bulimia is most common in college-aged women who are about average in weight or not excessively overfat. Reports of bulimic behavior in young men involve the consumption of large quantities of beer and foods such as pizza followed by vomiting.

Although many people with bulimia are extroverts and socially active, they tend to have problems with interpersonal relationships. They suffer from low self-esteem and feel isolated because of their behavior. Bulimics believe that this behavior is disgusting and beyond their control. They become depressed and anxious, which in turn leads to more binging and purging episodes. In severe cases, bulimics become so obsessed with obtaining enough food and laxatives that they have little money for other needs. Sometimes they are arrested in the act of shoplifting these items from stores.

Getting Help for Bulimia

If untreated, the purging episodes can damage the body. The depressed bulimic may decide that suicide is the only solution to this abnormal behavior. If you know someone who seems to be able to eat huge amounts of food, is not physically active, yet is not gaining weight, you may suspect this disorder. It often helps to discuss the possibility of bulimia with them and to encourage them to obtain counseling. Treatment should focus on the causes of the behavior, including reasons for the low self-esteem and how to build supportive relationships. Individuals benefit from counseling that teaches how to cope with stress in a more constructive manner than binging and purging. Success is often measured in reducing the behavior rather than totally eliminating it. Thus it is essential to be realistic about changing bulimic behaviors; habits take time to change.

ANOREXIA NERVOSA

Anorexia nervosa is a psychological disease in which a person develops an aversion to food and a distorted body image. Over a period of time, the person loses a considerable amount of body weight so that health and life are threatened. Recently, anorexia nervosa has become a more widespread problem, although not as widespread as bulimia. About 90 percent of people with anorexia nervosa are female, and

anorexia nervosa: a psychological disease in which a person develops an aversion to food and a distorted body image the disorder usually begins around puberty. It is very obvious that these individuals are anorexic. They are so thin that they appear to have a terminal disease such as cancer. The subcutaneous fat layer is nearly absent, so veins can be seen on arms and legs. The typical feminine shape that is due to body fat deposits is absent. Extreme physical activity behaviors are also characteristic of the illness; the anorexic may jog or work out tirelessly. The normal female hormonal cycle depends on a certain minimal level of body fat; most of these women fail to menstruate.

In certain players of sports, as well as in dancers, anorexic behaviors may be apparent, particularly for those individuals who think a thin appearance is important. These sports include gymnastics, wrestling, dancing, ballet, cheerleading, track, and, to some degree, tennis. This has been called *anorexia athletica.* These athletes seem to associate a slender appearance with the ability to perform successfully and appear more attractive.

In many instances the condition begins as an attempt to reduce body fat through caloric reduction and increased exercise. Instead of being satisfied with reaching a healthy goal weight, these individuals become obsessed with the ability to control body weight and continue the effort. They may fast, but often they eat small, precisely measured quantities of food that do not supply enough calories to fuel the high energy demands of their physical activity and maintain a reasonable amount of body fat. Reports of a combination of anorexia nervosa and bulimic behaviors are not uncommon. This is often called *bulimia nervosa.* An estimated 20 percent of those affected with this psychological disease die from the effects of severe malnutrition or the chemical imbalances created by purging.

Getting Help for Anorexia

Individuals with anorexia nervosa cannot be convinced that they are "too thin." Their body image is so distorted that even while looking at themselves in a mirror, they think they could lose some more weight. Therefore treating the condition is beyond the abilities of a health or physical educator. Simply referring the person to a health clinic is not effective unless specialists are on staff who are qualified to deal with these cases. Anorexics should be referred to a licensed psychologist or a medical doctor who specializes in treating such cases. In severe cases, long-term hospitalization is necessary. The key to treatment is getting patients to realize that they can gain control over their lives in ways that do not involve dieting. Unfortunately, many of those who do survive do not fully recover but remain underweight and fearful of any future weight gain.

FEMALE ATHLETE TRIAD SYNDROME

For many years the female athlete triad has been defined as a syndrome consisting of three necessary components: disordered eating, amenorrhoea, and osteoporosis. More recent descriptions of the triad have relaxed the criteria. For example, the definition of disordered eating has been expanded to include "abnormal eating behaviors"; amenorrhoea has been expanded to include menstrual cycle alterations; and osteoporosis includes a continuum of osteopenia, low bone mineral density, and other measures of bone metabolism. Therefore an individual does not necessarily have to have progressed to a clinically diagnosed eating disorder, amenorrhoea, and/or osteoporosis to be classified as having met the criteria for the female athlete triad. Unfortunately, this new definition of the triad may have extended the classification so broadly that almost any woman could be considered to have this syndrome. Disordered eating is likely the single most critical component since menstrual dysfunction and bone loss commonly result.

SUMMARY

- Body composition analysis indicates the percentage of total body weight composed of fat tissue versus the percentage composed of lean tissue.
- The size and number of adipose cells determine percent body fat, which can be measured by measuring the thickness of the subcutaneous fat with a skinfold caliper at specific areas.
- Changes in percent body fat are caused almost entirely by a change in caloric balance, which is a function of the number of calories taken in and the number of calories expended.
- Caloric expenditure may be calculated by maintaining accurate records of the number of calories expended for metabolic needs and in activities performed during the course of a day. Caloric intake measurement requires recording the number of calories consumed.
- Body fat can be lost either by increasing caloric expenditure through exercise or by decreasing caloric intake through reducing food intake. Most effective is a combination of moderate caloric restriction and a moderate increase in physical exercise during the course of each day.
- Fat loss should be accomplished gradually over a long period.
- Weight gain should be accomplished by increasing caloric intake and engaging in a weight-training program to increase lean body mass.
- Bulimia nervosa is an eating disorder that involves periodic binging and subsequent purging.
- Anorexia nervosa is a form of mental illness in which a person reduces food intake and increases energy expenditure to the extent that the loss of body fat threatens health and life.

SUGGESTED READINGS

Barnes, D. E. 2004. Eating well and controlling your weight. In *Action plan for diabetes,* edited by D. E. Barnes. Champaign, IL: Human Kinetics.

Beals, K. A. 2004. *Disordered eating among athletes: A comprehensive guide for health professionals.* Champaign, IL: Human Kinetics.

Beals, K., and A. Hill. 2006. The prevalence of disordered eating, menstrual dysfunction, and low bone mineral density among US collegiate athletes. *International Journal of Sport Nutrition and Exercise Metabolism* 16(1):1.

Black, D. and L. Leverence. 2009. *Physiological Screening Test (PST) manual for eating disorders/disordered eating among female collegiate athletes.* Monterey, CA: Healthy Learning.

Brownell, K., and C. Fairburn. 2005. *Eating disorders and obesity: A comprehensive handbook.* New York: Guilford Press.

Brownell, K., and K. Horgen. 2004. *Food fight: The inside story of America's obesity crisis—and what we can do about it.* New York: McGraw-Hill.

Burke, L. (ed.) 2009. *Clinical sports nutrition.* 4th ed., Sydney: McGraw-Hill.

Byrne, S., and N. McLean. 2001. Eating disorders in athletes: A review of the literature. *Journal of Science and Medicine in Sport* 4(2):145–59.

Campbell, C., T. Campbell, and H. Lyman. 2006. *The China study: The most comprehensive study of nutrition ever conducted and the startling implications for diet, weight loss, and long-term health.* Dallas, TX: BenBella Books.

Claude-Pierre, P. 1999. *The secret language of eating disorders.* New York: Vintage Books.

Coleman, E. 2002. The ACSM weight-loss position stand. *Sports Medicine Digest* 24(3):29, 31.

Fulton, J. E., M. T. McGuire, C. J. Caspersen, and W. H. Dietz. 2001. Interventions for weight loss and weight gain prevention among youth: Current issues. *Sports Medicine* 31(3):153–65.

Herriot, A., D. Thomas and K. Hart. 2008. A qualitative investigation of individuals' experiences and expectations before and after completing a trial of commercial weight loss programmes. *Journal of Human Nutrition and Dietetics* 21(1):72.

Heyward, V., and D. Wagner. 2004. *Applied body composition assessment.* Champaign, IL: Human Kinetics.

Jakicic, J. M., K. Clark, E. Coleman, and J. E. Donnelly. 2001. Appropriate intervention strategies for weight loss and prevention of weight regain for adults. *Medicine and Science in Sports and Exercise* 33(12):2145–56.

Karinch, M., ed. 2002. *Diets designed for athletes.* Champaign, IL: Human Kinetics.

Karinch, M. 2002. Gaining or cutting weight. In *Diets designed for athletes,* edited by M. Karinch. Champaign, IL: Human Kinetics.

Kruskall, L. J., L. J. Hohnson, and S. L. Meacham. 2002. Eating disorders and disordered eating—Are they the same? *ACSM's Health and Fitness Journal* 6(3):6–12.

Lebrun, C. M., and J. S. Rumball. 2002. Female athlete triad. *Sports Medicine and Arthroscopy Review* 10(1):23–32.

Levenkron, S. 2001. *Anatomy of anorexia.* New York: W. W. Norton & Co.

Litt, A. 2004. Lessons on losing weight. In *Fuel for young athletes,* edited by A. Litt. Champaign, IL: Human Kinetics.

Loucks, A. B. 2004. Energy balance and body composition in sports and exercise. *Journal of Sports Sciences* 22(1):1–14.

Manore, M., L. Kam, and A. Loucks. 2007. The female athlete triad: Components, nutrition issues, and health consequences. *Journal of Sports Sciences* 25(Supplement 1):61.

McArdle, W., F. Katch, and V. Katch. 2009. *Exercise physiology, energy, nutrition and human performance.* Baltimore: Lippincott Williams, & Wilkins.

McGraw, P. 2004. *The ultimate weight solution: The 7 keys to weight loss freedom.* New York: Simon and Schuster Adult Publishing.

Miller, W. C. 2001. Effective diet and exercise treatments for overweight and recommendations for intervention. *Sports Medicine* 31(10):717–24.

Montenegro, S. 2006. Disordered eating in athletes. *Athletic Therapy Today* 11(1):60.

Nelson, C. 2003. In female athlete "triad," amenorrhea not necessary for poor bone quality: Is "disordered eating" the culprit? *Sports Medicine Digest* 25(6):61, 63–66, 70–71.

Ode, J., J. Pivarnik, and M. Reeves. 2007. Body mass index as a predictor of percent fat in college athletes and nonathletes. *Medicine and Science in Sports and Exercise* 39(3):403–9.

Pollan, M. 2009. *In defense of food: An eater's manifesto.* New York: Penguin Books.

Pollan, M. 2009. *Food rules: An eater's manual.* New York: Penguin Books.

Schmitz, K. H. 2001. Effects on obesity of exercise- and diet-induced weight loss. *Clinical Journal of Sports Medicine* 11(2):130.

Schnirring, L. 2001. Body fat testing: Evaluating the options. *Physician and Sports Medicine* 29(5):13–14, 16.

Schultz, S. 2001. Disordered eating. In *Sports medicine handbook,* edited by S. J. Shultz et al. Indianapolis: National Federation of State High School Associations.

Sharkey, B. J. 2006. Weight-control programs. In *Fitness and health,* 5th ed., edited by B. J. Sharkey. Champaign, IL: Human Kinetics.

Swain, D. P., and B. C. Leutholz. 2007. Exercise prescription for weight loss. In *Exercise prescription: A case study approach to the ACSM guidelines,* edited by D. P. Swain and B. C. Leutholtz. Champaign, IL: Human Kinetics.

Thompson, J. 2003. *Handbook of eating disorders* and obesity. Hoboken, NJ: John Wiley & Sons.

Tribole, E. 2004. Losing and maintaining weight. In *Eating on the run,* edited by E. Tribole. 3rd ed., Champaign, IL: Human Kinetics

Van Marken Lichtenbelt, W. D., and F. Hartgens. 2004. Body composition changes in bodybuilders: A method comparison. *Medicine and Science in Sports and Exercise* 36(3):490–97.

Weyers, A. M., et al. 2002. Comparison of methods for assessing body composition changes during weight loss. *Medicine and Science in Sports and Exercise* 34(3):497–502.

Wong, S. L., P. T. Katzmarzyk, and M. Z. Nichaman. 2004. Cardiorespiratory fitness is associated with lower abdominal fat independent of body mass index. *Medicine and Science in Sports and Exercise* 36(2):286–91.

SUGGESTED WEB SITES

Food and Nutrition Center

Provides information on nutrition and safe dieting from WebMD.
http://my.webmd.com/nutrition

National Association of Anorexia Nervosa and Associated Disorders (ANAD)

This is the oldest nonprofit organization helping victims of eating disorders and their families.
www.anad.org

National Eating Disorders Organization

Get answers to any questions about eating disorders and their prevention. If you have an eating disorder (or know someone who has), NEDO has information that may help.
http://eatingdisorders.laureate.com

Calculating Body Mass Index (BMI)

_____   _____   _____
Name   Section   Date

PURPOSE   To determine body mass index (BMI) as a means of examining overweight and obesity.

PROCEDURE
1. Write down your weight in pounds.
2. Divide your weight by your height in inches.
3. Divide Ratio A from step 2 by your height in inches.
4. Then multiply the Answer A from step 3 by 703.
5. The resulting answer is your BMI.

1. _____
   Weight in Pounds

2. _____ ÷ _____ = _____
   Weight in Pounds   Height in Inches   Ratio A

3. _____ ÷ _____ = _____
   Ratio A   Height in Inches   Answer A

4. _____ × 703 = _____
   Answer A   Body Mass Index

INTERPRETA-TION   Health risks from obesity for men and women begin when BMI exceeds 25. At 27 the risk of diabetes and hypertension begins to rise. A BMI above 30 indicates an even greater health risk and is used as a cutoff for obesity. A BMI above 40 represents an exceedingly high risk for health problems.

Name   Section   Date

PURPOSE   To calculate percent body fat using a skinfold caliper.

PROCEDURE   1. Measure skinfold thickness in millimeters at the following sites:
- Thigh skinfold (males and females): A vertical fold on the anterior aspect of the thigh midway between the patella plateau and the inguinal line or fold (Figure 8-5, *A* on p. 235).
- Triceps skinfold (females only): A vertical skinfold located midway between the tips of the acromion and olecranon processes. The elbow should be relaxed and extended (Figure 8-5, *B*).
- Suprailiac skinfold (females only): Palpate the crest of the ilium and then lift a diagonal fold over the highest point of the crest (Figure 8-5, *C*).
- Abdominal skinfold (males only): A vertical skinfold at the midclavicular line horizontal to the umbilicus (about 2 centimeters from the umbilicus) (Figure 8-5, *D*).
- Chest skinfold (males only): A diagonal skinfold located midway between the axillary crease and the nipple (Figure 8-5, *E*).

A. Use the following measuring techniques:
- All measurements should be taken from the right side of the body. The skinfold site should be marked with a black felt-tip pen.
- Pick up the skinfold with your left index finger and thumb. Be sure you have two layers of skin and the underlying fat. To make sure it is a true skinfold and not muscle, check by having the subject contract the underlying muscle as you are grasping the skin—and then relax before taking a reading.
- The calipers should be held in the right hand perpendicular to the fold, with the dial face-up and easy to read. The calipers should be placed 1/4 to 1/2 inches away from the fingers holding the skinfold, so that the pressure of the calipers will not be affected.
- Apply the calipers about 1 centimeter below the fingers. It should be applied where the two surfaces of the folds are parallel. Do not apply the calipers where the fold is rounded near the top, or where it is broader near its base. Keep holding as the skin measures are read.
- Measure all skinfolds to the nearest 0.5 millimeter as you continue to grasp the skin. Measure one site once, then the next

261

site once, and so on until you have measured all sites once. Then repeat the cycle a minimum of three times at each site. Use the average of the scores at each site for the final skinfold score. If there is a question as to the accuracy of the measure, discard that measure and remeasure.

- During the measurement, maintain constant pressure with the thumb and forefinger.

2. Calculate the body density (Db) according to the following formulas:
   A. For Females

   $Db = 1.0994921 - (0.0009929 \times$ sum of the triceps, iliac crest, and thigh skinfolds$) + (0.0000023 \times$ [sum of triceps, iliac crest, and thigh skinfolds]2$) - (0.0001392 \times$ age$)$.

   B. For Males

   $Db = 1.0938 - (0.0008267 \times$ sum of chest, abdomen, and thigh skinfolds$) + (0.0000016 \times$ [sum of chest, abdomen, and thigh skinfolds]2$) - (0.0002574 \times$ age$)$.

3. Use the following equation to compute percent body fat in both males and females. Plugging density (Db) into the following equation will give you percent body fat.

   _____ Percent fat = $\underline{4.570} - 4.142 \times 100$ Db

4. Consult Table 8-2 to determine the classification of your total percent body fat.

INTERPRETA-TION

Ideal body composition consists of low fat and high muscle mass. Height–weight tables assess only one's weight in relation to insurance risk; they do not accurately reflect ideal body composition.

Your percent body fat can be estimated from skinfold measures. It is recommended that women stay within 17 to 25 percent fat and men within 9 to 17 percent fat.

Too little body fat may be just as detrimental to your health as too much fat. The critical level for women is no less than 12 percent and for men no less than 5 percent.

Worksheet for Calculating Percent Body Fat

Name _____   Section _____   Date _____

1. Thigh skinfold thickness in mm _____
2. Triceps skinfold thickness in mm _____
3. Suprailiac skinfold thickness in mm _____
4. Abdominal skinfold thickness in mm _____
5. Chest skinfold thickness in mm _____

Calculation of Percent Body Fat

1. Use the following formulas to determine body density (Db)
   Females

   Db = 1.0994921 − (0.0009929 × sum of the triceps, iliac crest, and thigh skinfolds) + (0.0000023 × [sum of triceps, iliac crest, and thigh skinfolds]2) − (0.0001392 × age).

   Db= _____

   Males

   Db = 1.0938 − (0.0008267 × sum of chest, abdomen, and thigh skinfolds) + (0.0000016 × [sum of chest, abdomen, and thigh skinfolds]2) − (0.0002574 × age).

   Db= _____

2. Use the following equation to compute percent fat in both males and females. Plugging density (Db) into the following equation will give you percent body fat.

   _____ Percent fat = 4.570 − 4.142 × 100 Db
                                  ‾‾‾‾‾

3. Using Table 8-2, find your gender and age range category. Take the percentage determined above, and determine which health rating you are in. For example, if your percentage is 23 and you are a 22-year-old woman, your health rating is fair.

Worksheet for Calculating Desired Body Weight

Work Sheet

1. Present body weight _____lbs

2. Present percentage body fat _____%

3. Desired percentage body fat _____%

4. _____% − _____ = _____%
   Present % body fat   Desired % body fat   % body fat to be lost

5. _____ × _____ = _____lbs
   % body fat to be lost*   Present body weight   Pounds to be lost

6. _____ − _____ = _____
   Present body weight   Pounds to be lost   Desired body weight

Alternative Method

4. _____lbs × _____% = _____lbs
   Present body weight   Percentage body fat   Present fat weight

5. _____lbs − _____lbs = _____lbs
   Present body weight   Fat weight   Fat-free weight

6. _____lbs × _____% = _____lbs
   Present body weight   Desired % body fat   Desired fat weight

7. _____lbs + _____lbs = _____lbs
   Fat-free weight   Desired fat weight   Desired body weight

Determining Your Basal Metabolic Rate (BMR)

Name ______________________ Section ____________ Date ____________

PURPOSE To determine your basal metabolic rate.

PROCEDURE

1. Use Figure 8-11 to determine your body surface area. Using a ruler, draw a straight line from your height to your weight. The point at which that line crosses the middle column shows your surface area in square meters (m^2). Record this number beside "Estimated Body Surface

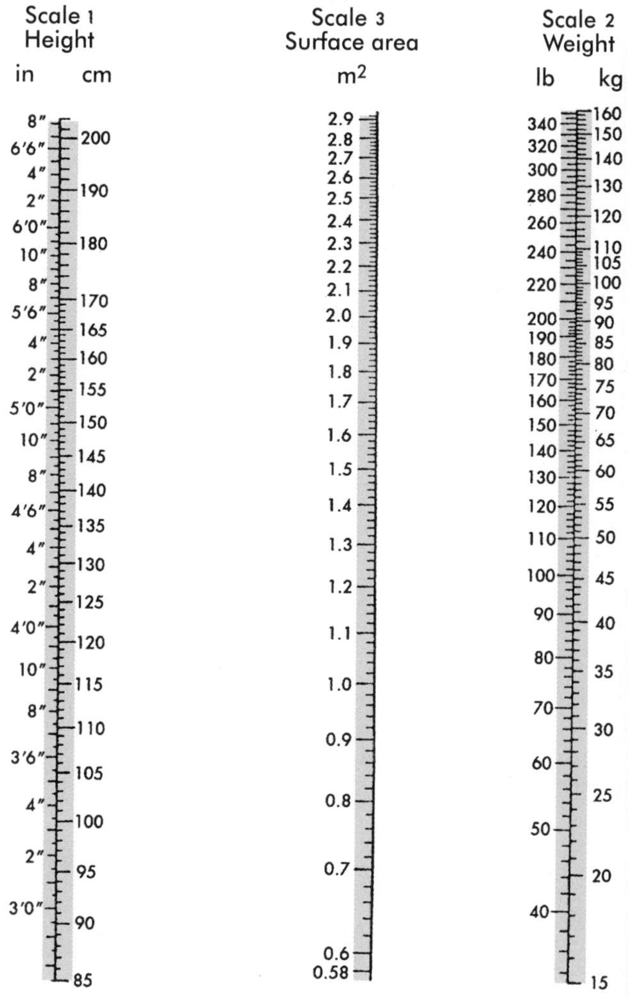

FIGURE 8-11. ESTIMATING TOTAL BODY SURFACE AREA. *Locate your height on scale 1 and then your weight on scale 2. Using a straight edge, connect the two points with a line. The intersection of the line on scale 3 is your body surface area.*

Determining Your Basal Metabolic Rate (BMR)

Area" on the worksheet. For example, for a 20-year-old man whose height is 6 feet (180 cm) and weight is 170 pounds (77.3 kg), his body surface area on the nomogram would be 1.99 square meters.

2. Next use Table 8-3 find the factor for your sex and age, and multiply your surface area by this factor. Record this number for "BMR factor" on the worksheet below. For example, for a 20-year-old man, the factor is 39.9 kcal per square meter per hour (kcal/m²/h).

TABLE 8-3
BASAL METABOLIC RATE ACCORDING TO AGE AND SEX

Age	BMR (kcal/m²/h) Men	Women	Age	BMR (kcal/m²/h) Men	Women
10	47.7	44.9	29	37.7	35.0
11	46.5	43.5	30	37.6	35.0
12	45.3	42.0	31	37.4	35.0
13	44.5	40.5	32	37.2	34.9
14	43.8	39.2	33	37.1	34.9
15	42.9	38.3	34	37.0	34.9
16	42.0	37.2	35	36.9	34.8
17	41.5	36.4	36	36.8	34.7
18	40.8	35.8	37	36.7	34.6
19	40.5	35.4	38	36.7	34.5
20	39.9	35.3	39	36.6	34.4
21	39.5	35.2	40–44	36.4	34.1
22	39.2	35.2	45–49	36.2	33.8
23	39.0	35.2	50–54	35.8	33.1
24	38.7	35.1	55–59	35.1	32.8
25	38.4	35.1	60–64	34.5	32.0
26	38.2	35.0	65–69	33.5	31.6
27	38.0	35.0	70–74	32.7	31.1
28	37.8	35.0	75+	31.8	

3. Next, multiply "Estimated body surface" by the "BMR factor" and record on the worksheet.
4. Finally, multiply this product by 24 hours per day to find your BMR needs per day.

Worksheet for Calculating Basal Metabolic Rate (BMR)

1. Estimated body surface area (see Figure 8-11) = _____

2. BMR factor (see Table 8-3) = _____

3. _____ $\times$ _____ = _____
   Estimated body surface area   BMR factor   BMR

4. _____ = _____ $\times$ 24 hours
   Basal metabolic needs for 1 day   BMR

Name   Section   Date

PURPOSE   To keep a 24-hour log of all activities done during the day: everything from eating breakfast to biking to school or work, recreational activities, and so forth.

PROCEDURE
1. Consult Table 8-5 (page 270), Energy Expenditure during Physical Activity. Use the guidelines in Table 8-4 below for activities not included in Table 8-5.
2. Record your activities on the worksheet provided, listing the following:*
   a. Clock time—Specify the time of day.
   b. Activity—The type of activity you were involved in.
   c. Total number of minutes spent in the activity.
   d. Total calories/min—Multiply the cal/min/lb from Table 8-5 by the total number of pounds (your body weight).
   e. Total calories expended—Multiply total number of minutes by total calories/min.
3. To calculate expenditure during sleep, multiply the number of hours you slept by the BMR calculated in Lab Activity 8-2.
4. Total the calories expended during activities on the worksheet.
5. Add in the calories expended in basal metabolism during a 24-hour period as calculated in Lab Activity 8-2.

*Every minute of the day should be accounted for.

TABLE 8-4
GENERAL GUIDELINES FOR ENERGY EXPENDITURE

Activity	cal/min/lb
Very light (such as typing, driving)	0.010
Light (such as shopping)	0.021
Moderate (such as dancing, bowling)	0.032
Heavy (such as football, running)	0.062

TABLE 8-5
ENERGY EXPENDITURE DURING PHYSICAL ACTIVITY

Activity	Cal/min/lb	Activity	Cal/min/lb
Archery	.030	Dancing	
Badminton	.044	Aerobic, medium	.047
Baseball	.031	Aerobic, intense	.061
Basketball	.063	Ballroom	.023
Billiards	.018	Eating (sitting)	.010
Boxing (sparring)	.062	Field hockey	.061
Canoeing		Fishing	.028
Leisure	.020	Football	.060
Racing	.047	Gardening	
Circuit training		Digging	.057
Hydra-Fitness	.060	Mowing	.051
Universal	.053	Raking	.025
Nautilus	.042	Golf	.039
Free weights	.039	Gymnastics	.030
Climbing hills	.055	Handball	.063
Croquet	.027	Hiking	.042
Cycling		Horseback riding	
5.5 mph	.029	Galloping	.062
9.4 mph	.045	Trotting	.050
Racing	.079	Walking	.019

Continued

Data from Bannier EW, Brown SR: The relative energy requirements of physical activity. In Falls HB, editor: *Exercise physiology,* New York, 1968, Academic Press; Howley ET, Glover ME: The caloric costs of running and walking one mile for men and women, *Med Sci Sports* 6:235, 1974; Passmore R, Durnin JVGA: Human energy expenditure, *Physiol Rev* 25:801, 1955.

TABLE 8-5
ENERGY EXPENDITURE DURING PHYSICAL ACTIVITY—CONT.

Activity	Cal/min/lb	Activity	Cal/min/lb
Ice hockey	.095	Downhill	.064
Jogging	.069	Water	.052
Judo	.089	Skindiving	
Jumping rope		Considerable motion	.125
70 per min	.074	Moderate motion	.094
80 per min	.075	Soccer	.059
125 per min	.080	Squash	.096
145 per min	.089	Swimming	
Lacrosse	.095	Backstroke	.077
Lying at ease	.010	Breast stroke	.074
Painting (outside)	.035	Butterfly	.078
Racquetball	.081	Crawl, slow	.070
Running		Crawl, fast	.071
11.5 min per mile	.061	Side stroke	.055
9 min per mile	.088	Treading, fast	.077
8 min per mile	.095	Treading, normal	.028
7 min per mile	.104	Table tennis	.031
6 min per mile	.115	Tennis	.050
5.5 min per mile	.131	Volleyball	.023
Cross-country	.074	Walking (normal pace)	.036
Sailing	.002	Weight training	.032
Sitting quietly	.009	Wrestling	.085
Skiing		Writing (sitting)	.013
Cross-country	.074		

Worksheet for Calculating Total Daily Energy Expenditure (Daily Activity Log)				
Clock Time	Activity	Total Minutes Spent in Activity	Total Calories/ min	Total Calories Expended

Total calories expended during activities _____

Add calories expended in basal metabolism during sleeping only _____

Total calories expended _____

Name _____   Section _____   Date _____

PURPOSE   To determine your daily caloric intake.

PROCEDURE

1. A daily food intake log such as the one in the worksheet on page 274 can be kept over a period of several days to let you know about how many calories you consume during the average day. College students are notorious for skipping meals and eating multiple snacks. Thus, it is important to record everything you consume during the entire 24-hour period. Don't neglect to record extras such as mustard and pickles that you include on a hamburger. Those columns that deal with hunger level and mood may help you to determine what causes you to eat when you do.

2. As with caloric expenditure, adding up the caloric values of all foods consumed during a 24-hour period can give you a reasonably accurate estimate of daily caloric intake.

Worksheet for Calculating Calorie Intake (Daily Food Intake Log)

Time	Food Eaten	Amount	Number of Calories	How Cooked	Meal or Snack	Hunger Level* (0–3)	Activity and Location when Eating	Mood† (1–3)

Total number of calories consumed =

*Hunger rating: 0, not hungry; 3, very hungry
†Mood: 1, good, happy; 2, fair, OK; 3, upset.

Worksheet for Estimating Caloric Balance

_____ _____ _____
Name   Section   Date

PURPOSE   To help you estimate whether you are in caloric balance, based on your assessment of a day's caloric intake and expenditure.

PROCEDURE   1. Consult Lab Activity 8-3 for estimated BMR caloric needs. Fill in below. Consult Lab Activity 8-4 for your estimation of activity caloric needs. Fill in below. Add the two numbers together.

   _____ + _____ = _____ Total calories
   BMR calories   Activity calories

2. Multiply the sum from step 1 by 0.1 to estimate the number of calories that are needed for the thermic effect of food (10% of BMR + Activity calories).

   _____ $\times$ 0.1 = _____ calories

3. Add the sum of calories from step 1 with the number obtained in step 2 to obtain an estimate of a day's caloric needs.

   _____ + _____ = _____ Total calories
   Step 1 calories   Step 2 calories

4. Consult Lab Activity 8-5 for an estimation of your caloric intake. Record the number below.

   _____ calories

5. Compare the total number of energy expenditure calories obtained in step 3 with the total for intake in step 4.

   Check which situation applies:

   a. Caloric intake is greater than expenditure   _____
   b. Caloric expenditure is greater than intake   _____
   c. Caloric expenditure equals intake   _____

   Is this day's energy situation in balance, in negative balance, or in positive balance? _____

CHAPTER 9

Practicing **Safe Fitness**

Objectives

After completing this chapter, you should be able to do the following:

- Realize that participation in physical activity sometimes creates situations in which injuries may occur.
- Discuss the principles and guidelines of injury prevention.
- Describe fractures, contusions, ligament sprains, muscle strains, muscle soreness, tendinitis, and bursitis.
- Identify the causes of low back pain and describe how such pain can best be avoided.
- Describe the RICE approach to the initial treatment of injuries.
- Identify exercises that may be dangerous or contraindicated.
- Discuss the precautions that should be exercised when working out in either a hot or a cold environment.

HOW CAN YOU PREVENT INJURIES?

Certainly, you don't participate in physical activities with the idea that you are going to be injured. Ironically, the nature of participation in any type of physical activity increases the possibility that injury will occur. Fitness programs will hopefully make you more fit and should ultimately reduce the possibility of injury. The overload demands placed on the body during exercise enable it to handle added stresses and strains that occur during physical activity. Thus the first step in practicing "safe fitness" and in preventing injuries associated with physical activity involves designing a well-planned

fitness program based on the principles of overload, progression, consistency, individuality, and safety.

If you are involved in some physical activity and realize that a specific part of your body is causing discomfort or pain that affects your performance, it is strongly recommended that this problem be evaluated immediately. Injuries should be evaluated by persons experienced in dealing with sport-related injuries, such as physicians, physical therapists, or athletic

KEY TERMS

low back pain
RICE

heat-related illness
hypothermia

277

trainers (Figure 9-1). Safe Tip 9-1 provides recommendations about when a health care professional should be consulted. The sooner an injury is diagnosed and treatment begun, the less chance there is that continued activity will make the problem worse. The popular quote "no pain, no gain" holds no credibility with regard to an activity program.

Pain indicates that something is wrong. You should stop activity immediately and determine what is producing the pain. There is a great difference between overloading the system while you are working hard during exercise and pushing yourself to exercise when you are hurt. When you are dealing with injuries, common sense is of prime importance. Injuries are to a large extent preventable, and paying attention to some simple guidelines can make exercise safer and more enjoyable.

Perhaps the biggest mistake that people make when beginning a physical activity pro-

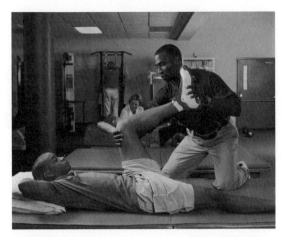

FIGURE 9-1. HEALTH CARE PROFESSIONAL.
It is wise to have injuries evaluated by a trained health care provider.

gram is starting at a level that is too advanced and then trying to progress too quickly. If you are physically inactive, you must begin at a much lower level and gradually increase

SAFE TIP 9-1

Basic Self-Treatment Guidelines

When trying to determine whether a health problem requires attention from a health care provider, ask yourself the following questions. If you answer *yes* to any of them, consult a professional.

Generally:

- Is this injury or pain so severe that I can't carry out my usual activities? Does it represent a threat to my health?
- Is this a strange sign or symptom, something that I have not experienced before?
- Is this condition worsening rather than improving?
- Have I had this condition too long?
- Have I had this condition in the past and it keeps recurring?

Specifically:

- Is there blood in my bowel movement or urine?
- Am I unable to control this bleeding?
- Do I have a high fever (102°F or above)?
- Am I becoming dehydrated?
- Do I have a stiff neck and a fever?
- Am I having a crushing sensation in my chest?
- Am I experiencing vomiting or diarrhea that just won't quit?

SAFE TIP 9-2

Injury Prevention

- Always warm up properly before engaging in any activity.
- Do not neglect the cool-down period after exercise.
- Make certain that muscles are stretched sufficiently. Use full range-of-motion static stretching during an active warm-up period and vigorous stretching during the cool-down period.
- Avoid passive overstretching to reduce the possibility of injury to the ligaments or joint capsule.
- Avoid any movements, exercises, or activities that produce compression or impingement of joint motion.
- Begin at a low intensity and progress within your individual limits to higher intensities. Do not try to do too much too soon.
- Avoid holding your breath and straining too hard during intense activity.
- Choose a level of intensity that is compatible with your abilities in terms of strength, power, and endurance.
- Select the appropriate clothing for exercising in hot or cold environments.
- Make sure you are acclimated to the environment in which you are exercising, regardless of whether it is extremely hot or cold.
- Select and use high-quality equipment when engaging in any physical activity. Breakdown of cheap or low-quality equipment may prove to be more expensive in the long run should injury occur.
- Listen to what your body is telling you. If you experience pain during activity, stop immediately.
- Do not engage in any activity that you think may have the potential to result in injury.

your level of activity. Some people stop exercising for a variety of reasons, and when they start exercising again, they have a tendency to try to begin where they left off. They do too much, too fast, too soon. Safe Tip 9-2 provides you with some tips for practicing "safe fitness."

WHAT TYPES OF INJURIES MIGHT OCCUR IN AN EXERCISE PROGRAM?

Several different types of injuries typically occur through participation in physical activity. These injuries are briefly identified here.

Fractures—Cracks or breaks in bones that usually require some type of immobilization in a cast.

Contusions—A bruise of the skin, fat, or muscle tissue.

Sprains—Damage to a ligament, which connects bone to bone, thus providing a support to a joint.

Strains—Separation or tearing of muscle fibers.

Muscle soreness—Delayed onset pain in muscle following physical activities that you are not accustomed to.

Tendinitis—Inflammation of a tendon, which connects muscle to bone.

Bursitis—Inflammation of a bursa, which is a membrane that functions to reduce friction between bone and muscle, ligament and bone, muscle and ligament, etc.

Skin conditions—Blister and sunburn are the most common skin problems in a physically active individual.

A detailed discussion of the many injuries, both acute and chronic, that can occur with participation in physical activity is beyond the scope of this text. However, a few injuries seem to occur frequently with physical activity. Table 9-1 provides a brief description of the causes and signs of the more common injuries.

TABLE 9-1
SUMMARY OF COMMON INJURIES ASSOCIATED WITH PHYSICAL ACTIVITY

Injury	Cause/Signs and Symptoms
Achilles tendinitis	A chronic tendinitis of the "heel cord" or muscle tendon located on the back of the lower leg just above the heel. It may result from any activity that involves forcefully pushing off of the foot and ankle, such as running and jumping. This inflammation involves swelling, warmth, tenderness to touch, and pain during walking and especially running.
Ankle sprains	Stretching or tearing of one or several ligaments that provide stability to the ankle joint. Ligaments on the outside or lateral side of the ankle are more commonly injured by rolling the sole of the foot downward and to the inside. Pain is intense immediately after injury followed by considerable swelling, tenderness, loss of joint motion, and some discoloration over a 24- to 48-hour period.
Athlete's foot	A fungal infection that most often occurs between the toes or on the sole of the foot and that causes itching, redness, and pain. If the skin breaks down, a bacterial infection is possible. It may be prevented by keeping the area dry; using powder; and wearing clean, dry socks that do not hold moisture. It is best treated using over-the-counter medications (e.g., Micatin) that contain the active ingredient miconazole.
Blisters	Friction blisters can occur anywhere on the skin where there is friction or repetitive rubbing, but they most often occur on the hands or feet. The blister takes on a reddish color, becoming raised and filling with fluid. It can be quite painful, and if it occurs on the foot it may be disabling. Taking measures to reduce friction, such as wearing gloves, breaking in new footwear, and wearing appropriately fitting socks, is helpful in preventing blisters.
Groin pull	A muscle strain that occurs in the muscles located on the inside of the upper thigh just below the pubic area resulting either from an overstretch of the muscle or from a contraction of the muscle that meets excessive resistance. Pain will be produced by flexing the hip and leg across the body or by stretching the muscles in a groin stretch position.
Hamstring pull	A muscle strain of the muscles of the back of the upper thigh that most often occurs while sprinting. In most cases, severe pain is caused simply by walking or in any movement that involves knee flexion or extension of the hamstring muscle. Some swelling, tenderness to touch, and possibly some discoloration extending down the back of the leg may occur in severe strains.
Patellofemoral knee pain	Nonspecific pain occurring around the knee, in particular the front part of the knee, or kneecap (patella). Pain can result from many causes, including improper movement of the kneecap in knee flexion and extension; tendinitis of the tendon just below the kneecap caused by repetitive jumping; bursitis (swelling) either above or below the kneecap; and osteoarthritis (joint surface degeneration) between the kneecap and thigh bone. This may possibly involve inflammation with swelling, tenderness, warmth, and pain with movement.

TABLE 9-1
SUMMARY OF COMMON INJURIES ASSOCIATED WITH PHYSICAL ACTIVITY—CONT.

Injury	Cause/Signs and Symptoms
Plantar fascitis or arch pain	Chronic inflammation and irritation of the broad ligament that runs from the heel to the base of the toes, forming part of the long arch on the bottom of the foot. It most often occurs in runners or walkers. It is frequently caused by wearing shoes that do not have adequate arch support. At first, pain is localized at the attachment on the heel; it then tends to move more onto the arch. It is most painful when you first get out of bed and then in the evening when you have been on your feet for long periods.
Quadriceps contusion, "charlie horse"	A deep bruise of the muscles in the front part of the thigh caused by a forceful impact or by some object that results in severe pain, swelling, discoloration, and difficulty flexing the knee or extending the hip. Small calcium deposits may develop in the muscle without adequate rest and protection from additional trauma.
Racquetball or golfer's elbow	Similar to tennis elbow, except the pain is located on the medial or inside surface of the arm just above the elbow at the attachment of the wrist and finger flexor muscles. It occurs in those activities that involve repeated forceful flexion of the wrist, such as hitting a forehand stroke in racquetball. Golfers also develop this inflammation in the trailing arm from too much wrist flexion in a golf swing.
Shin splints	A "catch-all" term used to refer to any pain that occurs in the front part of the lower leg or shin, most often caused by excessive running on hard surfaces. Pain is usually caused by muscle strains of those muscles that move the ankle and foot at their attachment points in the skin. It is usually worse during activity. In more severe cases it may be caused by stress fractures of the long bones in the lower leg, with the pain being worse after activity is stopped.
Shoulder impingement	Chronic irritation and inflammation of muscle tendons and a bursa underneath the tip of the shoulder, which results from repeated forceful overhead motions of the shoulder such as in swimming, throwing, spiking a volleyball, or a tennis serve. Pain is felt when the arm is extended across the body above shoulder level.
Sunburn	An extremely common problem for anyone who exercises outside. Overexposure to the sun can ultimately cause certain types of skin cancer. It is critical to protect yourself from the sun by applying sunscreens and paying attention to the SPF (sun protection factor). Wearing a hat and other protective clothing to cover the skin can further help to minimize overexposure to ultraviolet light.
Tennis elbow	Chronic irritation and inflammation of the lateral or outside surface of the arm just above the elbow at the attachment of the muscles that extend the wrist and fingers. It results from any activity that requires forceful extension of the wrist. This typically occurs in tennis players who are using faulty techniques hitting backhand ground strokes. Pain is felt above the elbow after forcefully extending the wrist against resistance or applying pressure over the muscle attachment above the elbow.

LOW BACK PAIN

There is no question that **low back pain** is one of the most common, annoying, and disabling ailments known. Many causes and cures for low back pain have been proposed. However, so many different things can cause pain in the lower back that no single incriminating cause or absolute cure can be identified.

▶ Causes of Low Back Pain

Of all the causes of low back pain, none is more common than imbalances between the strength and flexibility of the various muscle groups associated with the lower back. In most cases, the abdominal muscles are weak and stretched out, the spinal muscles are tight and inflexible, and the hamstring muscles are also tight. Therefore an exercise program that attempts to increase the strength and the tone of the abdominal muscles, improve the flexibility of the spinal muscles in the lower back, and stretch the tight hamstring muscles may alleviate many complaints of low back pain. Health Link 9-1 details some of the causes.

low back pain: pain in the lower back caused by muscle imbalances, muscle strain, ligament sprain, or disk degeneration

▶ Prevention of Low Back Pain

Some knowledge of the source of low back pain is important to treat the injury, but it is more important to understand how low back pain can be avoided. To prevent low back pain, the practice of avoiding unnecessary stresses and strains should be integrated into your daily life. The back is subjected to these stresses and strains when one is standing, lying, sitting, lifting, and exercising. Care should be taken to avoid postures and positions that can cause injury. Figure 9-2 shows examples of safe postures.

Exercises for Treating Low Back Pain. The specific exercises used to treat low back pain will vary depending upon the specific conditions causing the pain. In general, back pain may be caused by tightness or a lack of flexibility in a number of different muscle groups related to movement of the low back. Flexibility exercises for muscle groups that may need to be stretched in treating low back pain were discussed and illustrated previously in Chapter 6 (see Figures 6-9 through 6-15). Strengthening exercises can involve either flexion or extension exercises. Flexion exercises are used to strengthen the abdominal muscles and to stretch the low back muscles (see Figures 5-33, 5-36, and 5-37). Extension exercises are used to strengthen back extensors and to stretch the abdominal muscles (see Figures 5-39*B* and 5-42). Core stabilization exercises discussed previously in Chapter 5 are widely used to treat low back pain (see Figure 5-42).

HEALTH LINK 9-1

Causes of Low Back Pain

Low back pain may result from the following associated problems:

1. Disk degeneration and rupture (herniation).
2. A sprain of the intervertebral ligaments in the lumbosacral region of the spine.
3. A sprain of the ligaments in the sacroiliac region.
4. Muscle imblances—weak abdominal muscles/tight low back muscles/tight hamstrings.

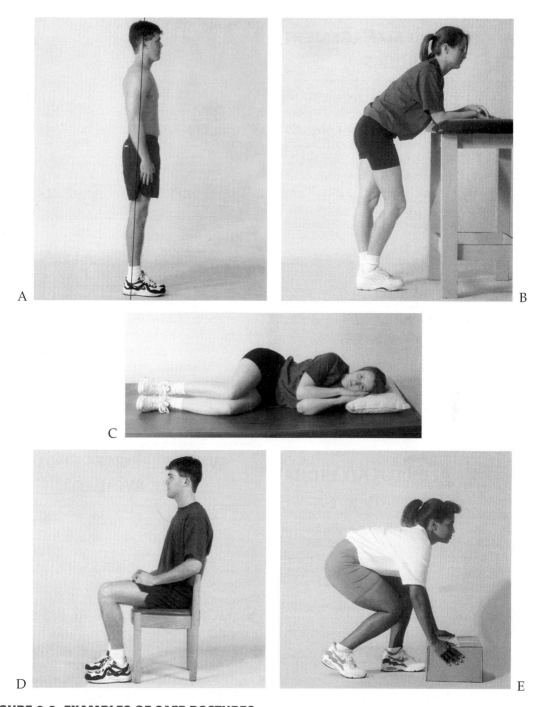

FIGURE 9-2. EXAMPLES OF SAFE POSTURES.

A, Ideal standing posture. *B, Correct leaning posture.* *C, Correct sleeping position.*
D, Ideal sitting position. *E, Correct lifting position.*

TREATMENT AND MANAGEMENT OF INJURIES

Initial first-aid and management techniques for most fitness injuries associated with physical activity are fairly simple and straightforward. Regardless of which type of injury we are talking about, there is one problem they all have in common—swelling. Swelling is most likely during the first 72 hours after an injury. Once swelling has occurred, the healing process is significantly retarded. The injured area cannot return to normal until all the swelling is gone. Therefore everything that is done in terms of first-aid management of any of these conditions should be directed toward controlling the swelling. If the swelling can be controlled initially in the acute state of injury, it is likely that the time required for rehabilitation will be significantly reduced.

To control and most effectively limit the amount of swelling, the RICE principle can be applied. **RICE** stands for Rest, Ice, Compression, and Elevation (Figure 9-3). Each factor plays a critical role in limiting swelling, and all four methods should be used simultaneously.

> *Rest*—You should rest the injured body part for approximately 72 hours before beginning a rehabilitation program.
>
> *Ice*—Ice should be applied to the injured area in a plastic bag to slow bleeding and decrease pain.
>
> *Compression*—The purpose of compression is to reduce the amount of space available for swelling by applying pressure around the injured area using an elastic wrap (such as an Ace bandage).
>
> *Elevation*—The injured part, particularly an extremity, should be elevated to eliminate the effects of gravity on blood pooling in the extremities.

RICE: initial first-aid technique for treating injuries including rest, ice, compression, and elevation

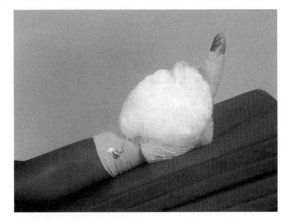

FIGURE 9-3. RICE.
Rest, ice, compression, elevation technique for treatment of a sprained ankle.

The goal of rehabilitation should be to return the person to the usual physical activities as quickly and as safely as possible. Long-term rehabilitation programs require the supervision of a trained professional if they are going to be safe and effective. An injury that is not given proper rehabilitation may continue to cause many problems with increasing age.

WHAT EXERCISES SHOULD BE AVOIDED?

Throughout this text, an effort has been made to recommend specific exercises that are both effective and safe. Over the years, other sources have recommended and widely used a number of exercises that place abnormal stresses, strains, or compression forces on particular muscles or joints. Such exercises potentially predispose these structures to injury. Appropriate stretching, strengthening, conditioning, and in some cases corrective exercises are described in detail within individual chapters. Figures 9-4 through 9-15 identify a series of exercises that for one reason or another are *not* recommended as being safe and may potentially result in injury.

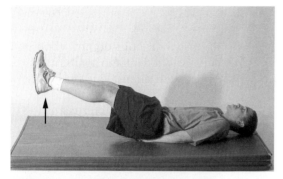

FIGURE 9-4. STRAIGHT-LEG LIFTS.
Used for strengthening abdominal muscles and hip flexors. Tends to tilt the pelvis forward, thus causing hyperextension of the lower back, which compresses the intervertebral disks. Alternative safe exercises: See Figures 5-33, 5-36 to 5-38.

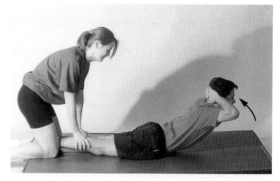

FIGURE 9-5. BACK HYPEREXTENSIONS.
Used to strengthen lower back muscles and stretch abdominal muscles. Causes compression of intervertebral disks with possible disk herniation or spinal nerve impingement. Alternative safe exercise: See Figure 5-42.

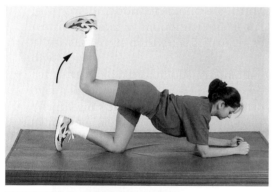

FIGURE 9-6. DONKEY KICKS.
Used to develop extensor muscles of the lower back. Involves a ballistic backward and upward kick with the leg and an extension of the neck. Causes compression of intervertebral disks and possible disk herniation or spinal nerve impingement. Alternative safe exercise: See Figure 5-39B.

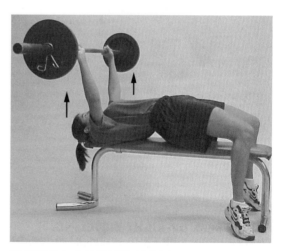

FIGURE 9-7. BENCH PRESS.
Used for strengthening pectoral and triceps muscles. This lift, when done with the feet on the floor and an arched back, hyperextends the lower back. Alternative safe exercise: See Figure 5-6.

TABLE 9-2
HEAT STRESS—SYMPTOMS, TREATMENT, AND PREVENTION

Disorder	Cause	Symptoms	Treatment	Prevention
Heat cramps	Hard work in heat; sweating heavily; imbalance between water and electrolytes	Muscle twitching and cramps, usually after midday; spasms in arms, legs, abdomen	Ingesting large amounts of water and salt, mild stretching, and ice massage of affected muscle	Acclimatize properly; provide large quantities of water; increase intake of sodium, calcium, and potassium
Heat exhaustion	Prolonged sweating; inadequate replacement of body fluid losses; diarrhea; intestinal infection	Excessive thirst, dry tongue and mouth; weight loss; fatigue; weakness; incoordination; mental dullness; small urine volume; slightly elevated body temperature; high serum protein and sodium; reduced swelling	Bed rest in cool room, immediate oral fluid replacement, increase fluid intake to 6 to 8 1/day; sponge with cool water	Supply adequate water and other liquids; provide adequate rest and opportunity for cooling
Heatstroke	Thermoregulatory failure of sudden onset	Abrupt onset preceded by headache, dizziness, and fatigue; flushed skin; relatively less sweating than seen with heat exhaustion; pulse rate increases; temperature rises rapidly to 104° F; person feels as if he or she is burning up; diarrhea, vomiting; circulatory collapse may produce death	Heroic measures to reduce temperature must be taken immediately (e.g., immerse the patient in a tub of ice water, or sponge cool water and air fan over body), transport to hospital as soon as possible	Ensure proper acclimatization, proper hydration; adapt activities to environment

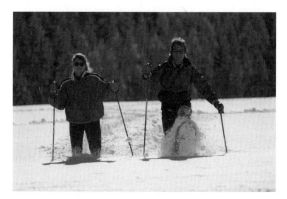

FIGURE 9-17. HYPOTHERMIA.
Exercising in cold environments can lead to hypothermia.

35°C (95°F). Essentially it is a breakdown in the body's ability to produce heat. Initially there is shivering followed by loss of coordination and difficulty speaking. As the body's temperature continues to drop, shivering stops, the muscles stiffen, and the person becomes unconscious. People who have hypothermia should be taken to the hospital for treatment, and all efforts should be directed toward elevating body temperature. Safe Tip 9-3 provides recommendations that may help reduce the chances of hypothermia.

PHYSICAL ACTIVITY DURING PREGNANCY

In the past, pregnancy was considered to be an abnormal condition. Today it is recognized as an altered physical state in which the woman's body undergoes a variety of changes to support the development of an unborn baby. The internal environment is very protective of the unborn baby. The developing baby is surrounded by the amniotic fluid, which acts as a shock absorber, dispersing the force of any direct blow to the mother's abdomen.

The type of exercise recommended will depend on the condition of the woman when her

SAFE TIP 9-3

Hypothermia Prevention

- Use common sense, and be aware of the environmental conditions that predispose to hypothermia.
- Wear a hat to reduce loss of body heat through the head.
- Dress in layers of clothing, which can be removed layer by layer to prevent sweating. Remember that dampness is one of the more critical factors. If possible, wear materials such as Gore-tex, which allow moisture to escape from the body while keeping out moisture from the environment.
- Wear sufficiently protective clothing on the feet, hands, ears, and neck to prevent frostbite.
- Gradually acclimate yourself to exercising in the cold. Acclimatization to exercising in the cold is just as important as acclimatization when exercising in a hot, humid environment.

pregnancy begins and the health of the pregnancy. The pregnant woman should avoid becoming overheated. When the woman's body temperature rises, the unborn baby's environment also heats up. This temperature increase has been linked to birth defects, especially if it occurs during the first 3 months of pregnancy.

The key to being able to exercise during pregnancy is to become fit before getting pregnant (Figure 9-18). It is advisable to curtail contact sports and sports that involve severe exertion, especially in highly competitive situations.

The following are suggested activities that can be done during pregnancy:

- Swimming seems to be suitable throughout the pregnancy. It is self-limiting, and the individual may perform at her own

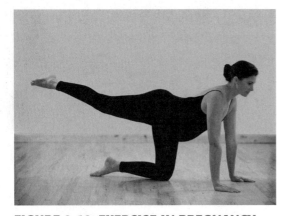

FIGURE 9-18. EXERCISE IN PREGNANCY.
There is no reason to avoid physical activity during pregnancy.

speed. Water is good for relaxation of muscles and provides a soothing effect. Pregnancy-induced changes in body composition make the female more buoyant, and swimming remains easy as pregnancy advances. Swimming may be started during pregnancy even though the woman had not been swimming before.

- Bicycling is another non-weight-bearing activity. A stationary bike may be preferable to standard cycling because of weight and balance changes during pregnancy. Also, it is possible to control climate indoors so that the expectant mother does not become overheated.
- Walking is an excellent activity during pregnancy, even though it is weight-bearing. Walking keeps the muscles of the trunk, pelvis, and legs in good tone during pregnancy. Like swimming and cycling, it offers aerobic benefits as well.
- Running is an activity of questionable value for the pregnant female. It is likely that few problems would develop during the first two trimesters of pregnancy. However, during the last trimester, running should be done with extra caution because of expected increases in body weight.

FIT LIST 9-1

Guidelines for Exercise During Pregnancy

- Consult your physician before starting an exercise program.
- It is better to modify your prepregnancy exercise program than to start a new one.
- Do not exercise to exhaustion.
- Avoid any activities that involve bouncing, jarring, or twisting motions.
- Avoid any activities that require rapid stops and starts.
- Do not perform any activity that puts the abdomen in jeopardy.
- Be aware that your body's center of gravity changes during pregnancy; it may be harder to keep your balance during some exercises.
- Do not exercise while lying on your back, particularly after the fourth month.
- Do not exercise during hot, humid weather.
- Drink plenty of fluids before, after, and sometimes during the workout.
- During your workout, make sure your temperature stays below 100°F and your heart rate does not exceed 140 beats per minute.

Modified from Alexander L. L. and J. H. LaRosa. 1994. *New dimensions in women's health,* Boston: Jones & Bartlett; and Agostini R., *Medical and orthopedic issues of active and athletic women.* Philadelphia: Hanley & Belfus.

- Aerobic exercise, like running, should be avoided during the third trimester, especially because it involves a considerable amount of bouncing.

The American College of Obstetrics and Gynecology has developed guidelines for pregnant women to follow when exercising. Fit List 9-1 summarizes guidelines designed to ensure the safety, health, and fitness of the pregnant woman and her developing baby.

SUMMARY

- Listen to what your body is telling you. The "no pain, no gain" mentality will likely worsen an existing injury. The best way to prevent injury is to pay close attention to the basic principles of training and conditioning.
- Low back pain can have many causes, but the most common are herniated disks, lumbosacral strains, sacroiliac sprains, excessive tightness of the hamstrings, and weak abdominal muscles.
- Low back pain can be prevented by paying attention to standing, lying, sitting, and lifting posture to prevent the lower back from being placed in potentially injurious positions.
- All injuries should be initially managed using rest, ice, compression, and elevation (RICE) to control swelling and thus reduce the time required for rehabilitation.
- It is important to understand the dangers involved in exercising in extreme environmental conditions.

SUGGESTED READINGS

Armstrong, L., D. Casa, and M. Millard-Stafford. 2007. Exertional heat illness during training and competition. *Medicine and Science in Sports and Exercise* 39(3):556–572.

Artal, R., and M. O'Toole. 2003. Guidelines of the American College of Obstetricians and Gynecologists for exercise during pregnancy and the postpartum period. *British Journal of Sports Medicine* 37(1):6–12.

Binkley, H. M., J. Beckett, and D. J. Casa. 2002. National Athletic Trainers' Association Position Statement: Exertional heat illness. *Journal of Athletic Training* 37(3):329–43.

Brown, W. 2002. The benefits of physical activity during pregnancy. *Journal of Science and Medicine in Sport* 5(1):37–45.

Brukner, P., and K. Khan. 2010. *Clinical sports medicine,* 3rd ed. Sydney, Australia: McGraw-Hill.

Campbell, J., and W. Sebastianelli. 2007. Athletics in extreme cold: Do's and don'ts. *Sports Medicine Update* 6(6):2–6.

Castellani, J., A.Yung and M. Ducharme. 2006. Prevention of cold injuries during exercise. *Medicine and Science in Sports and Exercise* 38(11):2012–29.

Clapp, J. 2002. *Exercising through your pregnancy.* Omaha, NE: Addicus Books.

Gallaspie, J., and D. May. 2001. *Signs and symptoms of athletic injuries.* St. Louis: McGraw-Hill.

2003. Heat illness symptoms and treatments. *JOPERD—The Journal of Physical Education, Recreation and Dance* 74(7):12–13.

2001. Heat-related illness. In *Sports medicine handbook,* edited by S. J. Shulz, Indianapolis: National Federation of State High School Associations.

Hinch, D. E., and M. W. Radomski. 2003. Exercise in the cold. *WellnessOptions* 4(11):43–44.

Howe, A., and B. Boden. 2007. Heat-related illness in athletes. *American Journal of Sports Medicine* 35(8):1384–95.

McGill, S. 2007. *Low back disorders: Evidence-based prevention and rehabilitation.* Champaign, IL: Human Kinetics.

Mellion, M. (ed.). 2002. *Sports medicine secrets.* Philadelphia: Lippincott, Williams & Wilkins.

Micheli, L., and M. Jenkins. 2001. *The sports medicine bible for the young athlete.* New York: Harper Perennial.

Moran, D. S. 2001. Potential applications of heat and cold stress indices to sporting events. *Sports Medicine* 31(13):909–17.

Nordahl, K., C. Petersen, and R. Jeffries. 2005. *Fit to deliver: An innovative prenatal and postpartum fitness program,*Vancouver: Hartley and Marks.

Pfeiffer, R., and B. Magnus. 2007. *Concepts of athletic training.* Boston: Jones & Bartlett.

Porterfield, J., C. Derosa, and M. Bilbas. 1998. *Mechanical low back pain: Perspectives in functional anatomy.* Philadelphia: W. B. Saunders.

Prentice, W. 2010. *Rehabilitation techniques in sports medicine and athletic training.* New York: McGraw-Hill.

Prentice, W. 2010. *Essentials of athletic injury management.* New York: McGraw-Hill.

Prentice, W. 2011. *Principles of athletic training.* New York: McGraw-Hill.

Rucker, K. S. 2001. *Low back pain: A symptom-based approach to diagnosis and treatment.* Burlington, MA: Butterworth-Heinemann.

Rush, S. 2001. Winter exercise. *ACSM's Health and Fitness Journal* 5(6):23–25.

Rush, S. 2002. Sports medicine approach to low back pain. *ACSM's Health and Fitness Journal* 6(2):22–24.

Shirreffs, S. M., L. E. Armstrong, and S. N. Cheuvront. 2004. Fluid and electrolyte needs for preparation and recovery from training and competition. *Journal of Sports Sciences* 22(1):57–63.

Thompson, D., L. 2007. Exercise during pregnancy. *ACSM's Health and Fitness Journal* 11(2):4.

Wallace, R., D. Kriebel and L. Punnett. 2005. The effects of continuous hot weather training on risk of exertional heat illness. *Medicine and Science in Sports and Exercise* 37(1):84–90.

Weiss, K. 2005. Practical exercise advice during pregnancy: Guidelines for active and inactive women. *Physician and Sportsmedicine* 33(6):24–30.

Vad, V., and H. Hinzmann. 2004. *Back Rx: A 15-minute-a-day yoga-and Pilates-based program to end low-back pain.* New York: Gotham.

SUGGESTED WEB SITES

American Orthopaedic Society for Sports Medicine

This site has a directory of doctors, publications, links to other sites, an ask the doctor section, and the *Sports Medicine Journal*.
www.sportsmed.org

ESPN.com: Training Room

This site has articles about fitness and conditioning, sports injuries, and sports nutrition.
http://espn.go.com/trainingroom

Gatorade Sport Science Institute

This site provides a wide range of information on exercise and nutrition.
www.gssiweb.com

Hughston Sports Medicine Hospital

This is the nation's first hospital specifically designed to treat patients suffering from activity-related injuries and disorders. It is in Columbus, Georgia.
www.hughstonsports.com

National Athletic Trainers' Association

Provides links to injury information, news about the organization, research and education, the *Journal of Athletic Training*, and other related topics.
www.nata.org

Spine-Health, your back pain and neck pain resource

This site presents in-depth information on back pain and neck pain, sciatica, scoliosis, herniated disc, degenerative disc disease, spinal stenosis.
www.spine-health.com/

Sports Injury Clinic

An interactive site that allows you to learn more about specific injuries.
http://www.sportsinjuryclinic.net/

Sportsmedicine.com

The Sports Medicine Network offers information on education, organizations, and topics about sports medicine, plus a chat room, mail list, and message board to connect people interested in sports medicine.
www.sportsmedicine.com

WebMD/Lycos-Article-Recommendations for Exercise in Pregnancy

WebMD provides recommendations for exercise during pregnancy. Prenatal exercise is a crucial part of staying healthy while you're pregnant.
www.americanpregnancy.org/pregnancyhealth/exerciseguidelines.html

CHAPTER 10

Becoming a Wise **Consumer**

Objectives

After completing this chapter, you should be able to do the following:

- Describe what is necessary to be a careful consumer of health and fitness products.
- Discuss the various types of exercise equipment that may be used in a health and fitness program.
- Explain how clothing should be selected for exercising in hot or cold environments.
- Identify special considerations for selecting a health or fitness club.
- Discuss what you should look for in health and fitness books and magazines.

ARE YOU A WISE CONSUMER OF FITNESS PRODUCTS?

To say that the emphasis on health and fitness in American society has increased significantly during the past decade is a gross understatement. The consumer of health and fitness products has become the target of an unprecedented media advertising blitz. The stereotypical image of the healthy and fit body appears in countless magazines at newsstands, on television, in infomercials, in newspaper ads, and on the Internet. Advertising includes everything from health foods and vitamins to exercise equipment, fitness centers, and weight-loss centers.

Further evidence of the magnitude of the interest in fitness and exercise is seen in the expenditures for sporting goods and exercise equipment, which have reached an all-time high. The sale of sporting goods has become big business. Sales of about $23 billion were recorded in the early 2000s. The athletic shoe business alone has become a $2.5 billion-a-year business. Recent sales figures show that close to $5 billion is being spent on athletic clothing annually. Sales of home exercise equipment have skyrocketed to about $3 billion today as individuals seek the convenience of being able to work out at home. Stationary bicycles, rowing machines, treadmills, stair climbers, and weight systems are the most popular items. Sales of diet and exercise books continue to rise. Corporate fitness programs and commercial health clubs have

KEY TERM

consumerism

attracted a record number of members. The list goes on and on. There is little doubt that a significant amount of misinformation is being disseminated in an effort to merchandise a lucrative health and fitness industry.

Marketing and advertising experts are extremely sensitive to the vulnerability of American consumers when it comes to buying products that promise to make them look and feel better. How can the consumer separate fact from hype when considering advertisements for health and fitness products? It is essential for consumers to educate themselves by taking a critical look at a product or service to be purchased. For example, if you are going to buy a new automobile, perhaps you begin by looking at advertisements. You may wish to consult an independent consumer magazine to look at performance specifications, maintenance records, and so on. Then you go to the dealers to find who can offer the best price along with a reputation for good service. Chances are that you will buy your new car from that dealer.

The point is that most people shop around and are careful when making a choice about a large purchase such as an automobile. They take the time necessary to learn everything they can about the product. The wise consumer will take a similar approach when buying health and fitness products. You should realize that it is easy to be "taken in" by advertisements that project an image that seems to be in demand by consumers. Practicing **consumerism** means that wise consumers will take the time to analyze the entire product and to decide if the outlay of money is necessary to reap the benefits they desire.

> **consumerism:** taking the time to analyze the entire product and to decide if the outlay of money is necessary to reap the desired benefits

WHAT TO CONSIDER WHEN BUYING FITNESS EQUIPMENT

The extent and variety of fitness and exercise equipment available to the consumer are at times mind-boggling. Prices of equipment can range from between $5 for a jump rope or Frisbee to $60,000 for certain computer-driven isokinetic devices. One of the most important facts that the consumer of health and fitness products and services must understand is that it is certainly not necessary to purchase expensive exercise equipment to see good results. You will achieve many of the same physiological benefits from using a $5 jump rope, an exercise mat, or dumbells as you will from running on a $10,000 treadmill. For the average college student, cost is a major consideration. The following discussion identifies some of the more popular pieces of exercise equipment.

FREE WEIGHTS VERSUS WEIGHT MACHINES

A discussion comparing the use of free weights including barbells and dumbbells to exercise machines can be found in Chapter 5 (pp. 124–125). There are advantages and disadvantages to both types of equipment. However, costs of purchasing free weights are substantially lower than the weight machines (Figure 10-1). Regardless of which type of equipment you use, the same principles of isotonic training may be applied.

STATIONARY EXERCISE BIKES

Many different exercise bikes are available to the consumer (Figure 10-2, *A*). Bicycle companies such as Schwinn or Ross, as well as Tunturi and Vitamaster, which specifically manufacture exercise equipment, are well-known name

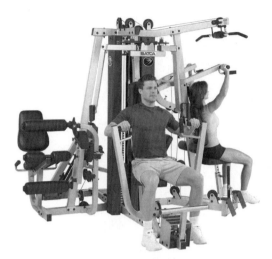

FIGURE 10-1. MULTISTATION EXERCISE MACHINE.

brands. Exercise bikes priced below $150 tend to be somewhat unstable. Most good models range between $150 and $700. Computerized exercise bikes used in health clubs may cost between $1,500 and $3,500.

There are essentially two types of exercise bikes. When you pedal a "single-action" model, resistance is created from a device such as a flywheel. With the flywheel you can change the resistance with a twist of a knob. The "dual-action" models also let you pump the handle-bars back with your arms. Most of these bikes use a fan to create resistance, which can be increased by pumping the arms and legs faster. The dual-action models allow you to rest your feet on coaster pedals and exercise only your arms. Obviously, those models that work both the upper and lower extremities require a higher energy expenditure. Most models have you sitting on a bicycle seat in a standard position. Some design variations allow you to sit in a recumbent position (Figure 10-2, *F*). This position on a recumbent bike exercises the hamstring muscles to a greater degree and is useful

for individuals who have back problems or poor balance.

Training stands hook a resistance device to your regular bicycle, allowing you to convert it to a stationary bike at relatively low cost. Features that are important to look for include a comfortable padded seat and some type of monitor that tells you how far you have pedaled or the time. Models with pedal straps will work your legs on the upstroke in addition to the downstroke.

Individuals who are unable to use their lower extremities on a regular exercise bike can use an upper-extremity bicycle ergometer (Figure 10-2, *H*).

TREADMILLS

An exercise treadmill is a belt stretched between two rollers (Figure 10-2, *B*). The belt may be driven manually in the least expensive models or by a motor in more expensive ones. Sears, Tunturi, Vitamaster, Voit, DP, Precor, and Proform are among the more common brands of treadmills manufactured for home use. Costs range from $400 to $1,000. More expensive machines have a bigger motor, a wider belt, and a faster top speed (up to about 5 mph). It is difficult to find a good motor-driven treadmill for under $500. Treadmills subjected to high use in health clubs cost between $1,000 and $12,000. Most of the more expensive motor-driven treadmills allow you to adjust both the speed of the belt and the incline angle to alter intensity. One of the big advantages of using treadmill with walkers is the ability to increase incline to increase heart work. For many new to fitness, walking on a track or on different elliptical type machines does not raise their heart rate into the aerobic zone. To avoid the stress on the knees and ankles of beginning exercisers, increasing the incline of a treadmill while maintaining a comfortable pace, such as 2 1/2 to 3 mph, increases heart rate into the proper workout zone.

Machine motors vary in both type and size. The type of motor can be either AC or DC. AC

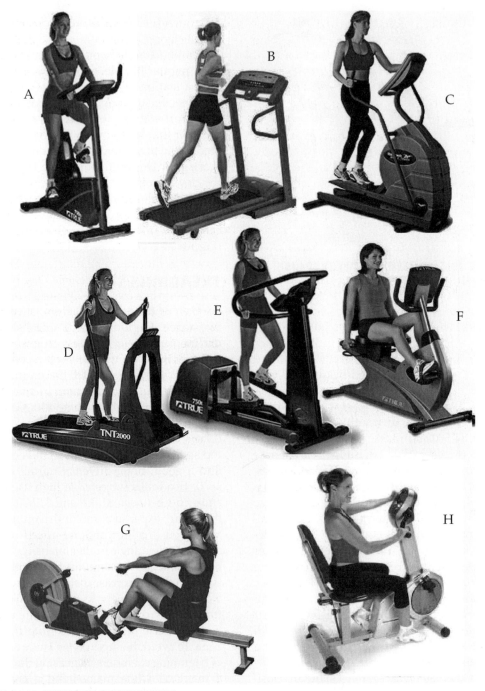

FIGURE 10-2. FITNESS EQUIPMENT.
A, Stationary bike; B, Treadmill; C, Stair climber; D, Cross-country ski machine; E, Elliptical exerciser; F, Recumbent bike, G, Rowing machine; H, Upper-extremity ergometer.

motors run at full speed, all the time, relying on a transmission-like pulley system to regulate speed. This means most models start up at full speed and can be somewhat dangerous when getting on. Treadmill motors that are DC can be run at different speeds, so start-up is not much of a problem. All models come with some type of speed control. Motor size varies from 1/2 horsepower to more than 1 horsepower. Bigger motors can handle heavier loads and higher speeds. A running gait requires that the treadmill is able to go at least 5 mph.

STAIR CLIMBERS

Stair climbers have become one of the more popular types of exercise machines (Figure 10-2, C). They are essentially a set of levers attached to some resistance device. Your legs pump the levers as if you are climbing stairs. Models vary in how they apply resistance, using either a flywheel, a hydraulic piston, a drive train, or wind resistance. In some models, the stairs are linked. As one goes down, the other automatically goes up. Dual-action models allow you to work both the arms and the legs simultaneously. The more expensive models have a series of stairs that rotate as if you were climbing the wrong direction on an escalator. Monitors on many models display information such as time, steps per minute, and energy expenditure. Some may be programmed to vary both the speed and the amount of resistance during the course of a workout. Sears, Tunturi, DP, and Precor are brand names of the typical home models. Stairmaster makes most of the more expensive units for commercial use. Stair-climbing machines cost between $200 and $3,000. Most of the home models are around $500. Programmable units cost a minimum of $800.

SKI MACHINES

A ski machine offers many of the aerobic benefits of cross-country skiing without having to worry about the snow. These machines have two flat boards, one for each foot, that slide back and forth in a groove on rollers. The arms are also involved, using either telescoping poles or a rope and pulley instead of the ski poles. The design of these machines allows you to simultaneously exercise both the upper and lower extremities. (Figure 10-2, D).

Ski machines have either dependent or independent leg motion. With a dependent machine, the leg boards are connected. As one goes forward, the other goes backward. On independent machines, the leg boards slide independently, making them somewhat more difficult to master but also affording you a better workout. Resistance on the ski machine comes from either an electromagnetic flywheel or from a belt wrapped around a flywheel that provides friction. Some models do not have variable resistance. More expensive models may also incline, increasing the stress on the quadriceps muscles in the front of the thigh. Most machines have some type of monitor that can show heart rate, resistance, speed, calories expended, and the like. Most of these machines can be folded and require little space for storage.

There are several manufacturers of ski machines, including NordicTrack, Precor, Proform, DP, Vitamaster, and Tunturi. Ski machines range in price from $300 to as high as $2,000 for health club models.

ELLIPTICAL EXERCISERS

Elliptical machines provide a new mode of cardiovascular exercise that makes use of a no-impact, elliptical-shaped stride (Figure 10-2, E). When using the machine, you stand upright while striding in a forward or reverse motion and holding handrails. An electronically adjustable ramp allows you to raise or lower ramp incline, adjust resistance, and use both forward and reverse motion. These options let exercisers simulate no-impact versions of their favorite exercise activities, such as walking, running, cycling, cross-country skiing, and stairclimbing. Lower ramp levels can simulate cross-country skiing or the walking or running options of a treadmill. Higher ramp levels can produce a safe, comfortable cycling or stair-climbing motion. Elliptical machines are manufactured by Vision Fitness, Life Fitness, Star Trac, Precor, NordicTrack, ICON Health and Fitness, Inc., Guthy-Renker, and Quantum Television. They range in price from $200 for home models to $3,500 for more sophisticated commercial models.

ROWING MACHINES

Rowing machines are designed to mimic the action of rowing a boat or sculling. Most brands have some type of movable handles, which are similar to oars, and a sliding seat. Exercise involves pressing against stationary footplates with the legs while sliding backward on the seat and simultaneously pulling on the handles to create a rowing motion. Rowing machines are similar to stair climbers in terms of their resistance mechanisms, which may include a flywheel, a hydraulic piston, or wind resistance. (Figure 10-2, *G*).

Sears, DP, and Tunturi are the most common home models of rowing machines. Costs range between $200 and $800 for home models. Rowing machines for health clubs range between $1,000 and $3,000.

PASSIVE EXERCISE DEVICES AND TECHNIQUES

Unfortunately, many consumers of health and fitness products are lured into thinking that there is some easy way to achieve physical fitness with little or no physical effort. The marketing of a variety of devices such as rubberized suits that let you sit around and sweat off weight, electrical devices that make muscles contract, and mechanical devices that

shake, vibrate, or roll fat off can seem to be very appealing shortcuts to getting fit. There are, however, no shortcuts.

▶ Passive Motion Machines

These machines have only been introduced into the health and fitness market in recent years. Passive motion machines are designed to exercise individual body parts by moving them for you with no effort on your part. You are simply required to lie or sit still while the machine does all the work. For example, one machine is designed to flex and extend your trunk and lower back, while another may flex and extend your hip and your knee. Manufacturers claim that these machines will help improve muscular endurance since a particular body part is moving repeatedly, improve flexibility by using slow continuous movement, and burn off fat while reducing cellulite in the exercised areas. All of these claims are totally ludicrous. The only potential benefit offered to healthy individuals by these machines may be relaxation. However, similar passive exercise devices, referred to as constant passive motion (CPM) machines, are widely and effectively used in rehabilitation for postsurgical patients to minimize development of scar tissue.

▶ Motor-Driven Exercise Bikes

Stationary exercise bikes or rowing machines that are motor driven may have some value in increasing circulation, particularly around joints. However, they are totally ineffective in elevating heart rate and thus stressing the cardiovascular system.

▶ Vibrating Belts and Rolling Machines

Vibrating belts placed around the trunk or the extremities that shake fat and muscle tissue or rolling machines that use movable wooden rollers to compress fat and muscle tissue in a rolling fashion have been promoted to break up fat tissue, thus making it easier to burn off. They also falsely claim to increase muscle tone and improve posture. The truth is that they do not "break up" fat, but they may damage connective tissue around joints and within a muscle. The rollers may also cause bruising of the skin and fat from repeated compression. Use of these machines should definitely be avoided by people with low back pain and by pregnant women.

▶ Massage

Massage can be an extremely effective therapeutic technique (Figure 10-3). It is most typically used for stimulating circulation, for inducing relaxation, and for loosening up muscles. However, as in the case of rolling machines, it will not selectively rub fat away from a specific spot.

▶ Rubberized or Inflatable Suits

Rubberized inflatable suits are also called sauna shorts or sauna sleeves. Promoters claim that the pressure created by the garment will help to break down fat tissue by squeezing it and that the rubber garment will help you "sweat off" fat. Once again these claims are ridiculous. Fat cannot be "squeezed off." Furthermore, sweating does not burn off a significant amount of fat.

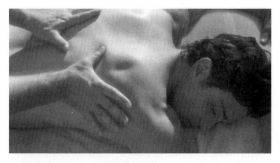

FIGURE 10-3. MASSAGE.
Massage can be an extremely effective therapeutic technique.

Wearing rubberized suits may help you lose body weight fairly quickly, but the weight loss represents the water weight of perspiration rather than loss of fat tissue. Elevation of body core temperature by wearing rubberized suits may predispose an individual to various forms of heat stress and can potentially be very dangerous for individuals with high blood pressure.

▶ Electrical Stimulating Devices

In general, electrical stimulating devices use low-amperage electrical current of sufficient intensity to cause involuntary muscle contraction. The technique involves connecting the electrodes to specific areas of the body and generating a weak electrical current to contract the muscles. (Promoters claim that the muscle contraction requires energy, thus calories will be used from stored fat to supply energy.) Once again, there is no credibility to the value of this technique for weight loss or fitness.

Electrical stimulating currents are routinely used by qualified rehabilitation specialists for treating many different musculoskeletal and neurological problems. When appropriate treatment limits are selected, electrical currents can be effectively used for pain control and muscle reeducation after injury, as well as to decrease muscle spasm and to reduce muscle atrophy. The indiscriminant use of electrical currents by untrained individuals is strongly discouraged and in many states is against the law.

SPAS, STEAM BATHS, SAUNAS

In the health and fitness industry, the use of spas (hot tubs), steam baths, and saunas is widespread. Most health and fitness clubs offer the use of at least one form of these to their members. Hot tubs and whirlpool baths are increasingly being installed in private homes.

Of all their therapeutic benefits, perhaps none is more important than the relaxation factor. Relaxation seems to be the primary reason why so many people are interested in using them. However, claims that sitting in either water or air at high temperatures will cause fat loss are again totally unfounded. Whatever weight is lost is due to a loss of water. Water loss should be immediately replaced through proper rehydration from beverages.

Saunas are likely to produce the greatest amount of body water loss because the air is hot and extremely dry. Thus significant amounts of water will be lost through the rapid evaporation of sweat. Temperatures in a sauna should not be higher than 180°F. You should limit yourself to no more than 15 minutes in the sauna at that temperature.

Steam baths, which should be no higher than 120°F., have a much lower temperature than saunas. However, the humidity in a steam bath is 100 percent. Thus individuals will appear to be sweating more heavily in a steam bath. Under humid conditions, sweat cannot evaporate to dissipate body heat, and body temperature rises rapidly. It is necessary to limit time in a steam bath to no longer than 10 minutes.

Spas or hot tubs involve full-body immersion in a whirlpool at a temperature that should be no higher than 100°F. for no longer than 10 minutes (Figure 10-4).

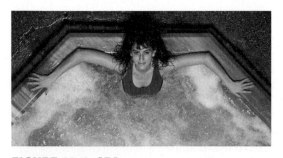

FIGURE 10-4. SPA.
A spa or hot tub is relaxing but it should not be used for the purpose of losing body fat.

Certain precautions should be taken when using any of these units:
1. If you have a heart condition or skin infection or are pregnant, you should avoid their use.
2. Do not use any of these without cooling down after exercise.
3. Wash off all oils or lotions before use.
4. Never drink alcohol before use.
5. If you feel faint for any reason, get out immediately.
6. Always have someone with you when using any of these.

TANNING BEDS

For years, having a deep, golden-brown tan was associated with being fit and healthy. During the past decade, artificial tanning beds have become very popular in the health and fitness club industry. These tanning salons, beds, and booths usually consist of an array of long tubes that produce ultraviolet light. The lights are positioned in some type of frame that allows for exposure of the entire body.

We now know beyond any doubt that prolonged or continuous exposure to ultraviolet light rays predisposes an individual to the development of skin cancer. Manufacturers of artificial tanning devices claim the ultraviolet light produced by tanning devices is safe. The Food and Drug Administration (FDA) has warned the public that sunlamps and tanning beds are dangerous. Besides the risk of skin cancer, long-term exposure to a form of ultraviolet light (UVA) causes premature aging of the skin with wrinkling and sagging. Production of UVA tanning beds is largely unregulated. Furthermore, there is generally no standard of training for people who operate these machines. Their knowledge of the tanning process and the danger of exposure to ultraviolet radiation may be limited at best. Therefore, extreme caution should be exercised whenever you are exposed to ultraviolet radiation, either from sunlight or from artificial sources.

HOW SHOULD YOU CHOOSE APPROPRIATE CLOTHING AND SHOES FOR EXERCISE?

CLOTHING FOR EXERCISING IN HOT, HUMID WEATHER

Guidelines for selecting clothing for exercising in hot, humid weather are relatively simple and straightforward. Clothing should allow for maximal dissipation of body heat through evaporation of sweat while minimizing the heat gained from the environment. By far the most effective means of heat loss involves the process of evaporation. If sweat remains on the skin, it will not produce heat loss. Thus the material worn must be lightweight and dry very quickly by permitting sweat to evaporate. The body area that has the greatest number of sweat glands is the upper back and shoulders. Consequently a tank top will allow for greatest exposure for evaporation. Radiation of heat from the sun or other hot surfaces such as pavement will cause the body to gain heat. Clothing should be a light color to reflect as much radiant heat energy as possible.

Wearing a hat will help block some of the radiant heat energy from the sun. However, it is critical that the hat be made of some type of mesh fabric to allow heat to be dissipated from the head.

It should be reemphasized that making certain you are well hydrated is the best way to minimize heat-related problems.

CLOTHING FOR EXERCISING IN COLD WEATHER

In situations where the weather is cold, the goal of wearing clothing is to create a "semitropical microclimate" for the body and to prevent chilling. The clothing should not restrict movement and should be as lightweight as possible. The material should permit free passage of sweat and body heat. Otherwise, sweat would accumulate on the skin or in the clothing and provide a chilling effect when activity ceases. This dampness, in combination with cold and wind, plays a critical role in the development of hypothermia. Individuals should routinely dress in thin layers of clothing that can be easily added or removed when the temperature increases or decreases. Constant adjustment of these layers will reduce sweating and the likelihood that clothing will become damp or wet.

Before exercise, during activity breaks, and after exercise, a warm-up suit or sweat clothes should be worn to prevent chilling. Activity in cold, wet, or windy weather poses some problem because such weather reduces the insulating value of the clothing. Consequently, the individual may be unable to achieve a level of metabolic heat production sufficient to keep pace with body heat loss. In cold weather, a hat should be worn to minimize excessive heat loss from the head. It is also a good idea to wear gloves to minimize the effects of cold and wind on the hands and fingers.

SHOE SELECTION

The athletic and fitness shoe manufacturing industry has become extremely sophisticated and offers a number of options when it comes to purchasing shoes for different activities. Terms like forefoot varus support or rearfoot valgus wedge are confusing to a person who simply wants to buy a pair of good running, aerobic, or court shoes. Most people are simply interested in finding a shoe that is designed for a specific activity that will last for a long time, and that will provide good support and comfort. For those individuals shopping for shoes who are searching for additional, more specific advice and/or assistance in finding the right shoe, there are several running shoe stores whose sales people are well trained and knowledgeable and can offer

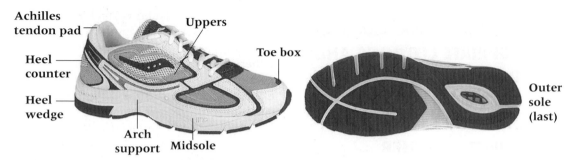

FIGURE 10-5. THE PARTS OF A WELL-DESIGNED SHOE.

good recommendations. Figure 10-5 shows the major parts of a shoe. For the average individual, the following guidelines can help you select the most appropriate shoe to fit your needs.

▶Toe Box

There should be plenty of room for your toes in the fitness shoe. Most experts recommend a 1/2- to 3/4-inch distance between toes and the front of the shoe. A few fitness shoes are made in varying widths. If you have a very wide or narrow foot, most shoe salespersons can recommend a specific shoe for your foot. The best way to make sure there is adequate room in the toe box is to have your foot measured and then try on the shoe. If the shoe feels too tight or there are areas of friction or pressure when trying the shoe in a store, it is likely that there will be some continuing problems with proper fit when you begin exercising.

▶Sole

The sole should possess two qualities. First, it must provide a shock-absorptive function; second, it must be durable. Most shoes have three layers on the sole: a thick spongy layer, which absorbs the force of the foot strike under the heel; a midsole, which cushions the midfoot and toes; and a hard rubber layer, which comes in contact with the ground. The average runner's feet strike the ground 1,500 to 1,700 times per mile. Thus it is essential that the force of the heel strike be absorbed by the spongy layer to prevent overuse-type injuries from occurring in the ankles and knees. "Heel wedges" are sometimes inserted on either the inside or the outside surface of the sole underneath the heel counter to accommodate and correct for various structural deformities of the foot that may alter normal biomechanics of the running gait. A flared heel may be appropriate for running shoes but is not recommended in aerobic or court shoes. The sole must provide good traction and must be made of a tough material that is resistant to wear. Most of the better-known brands of shoes tend to have well-designed, long-lasting soles.

▶Heel Counters

The heel counter is the portion of the shoe that prevents the foot from rolling from side to side at heel strike. The heel counter should be firm but well fitted (snug) to minimize movement of the heel up and down or side to side. A good heel counter may prevent ankle sprains and painful blisters.

▶Shoe Uppers

The upper part of the shoe is made of some combination of nylon and leather. The uppers should be lightweight, capable of quick drying, and well ventilated. The uppers should have some type of extra support in the saddle area, and there should also be some extra padding in the area of the Achilles tendon just above the heel counter. While running shoes are designed for straight ahead motion, court shoes and aerobic shoes have to absorb lateral motions and thus the uppers should be reinforced appropriately.

▶Arch Support

The arch support should be made of some durable yet soft supportive material and should smoothly join with the insole. The support should not have any rough seams or ridges inside the shoe, which may cause blisters.

▶Price

Unfortunately, for many people price is the primary consideration in buying running shoes. Running shoes and court shoes range from $40 to $160 per pair. Aerobic shoes tend to be less expensive, in the $30 to $80 range. When buying fitness shoes, remember that in many fitness activities, shoes are important for performance and prevention of injury. Thus it is worth a little extra investment to buy a quality pair of shoes.

WHAT TO LOOK FOR IN A HEALTH CLUB

It's easy to get caught up in a desire to join a health club. You walk in the front door and may immediately be greeted by an attractive, energetic receptionist who quickly introduces you to an attractive, energetic "fitness consultant," which is the term frequently used in fitness centers to label the salesperson. You may be escorted into a large exercise room with plush carpeting on the floor, mirrors on every wall, chrome-plated exercise equipment, and high-energy music coming from the sound system. Your eyes tend to ignore the overweight gentleman or the frail lady working on machines in the corner and go straight to the Adonis or Aphrodite working out in the center of the room. It is easy to think, "Hey, this place is beautiful, and if it can make me feel comfortable and look like that at the same time, I want to join—NOW." Unfortunately, in this situation the consumer has already decided to purchase the hype without investigating the facts.

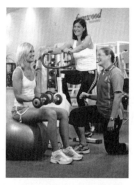

FIGURE 10-6. HEALTH CLUB INSTRUCTION.
Well-qualified instructors are an important factor to consider when selecting a health club.

Certainly it is possible to find health clubs that offer good-quality instruction and guidance (Figure 10-6) in addition to an aesthetically pleasing environment in which to work out. The guidelines described here are important for those individuals who are considering joining a health or fitness club. It should be strongly emphasized that you do not need to join a health club or a gym, nor do you need to hire a personal fitness trainer, to get fit or achieve your personal fitness goals. Certainly, these "luxuries" may not be affordable for most college students.

TYPES OF FACILITIES

Familiarize yourself with the many different types of facilities available, including spas, gyms, YMCA/YWCAs, and facilities at universities or high schools. Many times local schools or colleges will offer excellent facilities for public use at little or no cost. You can most often find a listing of facilities in the telephone book. It is important to contact all the available sources to get the most detailed information.

LOCATION OF FACILITY

Certainly the location of the facility is an important factor in deciding whether to join.

- Is it close or easily accessible to your home or apartment?

- Will you be stopping to exercise on your way to or from work or school?
- What is the traffic like near the facility at the times of day you are most likely to go?

EQUIPMENT AVAILABLE

Check the type of equipment available.

- Do they have weight equipment (free weights, exercise machines)?
- Is there a pool, whirlpool, sauna, steam room, running track, racquetball court, and aerobic exercise room?
- Is there sufficient available locker space, with showers and changing areas?
- Do they have the type of equipment necessary for your fitness program?

PROGRAMS OFFERED

Check the type and quality of programs offered, such as individualized and supervised weight training, aerobic exercise classes, spinning classes, kickboxing classes, jogging classes, yoga, weight-control programs, and cardiac rehabilitation programs. Do any of these cost extra?

HOURS OF OPERATION

- What are the hours of operation of the facility?
- Are they open 7 days per week?
- Is it a co-ed facility?
- Can both males and females work out there 7 days a week?
- What are the most crowded times?

QUALIFICATIONS OF PERSONNEL

You must be careful to consider the qualifications of the instructors. Many health and fitness clubs employ attractive, fit individuals whose primary function is to sell memberships to the club. Ask the salesperson the following questions:

- What is the background of the personnel who will be supervising your program?
- Do they have a background in physical education, exercise physiology, athletic training, or physical therapy?
- Are they certified by the American College of Sports Medicine as Exercise Leaders, Health/Fitness Instructors, or Exercise Specialists?
- Are they certified as aerobics instructors by the Aerobics and Fitness Association of America (AFAA), American Council on Exercise (ACE), Cooper Institute for Aerobics Research, or Exercise Safety Association (ESA)?
- Are they certified as personal trainers by the National Academy of Sport Medicine (NASM), the Aerobics and Fitness Association of America (AFAA), American Council on Exercise (ACE), Cooper Institute for Aerobics Research, Exercise Safety Association (ESA), International Fitness Institute, or the National Strength and Conditioning Association (NSCA)?

TYPES OF MEMBERSHIP CONTRACTS

Health and fitness clubs tend to offer a wide range of membership contract options, ranging from pay-by-the-visit to lifetime memberships. It is a good idea to avoid long-term contracts, especially in the beginning. Health clubs sell a lot of memberships because people tend to get caught up by the aesthetics of the facility and are manipulated by some very good salespeople. The firm commitment to consistently use the facility three to four times per week that is made in the sales office tends to become less important for most people over time. If all the people who bought memberships in a club were to show up at one time, it is likely that you would not be able to get in the door. If you do decide to join, check on various payment options that best suit your budget. Also check on additional fees that you may have to pay for extras, such as reserving racquetball courts or enrolling in aerobics classes.

TRIAL PERIODS

Before signing a contract, it is a good idea to spend several sessions working out at the club, talking with the instructors and with other club members. Current members can answer specific questions about the quality of the facility as well as identify its deficiencies. If there is some objection to doing this on the part of the management, then you should exercise extreme caution about signing a contract.

BE KNOWLEDGEABLE ABOUT FITNESS

It is probably wise to avoid the clubs or organizations that advertise programs, classes, equipment, or techniques that claim to result in "overnight" strength gains, weight loss, or improvements in appearance. You must realize that reaching your fitness goals requires selecting an activity you enjoy. The activity should not overload the body but progress within your individual limitations. Furthermore, by being consistent in your training program, you will accomplish your goals safely by paying attention to the basic principles outlined within this text.

RUNNING, BIKING, WALKING, TRIATHALON CLUBS

Over the years many clubs have organized both locally and nationally for individuals who have similar fitness interests and who enjoy specific types of fitness activity. There are running clubs, biking clubs, swimming clubs, walking clubs, and triathalon clubs, to name a few. Joining a special interest club has many benefits. It pro-

vides a great social environment where you can meet other like-minded people. Being part of a group makes it easier to train and can help motivate you to achieve your personal goals. You can get information about the latest equipment, training techniques, or good places to run, bike, or swim. Information about these clubs can easily be found on the Internet.

WHAT TO LOOK FOR IN FITNESS MAGAZINES, BOOKS, DVDS, AND WEB SITES

As with the various types of exercise equipment, consumer demand for literature and other media dealing with health and fitness issues makes publication in this area an extremely lucrative enterprise.

It is difficult, if not totally impossible, to pick up a popular magazine that does not contain at least one article about health and fitness. It is reasonable to assume that the majority of people in the United States obtain most of their health and fitness information while standing in line at the grocery store. This is certainly not to say that grocery store sources of health and fitness information are unreliable, but there is a tremendous amount of misinformation relative to health and fitness issues routinely spread through the popular media. Often, the articles in magazines are written by individuals with little or no health or fitness expertise who may interview fitness experts. Occasionally, you will find experts writing the articles. The same is true for so-called experts who appear on television or radio talk shows. These people have charming personalities but often lack reliable credentials.

A trip to the local bookstore, public library, or Internet booksellers to locate books dealing with health, wellness, fitness, exercise, sports, diet, and nutrition can be overwhelming. Many excellent, accurate books are available.

These books are written by health and fitness experts. Unfortunately, the majority of the best-selling books, and certainly the best-marketed ones, are written by celebrities who look fit and attractive. Some of these books contain excellent information. Others include some facts along with misinformation and border on being dangerous.

For anyone who has ventured into a video store, it is easy to see that celebrities also like to star or be featured in exercise DVDs. Again the available choices can be overwhelming. Many consumers choose to purchase exercise DVDs as an alternative to joining a health club. The convenience of having someone lead you through a workout at home certainly appeals to some people who have neither the time nor the motivation to leave home to participate in an exercise program. As is the case with books and magazines, the consumer must make informed choices when it comes to purchasing exercise DVDs. Remember, they don't always do exactly what the infomercials tell you they can do.

Throughout this text Web sites have been recommended at the end of each chapter that contain information pertinent to the information discussed in that chapter. As you are well aware there are literally millions of Web sites related to fitness that are at your fingertips. How do you know whether information presented in the popular media is reliable? Simply by being an informed consumer. The information presented in this text is accurate and up-to-date. The knowledge you have obtained from this text should make you a more informed consumer.

THE BOTTOM LINE FOR THE CONSUMER

Regardless of the type of exercise equipment, the aesthetics of a health club, or the claims of nutritional products, the bottom line is that the responsibility for getting fit and healthy ultimately lies with you. Remember, a commitment to a fitness program is first and foremost a commitment to yourself. Being cautious, asking a number of questions, and being well informed will help you make the best choice possible. Basing your physical activity program on the facts rather than on marketing techniques is the way to get fit. If you find that joining a health club or buying expensive exercise equipment in some way motivates you to adhere to your program, then by all means, do so. But never neglect the basic principles.

SUMMARY

- Be a conscientious and well-informed consumer when selecting products related to health and fitness.
- Don't be afraid to ask questions and fully investigate a health and fitness club before joining.
- An incredible amount and diversity of exercise equipment is available to the consumer.
- Deciding what type of equipment is best for you to use or purchase should be based primarily on individual interests and the goals of your physical activity program.
- Remember, there is no shortcut to fitness. Passive exercise devices are essentially useless when it comes to improvement in fitness levels.
- Spas, saunas, and steam baths should be used for relaxation and are not effective in reducing your percent body fat.
- The use of tanning beds and tanning booths is generally not recommended.
- Select appropriate clothing for exercising in either hot or cold environments to prevent heat stress or hypothermia.
- Selecting and purchasing a quality fitness shoe can reduce the likelihood of injury.
- Fitness books, magazine articles, DVDs, and Web sites should be critically analyzed by the informed and educated consumer of health and fitness products.

SUGGESTED READINGS

2004. Athletic shoes: The facts about fit. Forget the fancy gear and gadgets. All you really need for a great run or powerwalk is the right pair of shoes. *Active Woman Canada* 2(3):40–43.

Bender, M. 2002. Your guide to a good buy. *Health* 21 (6) : 63.

Burfoot, A. 2004. Treadmill nation: They help you lose weight, lower your race times, and stay fit wherever you are. Is it any wonder millions of Americans are running on treadmills? Here, the 20 best ways to make the most of your time inside. *Runner's World* 39(1):56–60.

Burke, E. 1996. *Complete home fitness handbook.* Champaign, IL: Human Kinetics.

Cardio Equipment. Cardio equipment. 2010. *Athletic Business* 34(3):49.

Chapan, C. 2007. Choosing the perfect fit: A guide for selecting running shoes. *Pro-Trainer Online.*

Coffman, S. 2007. Successful programs for fitness and health clubs: 101 profitable ideas, Champaign, IL: Human Kinetics.

Consumer Reports. 2010. *Consumer Reports 2010 buying guide.* New York: Consumer Reports.

2004. Creating together: Equipment, supplies and people provide the tools for successful programs. *IDEA Health and Fitness Source* 22(1):53–57.

Dickey, C. 2004. Tools for the trade: Books, looks, and stuff. *ACSM's Health and Fitness Journal* 8(2):32–33. 2004.

Editors of on Health and Consumer Report. 2008. *Consumer Reports diet, health, and fitness guide.* New York: Time Incorporated Home Entertainment.

Exercise equipment sales increase 3% in 2005. 2006. *NSGA Specialty Fitness News* 6(5): 2.

Faigenbaum, A. D. 2009. Weight machines. In Youth strength training: Programs for health, fitness and sport edited by A. D. Faigenbaum. Champaign, IL: Human Kinetics.

Fitness equipment warning use advisories to consumers. *Exercise Standards and Malpractice Reporter* 20(1):6.

Fitness Equipment. 2007. *Athletic Business* 31(2): 137–174.

Fitness Equipment. Fitness equipment. 2010. *Athletic Business* 34(2):103.

Forness, L. 2001. *Don't get duped: A consumer's guide to health and fitness.* Boston: Prometheus Books.

Gledhill, K. 2001. *Fitness and exercise sourcebook: Basic consumer health information about the fundamentals of fitness and exercise* (Health Reference Series). Detroit, MI: Omnigraphics.

Gormley, B. 2005. Understanding strength training equipment: Add some muscle to your strength equipment purchasing decisions. *Fitness Business Canada* 6(1):22–24.

Greene, W., and R. Fredericksen. 2007. Fall shoe guide. *Runner's World* 42(9):101.

Grisanti, S. 2002. *Industry of illusions: Health and fitness industry scams, frauds, fakes, and personal trainers exposed.* Rye, NY: Rivercat.

Hamilton, A. 2004. Rowers: Having looked at home-use bikes, treadmills and elliptical cross-trainers, it's time to consider rowers. Now you might think that a humble rowing machine, bereft of electronic gizmos, won't really cut the mustard when it comes to serious aerobic training, but you'd be wrong! *Ultra-FIT* 14(1):56–58.

Herbert, D. 2008. Standards for the certification of health fitness facilities on the horizon? *Exercise Standards & Malpractice Reporter* 22(6):81.

Holt, S. 2001. Mechanics of machines: Selecting the right piece of equipment. When choosing strength equipment, make sure the machine's mechanics replicate the members' body mechanics. *Fitness Management* 17(8):56–58, 60–61.

Howe, D. 2006. Finding a fitness trainer. *American Fitness* 24(1):9.

I've got only 30 minutes at the gym. Should I hit the elliptical machine or the treadmill? 2007. *Health.* 21(7):58.

Jung, A. P., and D. C. Nieman. 2000. An evaluation of home exercise equipment claims: Too good to be true. *ACSM's Health and Fitness Journal* 4(5):14–16, 30–31.

Karp, J. 2008. Show me the treadmill! *Fitness Management* 24(1):44.

Kreighbaum, E., and M. A. Smith (eds.). 1996. *Sports and fitness equipment design.* Champaign, IL: Human Kinetics.

Lombard, G. 2007. Best fitness advice from the year's top fitness books. *Health.* 21(10):44.

Multi-purpose fitness equipment. 2007. *Fitness Business Canada* 8(1):32.

Paris, S. 2009. A perfect fit: The top 12 running shoe buying tips. *American Fitness* 27(1):49.

Peterson, J. 2006. *American College of Sports Medicine health/fitness facility standards and guidelines.* Champaign, IL: Human Kinetics.

Porcari, J. P., et al. 2002. Effects of electrical muscle stimulation on body composition, muscle strength, and physical appearance. *Journal of Strength and Conditioning Research* 16(2):165–72.

Schroeder, J., and S. Dotan. 2010. 2010 IDEA fitness program and equipment trends. *IDEA Fitness Journal* 7(7):22.

Skinner, T., and M. Cardona. 2004. *Sneaker Book: 50 Years of Sports Shoe Design.* Atglen, PA: Schiffer Publishing, Ltd.

Stationary and recumbent bikes. 2006. *Fitness Business Canada* 7(5):18.

Tharrett, S., and J. Peterson. 2008. Fitness management: A comprehensive resource for developing, leading, managing, and operating a successful health/fitness club. *Healthy Learning.*

SUGGESTED WEB SITES

Exercise Equipment at Beyond Moseying

This site features exercise equipment, fitness machines, athletic equipment, gym apparatus, treadmills, ellipticals, versaclimbers, home gyms, bikes, steppers, and body building equipment.
www.fitnessstore.net

Fitness and Exercise Equipment Reviews

A resource of reviews on a wide variety of fitness and exercise equipment.
http://www.fitness-equipment-review.com/

Fitness Factory Outlet

This is a source for aerobic, strength training, and fitness equipment. It includes fitness tips, exercise charts, and the lowest prices on the highest quality health and fitness products available.
www.fitnessfactory.com

Healthrider

Find great treadmill deals, check your fitness age, buy equipment like treadmills, and check the weekly fitness special. Enjoy relaxation therapy, massage chairs, hydrotherapy, and spas.
www.healthrider.com

Nellies Exercise Fitness Equipment

This site presents a complete line of treadmills, home gyms, bikes, and pulse and heart monitors. It carries free weights and strength training and more.
www.nellies.com

NordicTrack Exercise Equipment Site

This site features the leading manufacturer of high-quality treadmill, cycle, skier, strength training, and other fitness equipment products. You can purchase conveniently online.
www.nordictrack.com

Precor USA

This is the industry leader in high-quality fitness equipment.
www.precor.com

APPENDIX

DIETARY REFERENCE INTAKES (DRIS): RECOMMENDED INTAKES FOR INDIVIDUALS, ELEMENTS
FOOD AND NUTRITION BOARD, INSTITUTE OF MEDICINE, NATIONAL ACADEMIES

Life-Stage Group		Calcium (mg/d)	Chromium (µg/d)	Copper (µg/d)	Fluoride (mg/d)	Iodine (µg/d)	Iron (mg/d)	Magnesium (mg/d)	Manganese (mg/d)	Molybdenum (µg/d)	Phosphorus (mg/d)	Selenium (µg/d)	Zinc (mg/d)	Potassium* (g/d)	Sodium (g/d)	Chloride (g/d)
Males	14–18 y	1,300*	35*	890	3*	150	11	410	2.2*	43	1,250	55	11	4.7*	1.5*	2.3*
	19–30 y	1,000*	35*	900	4*	150	8	400	2.3*	45	700	55	11	4.7*	1.5*	2.3*
	31–50 y	1,000*	35*	900	4*	150	8	420	2.3*	45	700	55	11	4.7*	1.5*	2.3*
	51–70 y	1,200*	30*	900	4*	150	8	420	2.3*	45	700	55	11	4.7*	1.3*	2.0*
	>70 y	1,200*	30*	900	4*	150	8	420	2.3*	45	700	55	11	4.7*	1.2*	1.8*
Females	14–18 y	1,300*	24*	890	3*	150	15	360	1.6*	43	1,250	55	9	4.7*	1.5*	2.3*
	19–30 y	1,000*	25*	900	3*	150	18	310	1.8*	45	700	55	8	4.7*	1.5*	2.3*
	31–50 y	1,000*	25*	900	3*	150	18	320	1.8*	45	700	55	8	4.7*	1.5*	2.3*
	51–70 y	1,200*	20*	900	3*	150	8	320	1.8*	45	700	55	8	4.7*	1.3*	2.0*
	>70 y	1,200*	20*	900	3*	150	8	320	1.8*	45	700	55	8	4.7*	1.2*	1.8*
Pregnancy	14–18 y	1,300*	29*	1,000	3*	220	27	400	2.0*	50	1,250	60	12	4.7*	1.5*	2.3*
	19–30 y	1,000*	30*	1,000	3*	220	27	350	2.0*	50	700	60	11	4.7*	1.5*	2.3*
	31–50 y	1,000*	30*	1,000	3*	220	27	360	2.0*	50	700	60	11	4.7*	1.5*	2.3*
Lactation	14–18 y	1,300*	44*	1,300	3*	290	10	360	2.6*	50	1,250	70	13	5.1*	1.5*	2.3*
	19–30 y	1,000*	45*	1,300	3*	290	9	310	2.6*	50	700	70	12	5.1*	1.5*	2.3*
	31–50 y	1,000*	45*	1,300	3*	290	9	320	2.6*	50	700	70	12	5.1*	1.5*	2.3*

NOTE: This table presents Recommended Dietary Allowances (RDAs) in **bold type** and Adequate Intakes (AIs) in ordinary type followed by an asterisk (*). RDAs and AIs may both be used as goals for individual intake. RDAs are set to meet the needs of almost all (97 to 98 percent) individuals in a group. For healthy breast-fed infants, the AI is the mean intake. The AI for other life stage and gender groups is believed to cover needs of all individuals in the group, but lack of data or uncertainty in the data prevent being able to specify with confidence the percentage of individuals covered by this intake.

SOURCES: *Dietary Reference Intakes for Calcium, Phosphorous, Magnesium, Vitamin D, and Fluoride* (1997); *Dietary Reference Intakes for Thiamin, Riboflavin, Niacin, Vitamin B₆, Folate, Vitamin B₁₂, Pantothenic Acid, Biotin. and Choline* (1998); *Dietary Reference Intakes for Vitamin C, Vitamin E, Selenium, and Carotenoids* (2000); *Dietary Reference Intakes for Vitamin A, Vitamin K, Arsenic, Boron, Chromium, Copper, Iodine, Iron, Manganese, Molybdenum, Nickel, Silicon, Vanadium, and Zinc* (2001); and *Dietary Reference Intakes for Water, Potassium, Sodium, Chloride, and Sulfate* (2004). These reports may be accessed via http://www.nap.edu.

A-1

DIETARY REFERENCE INTAKES (DRIS): RECOMMENDED INTAKES FOR INDIVIDUALS, VITAMINS

FOOD AND NUTRITION BOARD, INSTITUTE OF MEDICINE, NATIONAL ACADEMIES

Life-Stage Group	Vit A (µg/d)[a]	Vit C (mg/d)	Vit D (µg/d)[b,c]	Vit E (mg/d)[d]	Vit K (µg/d)	Thiamin (mg/d)	Riboflavin (mg/d)	Niacin (mg/d)[e]	Vit B6 (mg/d)	Folate (µg/d)[f]	Vit B12 (µg/d)	Pantothenic Acid (mg/d)	Biotin (µg/d)	Choline[g] (mg/d)
Males														
14–18 y	900	75	5*	15	75*	1.2	1.3	16	1.3	400	2.4	5*	25*	550*
19–30 y	900	90	5*	15	120*	1.2	1.3	16	1.3	400	2.4	5*	30*	550*
31–50 y	900	90	5*	15	120*	1.2	1.3	16	1.3	400	2.4	5*	30*	550*
51–70 y	900	90	10*	15	120*	1.2	1.3	16	1.7	400	2.4[i]	5*	30*	550*
>70 y	900	90	15*	15	120*	1.2	1.3	16	1.7	400	2.4[i]	5*	30*	550*
Females														
14–18 y	700	65	5*	15	75*	1.0	1.0	14	1.2	400[i]	2.4	5*	25*	400*
19–30 y	700	75	5*	15	90*	1.1	1.1	14	1.3	400[i]	2.4	5*	30*	425*
31–50 y	700	75	5*	15	90*	1.1	1.1	14	1.3	400[i]	2.4	5*	30*	425*
51–70 y	700	75	10*	15	90*	1.1	1.1	14	1.5	400	2.4[h]	5*	30*	425*
>70 y	700	75	15*	15	90*	1.1	1.1	14	1.5	400	2.4[h]	5*	30*	425*
Pregnancy														
14–18 y	750	80	5*	15	75*	1.4	1.4	18	1.9	600[j]	2.6	6*	30*	450*
19–30 y	770	85	5*	15	90*	1.4	1.4	18	1.9	600[j]	2.6	6*	30*	450*
31–50 y	770	85	5*	15	90*	1.4	1.4	18	1.9	600[j]	2.6	6*	30*	450*
Lactation														
14–18 y	1,200	115	5*	19	75*	1.4	1.6	17	2.0	500	2.8	7*	35*	550*
19–30 y	1,300	120	5*	19	90*	1.4	1.6	17	2.0	500	2.8	7*	35*	550*
31–50 y	1,300	120	5*	19	90*	1.4	1.6	17	2.0	500	2.8	7*	35*	550*

NOTE: This table (taken from the DRI reports, see www.nap.edu) presents Recommended Dietary Allowances (RDAs) in **bold type** and Adequate Intakes (AIs) in ordinary type followed by an asterisk (*). RDAs and AIs may both be used as goals for individual intake. RDAs are set to meet the needs of almost all (97 to 98 percent) individuals in a group. For healthy breastfed infants, the AI is the mean intake. The AI for other life stage and gender groups is believed to cover needs of all individuals in the group, but lack of data or uncertainty in the data prevent being able to specify with confidence the percentage of individuals covered by this intake.

[a] As retinol activity equivalents (RAEs). 1 RAE = 1 µg retinol, 12 µg β-carotene, 24 µg α-carotene, or 24 µg β-cryptoxanthin. The RAE for dietary provitamin A carotenoids is twofold greater than retinol equivalents (RE), whereas the RAE for preformed vitamin A is the same as RE.

[b] As cholecalciferol. 1 µg cholecalciferol = 40 IU vitamin D.

[c] In the absence of adequate exposure to sunlight.

[d] As α-tocopherol. α-Tocopherol includes RRR-α-tocopherol, the only form of α-tocopherol that occurs naturally in foods, and the 2R-stereoisomeric forms of α-tocopherol (RRR-, RSR-, RRS-, and RSS-α-tocopherol) that occur in fortified foods and supplements. It does not include the 2S-stereoisomeric forms of α-tocopherol (SRR-, SSR-, SRS-, and SSS-α-tocopherol), also found in fortified foods and supplements.

[e] As niacin equivalents (NE). 1 mg of niacin = 60 mg of tryptophan; 0–6 months = preformed niacin (not NE).

[f] As dietary folate equivalents (DFE). 1 DFE = 1 µg food folate = 0.6 µg of folic acid from fortified food or as a supplement consumed with food = 0.5 µg of a supplement taken on an empty stomach.

[g] Although AIs have been set for choline, there are few data to assess whether a dietary supply of choline is needed at all stages of the life cycle, and it may be that the choline requirement can be met by endogenous synthesis at some of these stages.

[h] Because 10 to 30 percent of older people may malabsorb food-bound B₁₂, it is advisable for those older than 50 years to meet their RDA mainly by consuming foods fortified with B₁₂ or a supplement containing B₁₂.

[i] In view of evidence linking folate intake with neural tube defects in the fetus, it is recommended that all women capable of becoming pregnant consume 400 µg from supplements or fortified foods in addition to intake of food folate from a varied diet.

[j] It is assumed that women will continue consuming 400 µg from supplements or fortified food until their pregnancy is confirmed and they enter prenatal care, which ordinarily occurs after the end of the periconceptional period—the critical time for formation of the neural tube.

CREDITS

Chapter 1

Figure 1-1, Karl Weatherly/Getty Images; Figure 1-2, Royalty-Free/CORBIS; Figure 1-3, Getty Images; Figure 1-4, PNC/Brand X Pictures/Jupiterimages; Figure 1-5, © Dynamic Graphics/Jupiterimages; Figure 1-6, © Corbis-All Rights Reserved; Figure 1-7, © Comstock Images/PictureQuest; Figure 1-8, © Stockbyte/PunchStock; Figure 1-10, Royalty-Free/CORBIS; Figure 1-11, Royalty-Free/CORBIS; Figure 1-12, © Ingram Publishing/Alamy; Figure 1-13, Royalty-Free/CORBIS; Figure 1-14, © Dynamic Graphics Group/PunchStock.

Chapter 2

Figure 2-1, Image Source/Getty Images; Figure 2-2, Getty Images; Figure 2-3, Asia Images/Getty Images; Figure 2-4, © Stockbyte/PunchStock; Figure 2-5, © Bob Mitchell/Corbis; Figure 2-6, Ryan McVay/Getty Images; Figure 2-7, Image Source/JupiterImages; Figure 2-9, Photodisc Collection/Getty Images; Figure 2-10, McGraw-Hill Companies, Inc/Gary He, photographer; Figure 2-11, Medioimages/PictureQuest; Figure 2-12, Royalty-Free/CORBIS; Figure 2-13, © BananaStock/PunchStock; Figure 2-14, Brand X Pictures.

Chapter 3

Figure 3-3, Brand X Pictures; Figure 3-4, Stockbyte/Getty Images; Figure 3-5a, © Beathan/Corbis; Figure 3-5b, © Dynamic Graphics Group/PunchStock.

Chapter 4

Figure 4-1, Stockbyte/Getty Images; Figure 4-6, Comstock Images/Getty Images; Figure 4-7, McGraw-Hill Companies, Inc/Gary He, photographer; Figure 4-8, © Ryan McVay/Getty Images; Figure 4-9 Comstock Images/JupiterImages; Figure 4-10, © liquidlibrary/PictureQuest; Figure 4-11, Digital Vision/Getty Images; Figure 4-13, Comstock Images/JupiterImages; Figure 4-14, © Karl Weatherly/Getty Images; Figure 4-16, ©Royalty-Free/Getty Images; Figure 4-17, © Royalty-Free/Getty Images.

Chapter 6

Figure 6-1, © Mark Andersen/Getty Images; Figure 6-4, Magnum Fitness Systems-South Milwaukee, Wisconsin.

Chapter 7

Figure 7-2a, Royalty-Free/CORBIS; Figure 7-2b, Getty Images; Figure 7-3a, BananaStock/Getty Images; Figure 7-3b, Allan Rosenberg/Cole Group/Getty Images; Figure 7-4, © Comstock/PunchStock; Figure 7-5, © Comstock Images/PictureQuest; Figure 7-6, © McGraw-Hill Companies/Jill Braaten, photographer; Figure 7-10, BananaStock/JupiterImages.

Chapter 8

Figure 8-1, Ingram Publishing/SuperStock; Figure 8-4a, Science Photo Library RF/Getty Images; Figure 8-4b, Comstock Images/Jupiterimages; Figure 8-6, Andersen Ross/Getty Images; Figure 8-7, Nancy R. Cohen/Getty Images; Figure 8-8, Royalty-Free/Corbis; Figure 8-9, © Stockbyte/PunchStock; Figure 8-10, ©BananaStock/PunchStock.

Chapter 9

Figure 9-1, Royalty-Free/CORBIS; Figure 9-17, C. Borland/PhotoLink/Getty Images; Figure 9-18, Ryan McVay/Getty Images.

Chapter 10

Figure 10-1, Batca Fitness; Figure 10.2, True Fitness; Figure 10-3, Suza Scalora/Getty Images; Figure 10-4, PhotoLink/Getty Images.

INDEX